$23.10

Advances in Neurosurgery 1

AF758250

Deutsche Gesellschaft für Neurochirurgie.

Brain Edema

Pathophysiology and Therapy

Cerebello Pontine Angle Tumors

Diagnosis and Surgery

Edited by
K. Schürmann · M. Brock · H.-J. Reulen · D. Voth

With 187 Figures

MOORE LIBRARY OF MEDICINE
MEDICAL COLLEGE OF PENNA.

Springer-Verlag
Berlin · Heidelberg · New York 1973

WL
348
D486b
1973

ISBN 3-540-06486-9 Springer-Verlag Berlin · Heidelberg · New York
ISBN 0-387-06486-9 Springer-Verlag New York · Heidelberg · Berlin

This work is subject to copyright. All rights are reserved, whether the whole or part of the material is concerned, specifically those of translation, reprinting, re-use of illustrations, broadcasting, reproduction by photocoping machine or similar means, and storage in data banks.

Under § 54 of the German Copyright Law, where copies are made for other than private use, a fee is payable to the publisher, the amount of the fee to be determined by agreement with the publisher.

The use of registered names, trademarks, etc. in this publication does not imply, even in the absence of a specific statement, that such names are exempt from the relevant protective laws and regulations and therefore free for general use.

© by Springer-Verlag Berlin · Heidelberg 1973. Library of Congress Catalog Card Number 73-14237.

Printed in Germany

Offsetprinting and Binding: Julius Beltz, Hemsbach/Bergstr.

RC386
D4

Preface

This volume contains the papers presented at the 24th Annual Meeting of the Deutsche Gesellschaft für Neurochirurgie, held in Mainz, Western Germany, on April 30 – May 3, 1973.

Deliberate choice was made of two crucial still hotly debated subjects which, for ages, have meant a source of constant worry, and nights without sleep to every neurosurgeon. Just as long as our special field exists, there have been the problems of how to control *brain edema* and of how to reduce lethality and the secondary lesions in surgery of *cerebello-pontine angle tumors.*

Concerning the first subject, new pathological, pathophysiological and chemical aspects, the mechanisms of brain edema formation and resolution are presented in the hope for better understanding. Furthermore, the relationship between brain edema, intracranial pressure, cerebral blood flow and metabolism are discussed. Finally, the therapeutical consequences as well as the results of experimental and clinical work are presented, and a comparison of effects between different methods (hypertonic solutions, diuretics, steroids, controlled hyperventilation, hyperbaric oxygen) is given.

Concerning the second main subject, any important contributions to the early diagnosis of cerebello-pontine angle tumors have been included. Nevertheless, it is of utmost interest for the neurosurgeon to know which approach he is to prefer for the different stages of tumor size and to be familiar with the trans-labyrinthine approach or the posterior craniotomy, as well as with the importance of the use of the microscope in neurosurgery, the preservation of the facial nerve and, in certain cases, its repair.

Therefore, we were particularly happy in obtaining the collaboration of experts from all over the world as discussants of these crucial questions from their very roots, so as to provide new insights with the aim of improving therapy.

Thus, this book surveys some aspects of our current knowledge on the prevention and therapy of brain edema and on the surgery of tumors of the cerebello-pontine angle.

The last chapter contains miscellaneous contributions from various fields of neurosurgery such as ultrasonic B-scanning and notes on surgical techniques.

The volume is closed by honoring OTFRID FOERSTER. The 1973 Annual Meeting is dedicated to the memory of OTFRID FOERSTER in celebration of the 100th anniversary of his birthday. Our special field is highly indebted to him.

OTFRID FOERSTER's achievement, the result of lifelong endeavour, will remain an obligation to honor and an example to follow. This centenary therefore supplies the Society with a deeply satisfying occasion for an appraisal of HUGO KRAYENBÜHL and the conspicuous service he has rendered to neurosurgery.

We must keep in mind that the work of every one of us rests on the achievements of our forerunners. We sincerely hope that our junior colleagues may become aware of such historic facts and their significance for the future development of the field they have chosen. May this not only stimulate individual achievement, but also encourage a sober view of the relative value of one's own efforts.

HUGO KRAYENBÜHL has been honored by the bestowing of the ORTFRID FOERSTER-Medal, the Society's highest mark of honor, on May 3, 1973.

Subsequently, the OTFRID FOERSTER-Memorial Lecture "The Treatment of Intramedullary Spinal Cord Tumors and Cervical Syringohydromyelia" has been included in this volume.

Editing has been restricted to rearrangements and small corrections. No homogeneity of style was attempted. The editors considered that rapid publication should be their main objective and preferred to publish as early as possible. Therefore, the texts submitted have been included almost in their original form.

We take great pleasure in expressing our thanks to Springer-Verlag for technical aid in the preparation of the first volume of the series of *Advances in neurosurgery,* for its prompt publication and its acceptable price, with the hope of success in the future.

Mainz, July 1973 KURT SCHÜRMANN

Contents

Chapter I. Pathophysiology of Brain Edema

Chapter II. Clinical Therapy of Brain Edema

Chapter III. Intracranial Pressure, Cerebral Blood Flow and Metabolism

Chapter IV. Diagnosis of Cerebello-Pontine Angle Tumors

Chapter V. Surgery of Cerebello-Pontine Angle Tumors

Chapter VI. Miscellaneous

Addendum

List of Contributors

AGNOLI, A.L.	Gießen, Neurochirurg. Univ.-Klinik
ALBERTI, E.	Heidelberg, Neurochirurg. Univ.-Klinik
ALTENBURG, H.	Erlangen, Neurochirurg. Univ.-Klinik
BAETHMANN, A.	München, Institut für Experiment. Chirurgie Chirurg. Univ.-Klinik
BAZIN, M.	Montpellier/Frankreich, Service de Neurochirurgie
BEKS, J.W.F.	Groningen/Niederlande, Neurochirurg. Univ.-Klinik
BILLET, R.	Paris/Frankreich, Centre Neurochirurgicale Hopital Sainte-Anne
BOCK, W.J.	Essen, Neurochirurg. Univ.-Klinik der Ruhr-Universität
BÖCK, F.	Wien/Österreich, Neurochirurg. Univ.-Klinik
BRENNER, H.	Wien/Österreich, Neurochirurg. Univ.-Klinik
BÜCKING, H.	Mainz, Neurolog. Univ.-Klinik
CERVOS-NAVARRO, J.	Berlin, Institut für Neuropathol., Klinikum Steglitz
CHODKIEWICZ, J.P.	Paris/Frankreich, Centre Neurochirurgicale Hopital Sainte-Anne
CZAJKOWSKA, D.	Warschau/Polen, Neurosurgery Unit
DIETZ, H.	Hannover, Med. Hochschule, Neurochirurg. Klinik
DORLAND, P.R.	Paris/Frankreich, Centre Neurochirurgicale Hopital Sainte-Anne
DRAKE, C.G.	London, Ontario/Canada, Departm. of Clinical Neurological Sciences

DÜNNEBEIL, K.	Wuppertal, Neurochirurg. Abtlg. (Bethesda)
ENTZIAN, W.	Bonn, Neurochirurg. Univ.-Klinik
ENZENBACH, R.	München, Neurochirurg. Klinik, Anaesthesiolog. Abteilung
FREREBEAU, Ph.	Montpellier/Frankreich, Service de Neurochirurgie
FROMM, H.	Frankfurt/M., Neurochirurg. Univ.-Klinik
FRONT, D.	Groningen/Niederlande, Departm. of Neuroradiology, University Hospital
FROWEIN, R.A.	Köln-Lindenthal, Neurochirurg. Univ.-Klinik
FUCHS, E.	Berlin, Neurochirurg. Klinik, Klinikum Westend
GOBIET, W.	Essen, Neurochirurg. Klinik der Ruhr-Universität
GROMEK, A.	Warschau/Polen, Neurosurgery Unit
GROS, C.	Montpellier/Frankreich, Service de Neurochirurgie
GROTE, J.	Mainz, Physiolog. Inst. der Universität
GROTE, W.	Essen, Neurochirurg. Klinik der Ruhr-Universität
GRUMME, Th.	Berlin, Neurochirurg. Klinik, Klinikum Westend
GRUNERT, V.	Wien/Österreich, Neurochirurg. Univ.-Klinik
GULLOTTA, F.	Bonn, Neuropatholog. Institut der Universität
HALVES, E.	Göttingen, Neurochirurg. Univ.-Klinik
HAMER, J.	Heidelberg, Neurochirurg. Univ.-Klinik
HAUSDÖRFER, J.	Tübingen, Inst. für Anaesthesiolog. der Universität
HELLER, W.	Tübingen, Neurochirurg. Univ.-Klinik
HIRSCHAUER, M.	Freiburg, Institut für Anaesthesiologie der Universität
HITSELBERGER, W.E.	Los Angeles/U.S.A., Incorp. Neurologic Surgery
HOLBACH, K.H.	Bonn, Neurochirurg. Univ.-Klinik
HOPMAN, E.	München, Neurochirurg. Univ.-Klinik
HOUSE, W.F.	Los Angeles/Calif., U.S.A., Otologic Medical Group

HOYER, S.	Heidelberg, Institut für Pathochemie und Neurochemie der Universität
JAUMANN, E.	München, Neurochirurg. Univ. -Klinik
JURKIEWICZ, J.	Warschau/Polen, Neurosurgery Unit
KARIMI-NEJAD, A.	Köln-Lindenthal, Neurochirurg. Univ. -Klinik
KAZNER, E.	München, Neurochirurg. Univ. -Klinik
KENDALL, B.	London/England, Departm. of Neurosurgical Studies, The National Hospital
KIENOW, I.	Frankfurt/M., Neurochirurg. Univ. -Klinik
KIVELITZ, R.	Homburg/Saar, Neurochirurg. Univ. -Klinik
KLATZO, I.	Bethesda/U.S.A., National Institute of Neurological Diseases and Stroke
KLEMANN, T.	Berlin, Institut für Neuropathologie, Klinikum Steglitz
KOLBERG, T.	Bonn, Neurochirurg. Univ. -Klinik
KONTOPOULOS, B.	Heidelberg, Neurochirurg. Univ. -Klinik
KOOS, W.	Wien/Österreich, Neurochirurg. Univ. -Klinik
KRAUS, H.	Wien/Österreich, Neurochirurg. Univ. -Klinik
KRAYENBÜHL, H.	Zürich/Schweiz, Zollikon, Schloßbergstraße 18
KÜHNER, A.	Montpellier/Frankreich, Service de Neurochirurgie
KUHN, H.	Mannheim, Neurolog. Klinik im Klinikum Mannheim der Universität Heidelberg
LIESEGANG, J.	Essen, Neurochirurg. Klinik der Ruhr-Universität
LINS, E.	Bonn, Neurochirurg. Univ. -Klinik
LOEW, F.	Homburg/Saar, Neurochirurg. Univ. -Klinik
MARKAKIS, E.	Hannover, Med. Hochschule, Neurochirurg. Klinik
MARX, P.	Mannheim, Neurolog. Klinik im Klinikum Mannheim der Universität Heidelberg
MATAKAS, F.	Berlin, Institut für Neuropathologie, Klinikum Steglitz

MEER, v., A.	München, Neurochirurg. Univ.-Klinik
METZEL, E.	Freiburg/Brsg., Neurochirurg. Univ.-Klinik
MIEHLKE, A.	Göttingen, HNO-Klinik der Universität
MILLER, D.	Glasgow/Scotland, Institute of Neurological Sciences
MOHR, G.	Frankfurt/M., Neurochirurg. Univ.-Klinik
MUNDINGER, F.	Freiburg/Brsg., Neurochirurg. Univ.-Klinik
OLDENKOTT, P.	Tübingen, Neurochirurg. Univ.-Klinik
OLTENAU-NERBE, v., V.	München, Neurochirurg. Univ.-Klinik
OVERGAARD, J.	Odense/Dänemark, Neurochirurg. Univ.-Klinik
PACKSCHIES, P.	Heidelberg, Anaesthesiolog. Institut der Universität
PENNING, L.	Groningen/Niederlande, Departm. of Neuroradiology, University Hospital
PENZHOLZ, H.	Heidelberg, Neurochirurg. Univ.-Klinik
PFIESTER, P.	Mannheim, Neurolog. Klinik im Klinikum Mannheim der Universität Heidelberg
POTTHOFF, P.	Günzburg/Ulm, Neurochirurg. Abtlg., Nervenkrankenhaus
PRIVAT, J.M.	Montpellier/Frankreich, Service de Neurochirurgie
PULEC, J.	Los Angeles/Calif., U.S.A., Neurologic Surgery
REULEN, H.J.	Mainz, Neurochirurg. Univ.-Klinik
RICHARD, K.G.	Köln-Lindenthal, Neurochirurg. Univ.-Klinik
RIEGER, H.	Mainz, Neuropsychiatr. Univ.-Klinik
ROQUEFEUIL, B.	Montpellier/Frankreich, Service de Neurochirurgie
RUF, H.	Frankfurt/M., Neurochirurg. Univ.-Klinik
RUNGE, P.	Wuppertal, Neurochirurg. Abtlg. (Bethesda)
SALAH, S.	Wien/Österreich, Neurochirurg. Univ.-Klinik

SEEGER, W.	Gießen, Neurochirurg. Univ. -Klinik
SEITZ, H. D.	Freiburg, Inst. für Anaesthesiologie
SPRING, A.	Hannover, Med. Hochschule, Neurochirurg. Klinik
SUNDER-PLASSMANN, M.	Wien/Österreich, Neurochirurg. Univ. -Klinik
SWOZIL, U.	München, Neurochirurg. Univ. -Klinik
SYMON, L.	London/England, Departm. of Neurosurgical Studies, The National Hospital
SCHAAF, W.	Mainz, Neurochirurg. Univ. -Klinik
SCHÄFER, M.	Frankfurt/M., Neurochirurg. Univ. -Klinik
SCHMIDT, R.	München, Neurochirurg. Univ. -Klinik
SCHMIEDEK, P.	München, Institut für Experiment. Chirurgie Chirurg. Univ. -Klinik
SCHRADER, H.	Freiburg, Neurochirurg. Univ. -Klinik
SCHUBERT, R.	Mainz, Neurochirurg. Univ. -Klinik
SCHÜRMANN, K.	Mainz, Neurochirurg. Univ. -Klinik
STEINHOFF, H.	München, Neuroradiolog. Abtlg., Neurochirurg. Univ. -Klinik
STERKERS, J. M.	Paris/Frankreich, Centre Neurochirurgicale Hopital Sainte-Anne
STOECKEL, H.	Heidelberg, Institut für Anaesthesiologie der Universität
STOLZ, Ch.	Tübingen, Institut für Anaesthesiologie der Universität
THOMALSKE, G.	Frankfurt/M., Neurochirurg. Univ. -Klinik
TROUPP, H.	Helsinki/Finnland, Neurokirurgiska Kliniken
TWEED, A.	Odense/Dänemark, Neurochirurg. Klinik
TZONOS, T.	Stuttgart, Neurochirurg. Klinik
VAPALAHTI, M.	Helsinki/Finnland, Neurokirurgiska Kliniken
VIGUIE, E.	Montpellier/Frankreich, Service de Neurochirurgie

VOGEL, B.	München, Neurochirurg. Univ.-Klinik
WALLENFANG, Th.	Mainz, Neurochirurg. Univ.-Klinik
WALTER, W.	Erlangen, Neurochirurg. Univ.-Klinik
WAPPENSCHMIDT, J.	Bonn, Neurochirurg. Univ.-Klinik
WEINERT, G.	Mannheim, Neurolog. Klinik im Klinikum Mannheim der Universität Heidelberg
WENDE, S.	Mainz, Neuroradiolog. Abtlg. der Neurochirurg. Univ.-Klinik
VAN DER WERF, A.J.M.	Abcoude/Niederlande, Neurochirurgie Amsterdam
WILCKE, O.	Köln-Lindenthal, Neurochirurg. Univ.-Klinik
WINKELMÜLLER, W.	Hannover, Med. Hochschule, Neurochirurg. Klinik
WÖRZ, R.	Mainz, Neuro-Psychiatr. Univ.-Klinik
WÜLLENWEBER, R.	Bonn, Neurochirurg. Univ.-Klinik
YASARGIL, M.G.	Zürich/Schweiz, Neurochirurg. Univ.-Klinik
ZIMMERMANN, H.	Freiburg, Universitätsklinik
ZIMMERMANN, W.E.	Freiburg, Chirurg. Univ.-Klinik

Chapter I.

Pathophysiology of Brain Edema

Pathophysiology of Brain Edema: Pathological Aspects

I. KLATZO

Accepting the definition of edema as an abnormal accumulation of a fluid in a tissue, two basic types of brain edema (BE) namely, vasogenic and cytotoxic have been recognized (5). This classification is based on recognition of two fundamentally different pathomechanisms involved, as well as, on predominance of extracellular or intracellular localization of the edema fluid in respective types.

As much as the vasogenic type of BE is clinically most important (it occurs as the complication of brain traumatic lesions, brain tumors, cerebro-vascular accidents, inflammatory lesions, etc.) it has been extensively studied in various experimental models, particularly in the one based on cold injury (4).

In view of recent reports, and great potential significance of biogenic amines, Dr. J. COSTA from our laboratory has examined these compounds in the model of cold lesion BE in cats. Both specific histofluorescent observations and quantitative assays were undertaken. Dopamine, norepinephrine, and serotonin were studied. For quantitative assays, (Fig. 1) blocks of brain tissue were taken from area of immediate cold lesion, edematous white matter, and control areas from the adjacent gyrus. Dr. COSTA's results indicated that dopamine values were similar in all blocks of the tissue examined. Norepinephrine was about 25% lower in area of cold lesion and in edematous white matter than in the adjacent control gyrus. On the other hand, serotonin in the area of cold lesion was about four times higher than in control gyrus and its levels in the edematous white matter were approximately equal to the control values. Specific histofluorescent observations according to the method of Flack and Owman (2) revealed in the area confined only to the cold lesion a striking yellow-green fluorescence of blood vessels, compatible in color to that described for serotonin. The final proof that serotonin was responsible for characteristic fluorescence of the blood vessels and thus accounted for high quantitative values of serotonin in area of lesion was obtained by the courtesy of Dr. DEMERJIAN at the Albert EINSTEIN College of Medicine, who performed specific microfluorometric measurements which unequivocally identified fluorescent substance as serotonin.

The discovery of the presence of serotonin in the injured blood vessels in the area of cold lesion acquires a special significance in view of the recent observations of Westergaard and Brightman from our laboratory which indicate that serotonin introduced via the cerebrospinal fluid into the brain parenchyma may increase the permeability of arterioles. It is thus conceivable that serotonin in injured blood vessels in our cold injury model, as well as in clinical cases of brain trauma associated with vascular injury, may present an important factor influencing the permeability of cerebral blood vessels and the dynamics of vasogenic brain edema.

The cytotoxic type of BE has been much less explored than the vasogenic one. Pathogenesis of cytotoxic edema is related to some toxic factor affecting directly cellular elements of brain parenchyma causing their swelling. Since in this case the essential event is the intracellular uptake of water, which itself passes freely through the blood-brain barrier, the permeability of cerebral blood vessels remains usually unchanged. The parameters of the cytotoxic type of BE have been evaluated in greater detail only in intoxications such as triethyltin (1) or hexachlorophene poisonings (6). Yet there has been a number of indications that the most clinically important cytotoxic edema may be related to an acute oxygen deficiency, and particularly it may be manifest in the cerebral ischemia. For example, swelling of brain parenchyma cells, particularly perivascular astrocytes, has been recognized for a long time to occur invariably as a postmortem change or following an imperfect fixation, i.e., conditions in which an acute oxygen deficiency constitutes a predominant feature.

Brain edema, following a regional ischemia, has been recently investigated in our laboratory using Mongolian gerbils (Meriones unguiculatus). In these animals, due to an anatomical pecularity of the circulus of Willis, a unilateral ligation of the common carotid produces ischemic infarction in the ipsilateral hemisphere in 30% of cases. According to studies of Dr. GO Visiting Scientist from the University of Groningen, Holland in which edema was evaluated on the basis of wet/dry weight ratios, BE becomes noticeable in the infarcted hemisphere already 3 hours after ligation and it reaches its peak at 18 hrs. interval (Fig. 2). Interestingly, only then, 18 hrs. after carotid ligation, there is a demonstrable alteration of the blood-brain barrier in the ischemic hemisphere as tested with the Evans Blue indicator. Such remarkable "resistance" of the blood-brain barrier following ischemia has been reported previously by HOSSMANN and OLSSON (1972); in the case of gerbils this indicates that vascular permeability to serum proteins remains unimpaired during the development of BE up to 18 hours after ischemic insult, and thus this period of edema appears to be of cytotoxic type. A further strong support for such assumption comes from the morphological observations of the ischemic brain areas in gerbils, which even in ordinary light microscopic preparations clearly showed that accumulation of the edema fluid is primarily in intracellular location (Fig. 3). The studies described thus indicate that ischemic BE is primarily of the cytotoxic variety and that only in the later stages severe injury to the cerebral blood vessels with breaking down of the blood-brain barrier may add a vasogenic component. Furthermore, these studies demonstrate how great is variety of pathophysiological events in the development of brain edema. It is only recently that we began to grasp the complexities of cerebral vasoregulation and how much it affects the supply of oxygen and transport of essential nutrients. We should know much more about the factors regulating water movement across the cellular membranes.

The progress in understanding of basic pathophysiology of BE is nevertheless impressive and here lies our best hope that continuation of these basic studies will eventually provide foundation for rational and effective clinical management of BE.

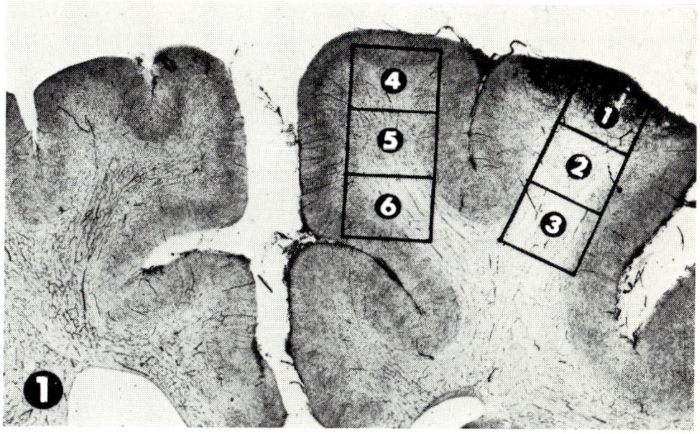

Fig. 1. Cold lesion injury in cat. Thenumbers represent blocks of tissue subjected to quantitative assay on biogenic amines. 1 - area of cold injury, 2 and 3 - edematous white matter, 4, 5 and 6 - control tissue from the adjacent gyrus

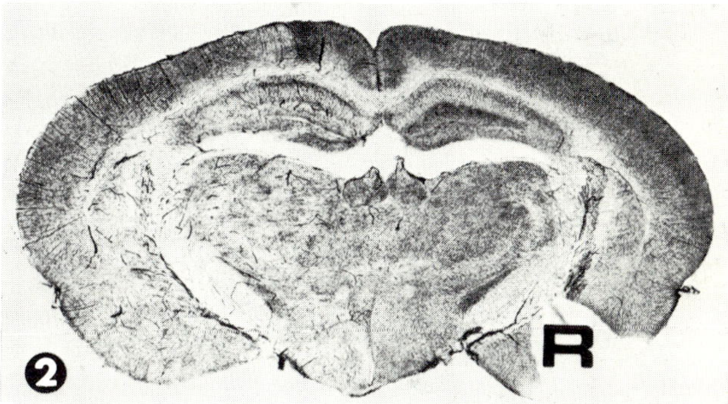

Fig. 2. Six hours ligation of the lett common carotid artery in gerbil. Pickworth-Lepehne stain for erythrocytes demonstrating a picture of passive hyperemia in the enlarged, edematous left hemisphere

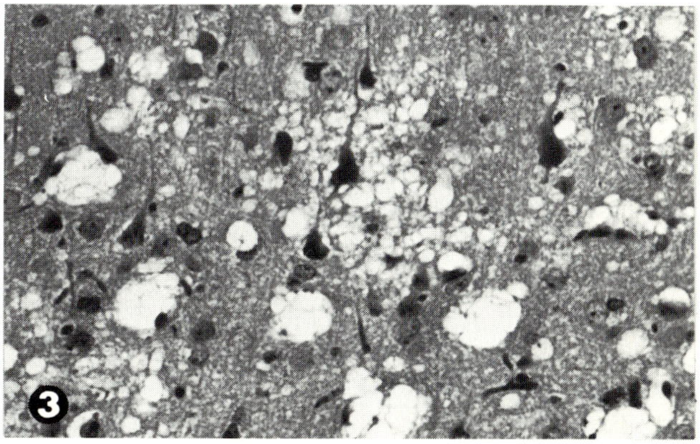

Fig. 3. Cerebral cortex of the left hemisphere of the gerbil subjected to six hours ligation of the left common carotid artery. Extensive vacuolation due to intracellular accumulation of the fluid. Hematoxylin and eosin; X 340

References

1. ALEU, F.P., R.KATZMAN and R.D.TERRY: Fine structure and electrolyte analysis of cerebral edema induced by alkyltin intoxication. J.Neuropath.Exp. Neurol. 22, 403-414 (1963)

2. FALCK, B. and C.OWMAN: A detailed methodological description of the fluorescense method for the cellular demonstration of biogenic monoamines. Acta Universitatis Ludensis 2, 1-23 (1965)

3. HOSSMANN, K.A. and Y.OLSSON: Functional aspects of abnormal protein passage across the blood-brain barrier. In REULEN, H.J. and K.SCHÜRMANN (Eds.): Steroids and Brain Edema. Berlin-Heidelberg-New York, Springer-Verlag, pp. 9-17 (1972)

4. KLATZO, I., A.PIRAUX and E.J.LASKOWSKI: The relationship between edema, blood-brain barrier, and tissue elements in local brain injury. J.Neuropath. Exp.Neurol. 17, 548-564 (1958)

5. KLATZO, I.: Neuropathological aspects of brain edema: Presidential Address. J.Neuropath.Exp.Neurol. 26, 1-14 (1967)

6. LAMPERT, P., J.O'BRIEN and R.GARRET: Hexachlorophene encephalopathy. Acta Neuropath. 23, 326-333 (1973)

Pathophysiology of Cerebral Edema: Chemical Aspects+)

A. BAETHMANN and P. SCHMIEDEK

Chemical or biochemical investigations in cerebral edema may be concerned with a variety of subjects, as e.g. the chemical composition of the edematous tissue, or the edema fluid itself, the distribution of the edema fluid within the tissue, and the metabolic tissue response to edema.

In the present paper it is attempted to analyze and compare changes of the electrolyte and water content, as well as other parameters in various forms of brain edema, which according to the definition as introduced by KLATZO (16) may be described as vasogenic or cytotoxic.

In Fig. 1 the electrolyte and water changes in three different experimental types of vasogenic edema, such as after cold lesion, tumor implantation, or acceleration concussion of the mobile skull (10, 20, 22) are shown. The net water-, sodium- and potassium increases in samples of gray and white matter or mixed cortical and white matter were calculated on dry weight basis according to the data published by the respective authors. In addition, the tissue swelling was computed in volume percent utilizing the ELLIOT and JASPER (8) equation $\frac{\Delta H_2O\,\%}{dw\,\%} \times 100$ where ΔH_2O is the difference in percent water content of control and experimental tissue and dw % the dry weight in percent of the edematous tissue. The figures on top of the Columns give the electrolyte concentrations of the edema fluid, which were calculated again on dry weight basis by $\frac{\Delta Na, K}{\Delta H_2O} \times 1000$, where ΔNa, or K or ΔH_2O signifies the difference of the control and experimental conditions of the respective parameters.

The variability in magnitude of the edema as well as the different susceptibility of gray and white matter can easily be concluded from the different experimental models shown. In the case of skull trauma in rats (acceleration concussion) no separation of gray and white substance was attempted. It is suggested that the rather small, but still significant changes found in non separated cerebral tissue after blunt skull injury may be due to a mixing of affected and unaffected tissue.

The calculation of the electrolyte concentration of the edema fluid, taken up by the brain, provides some clues concerning its origin. The figures obtained from PAPPIUS' s experiments suggest a close relationship of the edema fluid in the white

+) Supported in part by DFG-Sonderforschungsbereich 51 - Medizinische Molekularbiologie und Biochemie - and by US PHS Grants 1 FO 5 TWO 1688 and NB-07658

matter with plasma, whereas the Na-concentration of 57 meq/l of the edema fluid in the experiments of REULEN et al. bears no such similarities. However, it is impossible to exclude that a mixing of the two different tissues can be the cause for this. Since only the Na/K ratio was given in HERZOG's study, the respective edema concentration could not be calculated.

The Na- and K-concentration of the edematous white matter is more or less related with the tissue water content as indicated by Fig. 2, where the electrolyte concentrations were plotted versus the dry weight of the tissue. The regression lines symbolize a Na- or K-water relationship assuming the edema fluid to be whole plasma or a plasma-filtrate. The distribution of the individual values suggests the edema fluid to be more similar to a plasma-filtrate than to plasma itself. Studies in perifocal edematous brain tissue in man revealed virtually the same for the Na-water relation in white matter, however, not in edematous gray matter (24). The different Na-water regressions in gray and white matter may also be indicative for different properties of the edema in both tissues (Tab. I).

CLASEN et al. analyzed directly the fluid he was able to obtain from edematous white matter by centrifugation of the tissue (5). Table I gives the electrolyte and protein concentration or of protein equivalents such as EVANS blue or RIHSA of the edema fluid in experimental cerebral edema produced by cold injury. The corresponding data measured in the plasma of the same animals are given for comparison. The more or less constant relationship between the electrolytes or between the protein equivalents of the edema fluid and plasma should be noted. The similarity of the respective figures of the edema fluid which have been calculated from the data of PAPPIUS and GULATI, particularly of potassium, and the values which have been directly analyzed, is striking.

The edema fluid in the white matter to be protein-rich in the cold injury model can also be concluded from direct studies from the affected tissue as repeatedly in-

Table I. Chemical constituents of edema fluid in the white matter +)

	Edema Fluid	Plasma	E/P
Na^+	123.4 meq/l	143.0 meq/l	0.86
Cl^-	86.7 meq/l	110.0 meq/l	0.79
K^+	15.0 meq/l	-	-
Albumin	1.9 %	2.1 %	0.87
Evans Blue	16.4 mg%	31.8 mg%	0.52
RIHSA	7.5 cpm/mg	9.0 cpm/mg	0.83

+) from CLASEN, R.A. et al. (5); E/P: edema / plasma ratio

vestigated in different forms of edema (11, 12, 14, 15). RASMUSSEN and KLATZO (21) subjected edematous white matter to disc-gel-electrophoresis (Fig. 3) and found 24 hours after cold injury a marked increase of the albumin and pre-albumin content compared to the uninjured hemisphere. Five days later the albumin content was found normal, with the pre-albumin still slightly increased and a now more prominent γ -globulin profile.

The influence of the tissue blood content which in edematous white matter (cold injury) may be increased to a fivefold level compared to normal (29), should not be neglected in chemical analyses of edema-tissue, since it may affect the correlations of the various edema parameters, as e.g. between the tissue Na- and water-content, leading to erroneous conclusions. Other types of edema are shown in Fig. 4, which according to KLATZO can be characterized as cytotoxic or metabolic, since an initial involvement of metabolic derangements of cellular elements may be inferred from the biochemical effects of the edema inducing substances used.

Triethyltin (TET) is shown to inhibit mitochondrial metabolic activity (19). The TET edema accumulates mostly in the white matter within splits of the myelin lamellae, the grey matter remains virtually unaffected (2). 6-aminonicotinamide is a nicotinic acid compound, where in position 6 an amino-group replaces a proton. The homologous compound is utilized for the pyridine nucleotides NAD or NADP on account of the low specifity of the synthesizing enzyme (6). Dinitrophenol interferes with the oxydative production of energy-rich phosphate compounds rendering the cell deficient of metabolic available energy. The administration of the latter two compounds mentioned, also induces a significant, though more moderate electrolyte and water accumulation in the cerebral tissue (4, 23). The Na-concentration in the edematous gray matter after TET of 720 meq/l is quite different from plasma values, however, the white matter edema was found to have a concentration similar to plasma, of 133 meq/l which may be surprising in face of the blood brain barrier found intact to other plasma constituents such as vital dyes or RIHSA. The electrolyte concentrations as calculated in the edema fluid of the 6-AN-or dinitrophenol-edema differs considerably from plasma values which cannot be reconciled with an edema fluid representing a plasma-filtrate which accumulates simply within the extracellular space, provided the white and gray matter is equally affected in these edema types which however is not known.

Corresponding investigations on human cerebral edema have also been performed in autopsy material or in biopsy specimens taken during neurosurgery. In Fig. 5, changes of the water and electrolyte content and the resulting tissue swelling is shown in edematous grey and white matter surrounding tumors, or in malignant hypertensive encephalopathy. Again, in these edema types the white matter seems to be predominantly affected particularly as inferred from the post-mortem studies of STEWART-WALLACE or ADACHI et al. (1, 30) who, in addition, subjected their material to fixation before measuring the water content. When perifocal tissue was sampled in vivo from patients which were operated on, due to intracranial neoplasms, a more pronounced edema accumulation within the gray matter became apparent, although the white matter swelling still exceeds that of the gray matter by three times (24).

Biochemical tissue analyses of edema parameters can also be applied in order to evaluate the effects of therapeutical measures on cerebral edema more directly. This has been tried in Fig. 6, where from the chemical changes (e.e.: the difference between control and edema tissue) found in edematous white and gray matter obtained from the data of REULEN et al. (ref. Fig. 5), the differences in water,

Na- or K. content between a specifically pre-treated and an untreated group of patients have been subtracted. The therapy consisted of a 3-5 day pretreatment with 10 mg/day of aldosterone[x)] (i. m.) which is employed at the Department of Neurosurgery in Munich or of 24 mg/day of Dexamethasone[xx)] (i. m.) which is used at the Department of Neurosurgery in Mainz (25, 26). The columns surrounded by dotted lines with an arrow, thus respresent the amount of edema and of electrolytes being removed by the treatment, the solid white or black columns symbolize the remainder of the edema in the white and gray matter. We are aware of the limitations this kind of approach necessarily has, but we consider it permissible, since we were only comparing relative changes and not absolute figures.

The question where to localize the edema fluid within the tissue can also be studied by biochemical techniques. Table II gives a compilation of the uptake of plasma proteins equivalents, or of extracellular space labels in various forms of vasogenic or cytotoxic edema (Tab. II). In the vasogenic type, the accumulation of plasma

Table II. Blood - brain - barrier and extracellular space in brain edema

VASOGENIC		Vital dyes	Serum Protein	ECS-Substances
cold lesion	gray	(↗)	(↗)	(↗)
	white	➚	➚	➚
Tumor[+)]	gray	(↗)	(↗)	(↗)
Ballon				
P P D	white	➚	➚	➚
CYTOTOXIC				
Triethyltin	gray	∅	∅	↙
	white	∅	∅	↙
2.4 D N P		-	-	↙

+) from SCHEINBERG, L. C., I. HERZOG, J. M. TAYLOR and R. KATZMAN: Ann. N. Y. Acad. Sci. 159: 509-532 (1969)
PPD: the edema was produced by implantation of a purified protein derivative (PPD)

x) Aldocorten, CIBA AG, Wehr, Baden, W-Germany
xx) Decadron Phosphat, Sharp und Dohme, München, W-Germany

constituents or of ECS-labels is far more pronounced and distributes more widely in the white matter than in the gray matter. In the cytotoxic forms, as e.g. in the TET model, there is no uptake of vital dyes or plasma proteins, neither in gray nor in white matter. The uptake of ECS-markers such as sulphate or thiosulphate even when administered via ventriculo-cisternal perfusion (28) is significantly reduced. Therefore, the increased tissue water content in metabolic edema probably accumulates within the intracellular compartment simultaneously reducing the extracellular space. To our knowledge, the blood-brain-barrier properties have not been analyzed after administration of 2, 4 dinitrophenor 6-aminonicotinamide. An accumulation of edema fluid within the intracellular compartment appears to be supported by a great number of electronmicroscopical reports. However, the fixation techniques generally in use for electronmicroscopy may cause by themselves alterations of the ultrastructure, particularly of the intra-extracellular volume distribution, thus leading to erroneous interpretations of the morphological findings. Fixation by freeze-substitution which was shown to affect the intra-extracellular distribution of tissue fluid to a lesser extent (31), was applied in experimental brain edema produced by the nicotinic acid homologue 6-aminonicotinamide (4). Figure 7 is an electronmicrograph of the molecular layer of the cerebellar vermis of a control and edematous animal. This part of the cerebellar cortex is characterized by the abundancy of non-myelinated nerve fibers, synaptic contacts and processes of glial elements. In the control preparation the extracellular space can easily be recognized immediately under the pia-glia surface membrane, within the axon fields, or surrounding synaptic structures. The electron density of the cellular elements is more or less equal. The most pronounced feature in the edema preparation (lower pannel) is the appearance of swollen cellular elements, probably of glial origin, e.g. around the pre- and postsynaptic endings, rendering the axons closely packed. The extracellular space, however, is still visible in the edema preparation. From the preparation, it may be concluded that this type of cytotoxic or metabolic edema is intracellularly localized, however, without disappearance of the extracellular compartment. Impedance studies in the same experimental model in rats corroborate these findings as far as a moderate reduction of the extracellular compartment is concerned (4).

In the following, the biochemical response of the cerebral tissue to edema shall briefly be mentioned. An involvement of energy metabolism in the development of cerebral edema constitutes an attractive concept which is favoured either by experimental observations about edema production by metabolic inhibitors, some of them have been presented in this context, or by in vivo or in vitro findings on alterations of metabolic activity in edematous tissue (7, 9, 17). Also, in human cerebral edema this aspect has been scrutinized by several groups including ourselves (13, 18, 24, 27). In human cerebral edema, investigations of labile tissue metabolites, such as the energy-rich phosphates, or the lactic or pyruvic acid concentrations are impeded by the technical problem of tissue sampling under freeze-stop conditions. A substantial improvement has been achieved by SCHMIEDEK, who in collaboration with the Linde AG in Munich, developed a safe and sterile biopsy technique praticularly suited for studies in man. This device was applied in clinical studies on tissue concentrations of the energy-rich phosphate compounds or of glycolysis parameters. In Table III, the phosphocreatine content, the ATP/ADP ratio, or the energy charge potential are shown as measures of the energy state of the tissue (3), which may reflect the state of oxygen supply, as well as the lactic acid concentration and the lactate/pyruvate ratio of 26 biopsy specimen of cortical tissue adjacent to a brain tumor. Since for obvious reasons, human control material

Table III. Energy - metabolism in perifocal cerebral cortex

	CrP (μM/g fw)	ATP/ADP	Lactate (μM/g fw)	E C	Lac/Pyr
Edema n = 26	3.53 $\pm$0.34	2.68 $\pm$0.22	4.18 $\pm$0.56	0.78	20.48 $\pm$ 3.13
Controls (dog) n = 6	2.98 $\pm$0.15	4.00 $\pm$0.21	1.40 $\pm$0.13	0.85	4.32 $\pm$ 0.40

CrP = Phosphocreatine, ATP = Adenosinetriphosphate, ADP = Adenosinediphosphate
Lac/Pyr = Lactate - Pyruvate ratio, E C = energy charge potential (3)

$$= \frac{ATP + 0.5\ ADP}{ATP + ADP + AMP}$$

is almost inaccessible, metabolite data obtained from canine cortex under control conditions are shown for comparison. Therefore, we are aware of the fact that conclusions can only be drawn with some reservation. The parameters of the energy state, e.g. the ATP/ADP ratio or the energy charge potential are only slightly reduced in the perifocal tissue compared with control cortex, which is contrasted, however, by the considerably enhanced glycolytic activity as seen from the rise of lactic acid or of the lactate/pyruvate ratio. Consequently, direct edema parameters, as e.g. the tissue water content were found to correlate significantly with the lactic acid concentration ($r=0,52$; $p<0,01$) or the lactate/pyruvate ratio ($r=0,48$; $p<0,05$), whereas no correlations could be established between the energy state and the water content (27).

Conclusions

In the present paper, an attempt was made to demonstrate that chemical analyses of edematous tissue also support the concept advanced by KLATZO, of mainly two representatives of brain edema, namely the vasogenic and cytotoxic type. It appears safe to suppose that the clearcut definition of one type of edema only rarely applies to human brain edema but rather that a combination with a more pronounced vasogenic or more pronounced cytotoxic component prevails. The significance of the vasogenic edema type for human conditions may more easily be understood as being due to the more marked swelling, or the similarity of the chemical findings between experimental and clinical conditions. The role of cytotoxic brain edema in human edema forms is less evident, and can only indirectly be evaluated at the moment. However, the indirect evidence available seems to be convincing, as e.g. the production of brain edema by metabolic inhibitors, which may be paralleled in clinical situations by lowering the oxygen supply to the CNS due to local or general circulatory failures, or during general metabolic intoxications, for example in diabetic coma. The problem to understand the cytotoxic edema in man may be due to the fact that manifestations of cytotoxic edema are superimposed or even modified by the vasogenic component, and/or that the analytical approaches to study cytotoxic edema in man are more limited than for the vasogenic type.

REFERENCES

1. ADACHI, M., W.I.ROSENBLUM and I.FEIGIN: Hypertensive disease and cerebral edema. J.Neurol.Neurosurg.Psychiat. 29, 451-455 (1966)
2. ALEU, F.P., R.KATZMAN and R.D.TERRY: Fine structure and electrolyte analyses of cerebral edema induced by alkyl tin intoxication. J.Neuropath.Exp. Neurol. 22, 403-413 (1963)
3. ATKINSON, D.E.: The energy charge of the adenylate pool as a regulatory parameter. Interaction with feedback modifiers. Biochem. 7, 4030-4034 (1968)
4. BAETHMANN, A. and A. van HARREVELD: Water and electrolyte distribution in gray matter rendered edematous with a metabolic inhibitor. J.Neuropath.Exp. Neurol. (in press)
5. CLASEN, R.A., H.H.SKY-PECK, S.PANDOLFI, I.LAING and G.M.HASS: The chemistry of isolated edema fluid in experimental cerebral injury. In: KLATZO, I. and F.SEITELBERGER: Brain Edema, pp. 536-553, Springer, Wien-New York, (1967)
6. DIETRICH, L.S., I.M.FRIEDLAND and L.A.KAPLAN: Pyridine nucleotide metabolism: Mechanism of action of the niacin antagonist, 6-aminonicotinamide. J.Biol.Chem 233, 964-968 (1958)
7. DITTMANN, J., H.D.HERRMANN, F.LOEW and U.OBERMANN: Examination of the metabolism of edematous brain tissue. Part II. Acta neurochir. 26, 61-82 (1972)
8. ELLIOT, K.A.C. and H.JASPER: Measurement of experimentally induced brain swelling and shrinkage. Amer.J.Physiol. 157, 122-129 (1949)
9. FREI, H.J., Th.WALLENFANG, W.PÖLL, H.J.REULEN, R.SCHUBERT and M.BROCK: Regional cerebral blood flow and regional metabolism in cold edema. Acta neurochir. (in press)
10. HERZOG, I., W.A.LEVY and L.C.SCHEINBERG: Biochemical and morphologic studies of cerebral edema associated with intracerebral tumors in rabbits. J.Neuropath.Exp.Neurol. 24, 244-255 (1965)
11. KAPS, G.: Über elektrophoretische Untersuchungen an Hirngewebe insbesondere aus der Umgebung von Tumoren - zugleich ein Beitrag zur Pathogenese von Hirnschwellung und Hirnödem. Arch.Psychiatr.Nervenkr. 192, 115-119 (1954)
12. KARCHER, D. and A.LOWENTHAL: Hydrosoluble proteins of edematous human nervous tissue. In: KLATZO, I. and F.SEITELBERGER: Brain Edema, pp. 195-201, Springer, Wien-New York, (1967)
13. KIRSCH, W.M. and J.W.LEITNER: Glycolytic metabolites and co-factors in human cerebral cortex and white matter during complete ischemia. Brain Research 4, 358-368 (1967)
14. KIYOTA, K.: Electrophoretic protein fractions and the hydrophilic property of brain tissue - II. J.Neurochem. 4, 209-216 (1959)

15. KLATZO, I., A.PIRAUX and E.J.LASKOWSKI: The relationship between edema, blood-brain-barrier and tissue elements in a local brain injury. J.Neuropath. Exp.Neurol. 17, 548-564 (1958)

16. KLATZO, I.: Neuropathological aspects of brain edema. J.Neuropath.Exp. Neurol. 26, 1-14 (1967)

17. NELSON, S.R. and M.L.MANTZ: Energy reserve levels in edematous mouse brain. Exp.Neurol. 31, 53-59 (1971)

18. OLESEN, J.: Total CO_2, lactate and pyruvate in brain biopsies taken after freezing the tissue in situ. Acta Neurol.Scand. 46, 141-148 (1970)

19. OZAWA, K., H.ARAKI, K.SETA and H.HANDA: Comparison of the inhibitory actions of triethyltin on rat brain and liver mitochondria. J.Biochem 61, 411-413 (1967)

20. PAPPIUS, H.M. and D.R.GULATI: Water and electrolyte content of cerebral tissues in experimentally induced edema. Acta Neuropath. 2, 451-460 (1963)

21. RASMUSSEN, L.W. and I.KLATZO: Protein and enzyme changes in cold injury edema. Acta Neuropath. 13, 12-28 (1969)

22. REULEN, H.J., H.F.HOFMANN and A.BAETHMANN: Die Beeinflussung des experimentellen traumatischen Hirnödems bei der Ratte mit einer Nicotinsäurethophyllin-Verbindung. Zschr.ges.exp.Med. 138, 246-256 (1964)

23. REULEN, H.J. and A.BAETHMANN: Das Dinitrophenolödem. Ein Modell zur Pathophysiologie des Hirnödems. Klin.Wschr. 45, 149-154 (1967)

24. REULEN, H.J., F.MEDZIHRADSKY, R.ENZENBACH, F.MARGUTH and W. BRENDEL: Electrolytes, fluids and energy metabolism in human cerebral edema. Arch.Neurol. 21, 517-525 (1969)

25. REULEN, H.J., A.HADJIDIMOS and K.SCHÜRMANN: The effect of dexamethasone on water and electrolyte content and on rCBF in perifocal brain edema in man. In: REULEN, H.J. and K.SCHÜRMANN: Steroids and Brain Edema. pp. 239-252, Springer, Berlin-Heidelberg-New York, (1972)

26. SCHMIEDEK, P., A. BAETHMANN, E.SCHNEIDER, W.OETTINGER, R.ENZENBACH, F.MARGUTH and W.BRENDEL: The effect of aldosterone and an aldosterone-antagonist on the metabolism of perifocal brain edema in man. In: REULEN, H.J. and K.SCHÜRMANN: Steroids and Brain Edema, pp. 203-210, Springer, Berlin-Heidelberg-New York, (1972)

27. SCHMIEDEK, P., A.BAETHMANN, G.SIPPEL, W.OETTINGER, R.ENZENBACH, F.MARGUTH and W.BRENDEL: Energy state and glycolysis in human cerebral edema (in preparation)

28. SOHLER, K.: Thesis (in preparation)

29. STERN, W.E., M.L.ABBOTT and B.W.CHESEBORO: A study of the role of osmotic gradients in experimental cerebral edemas. J.Neurosurg. 24, 57-60 (1966)

30. STEWART-WALLACE, A.M.: A biochemical study of cerebral tissue, and of the changes in cerebral edema. Brain 62, 426-438 (1939)

31. van HARREVELD, A., J.CROWELL and S.K.MALHOTRA: A study of extracellular space in central nervous tissue by freeze-substitution. J.Cell.Biol. 25, 117-137 (1965)

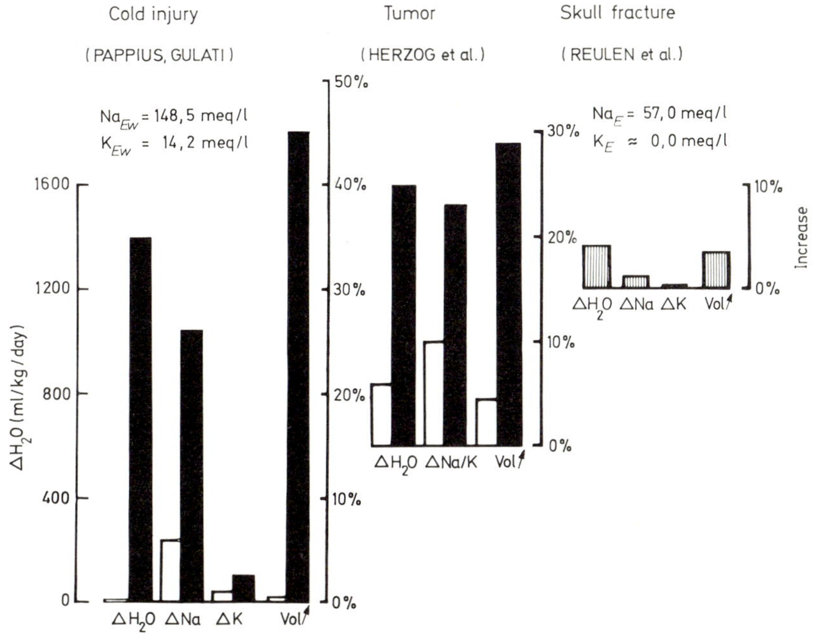

Fig. 1. Changes of the cerebral electrolyte and water content in brain edema after cold injury (Kältetrauma), in perifocal tissue surrounding an implanted tumor, and after acceleration concussion of the mobile skull of rats (stumpfes Schädeltrauma). The differences in electrolyte and water content have been calculated on dry weight (TG) basis. In perifocal tissue (HERZOG et al.) the changes of the molar Na/K ratio computed on fresh weight basis are given. The percent tissue swelling (Vol ↗, Schwellung) is obtained by the ELLIOT and JASPER equation. The grey and white matter is symbolized by white or black columns respectively. Na_{EW}, or K_{EW} gives the concentration of the electrolytes as computed in the white matter edema fluid by $\frac{\Delta Na, K(meq/kg\ dw)}{\Delta H_2O(ml/kg\ dw)} \times 1000$. Na_E, K_E is the electrolyte edema concentration in mixed gray and white matter after skull trauma in rats

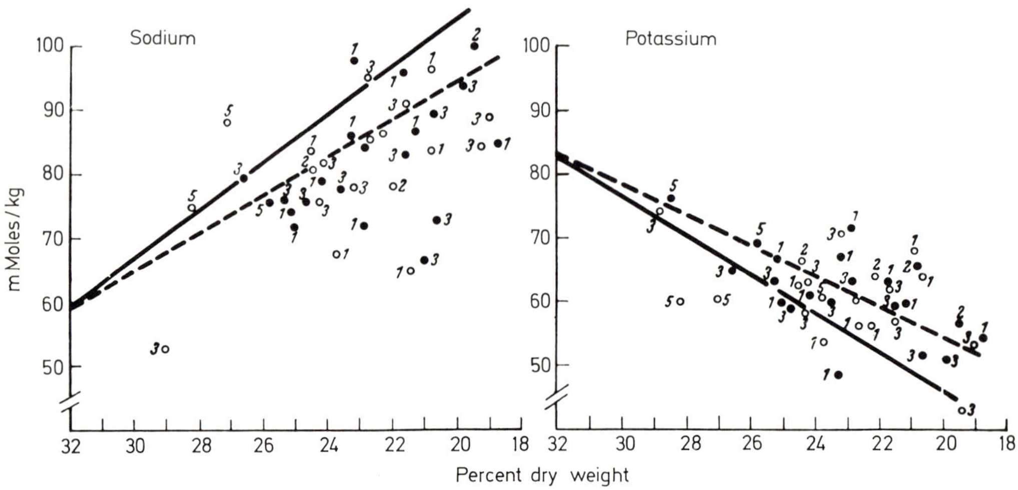

Fig. 2. Correlation diagram between the tissue Na- or K-concentration (meq/kg fw) and the percent dry weight of edematous white matter of the cat (cold injury). The solid lines and the dotted lines were computed assuming the edema fluid to be whole plasma or plasma filtrate
o = untreated, • = pretreated with cortisone
(from: PAPPIUS, H. and D.R. GULATI,[20])

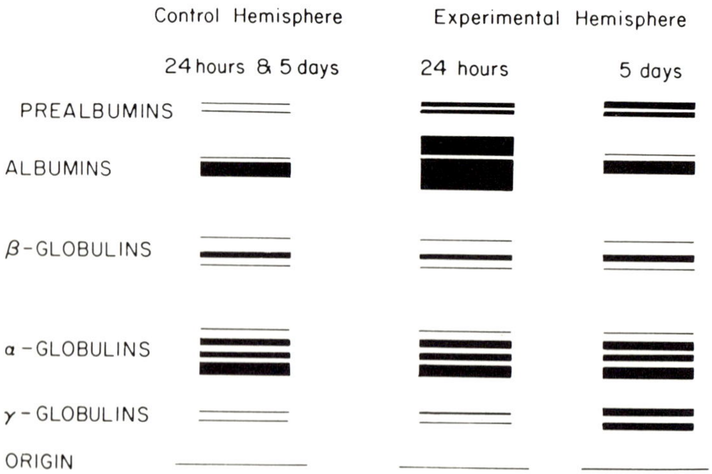

Fig. 3. White matter proteins of edematous tissue separated by disc gel electrophoresis. The edema was produced by cold injury of the exposed cortical surface. 5 days after traumatization the albumins returned to control levels, with a persistent elevation of the pre-albumins. The initially normal γ-globulins rose slightly after 5 days
(from: RASMUSSEN, L. E. and I. KLATZO,[21])

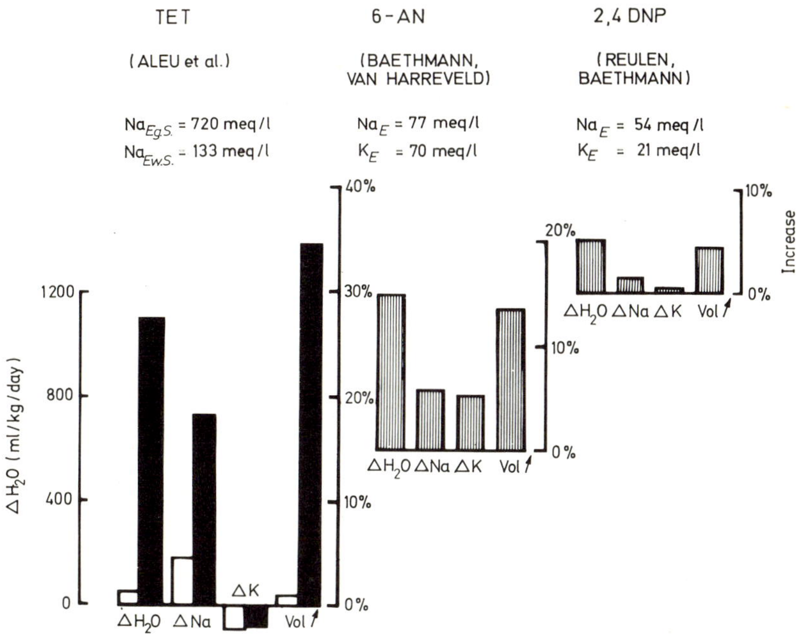

Fig. 4. Changes of the water and electrolyte content (difference between control and experimental animals) in cytotoxic brain edema calculated on dry weight (TG) basis from the data of ALEU et al. (2), BAETHMANN and van HARREVELD (4), and REULEN and BAETHMANN (23). The tissue swelling (Vol ↗, Schwellung) is given in percent volume (ref. to the text). Gray and white matter is symbolized by white and black columns, respectively. Mixed gray and white substance are shown as screened columns. Na $_{EgS.}$ =(Na^+) concentration of the edema fluid in the gray substance, $Na_{EwS.}$ =edema (Na^+) in the white substance, Na_E, K_E =edema electrolyte concentration in mixed gray and white matter. For calculation ref. to the text. TET = triethyltin, 6-AN = 6-aminonicotinamide, 2, 4 DNP = dinitrophenol

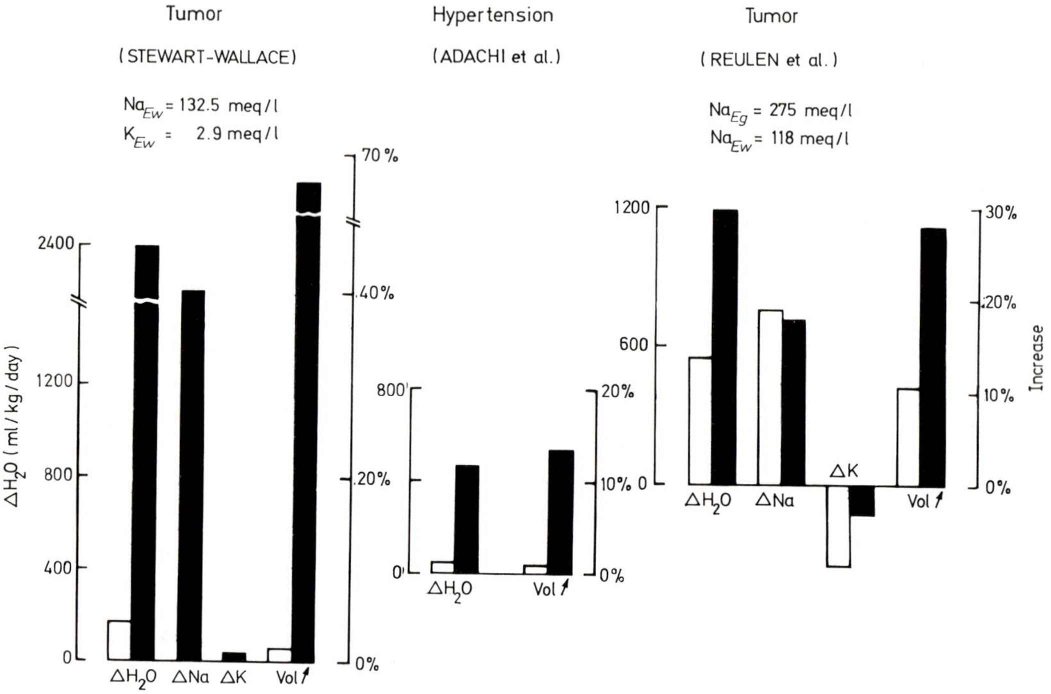

Fig. 5. Tissue swelling (Schwellung) and changes of the electrolyte and water content on dry weight basis (ref. also to Fig. 1 and 4) in human perifocal edema or in malignant hypertension, computed from the data of STEWART-WALLACE (30), ADACHI et al. (1) and REULEN et al. (24). Only the data of REULEN reflect in vivo conditions. The figures on top of the columns give the calculated electrolyte concentrations in the edema fluid of white matter (E_w) or gray matter (E_g) in milliequivalent per liter

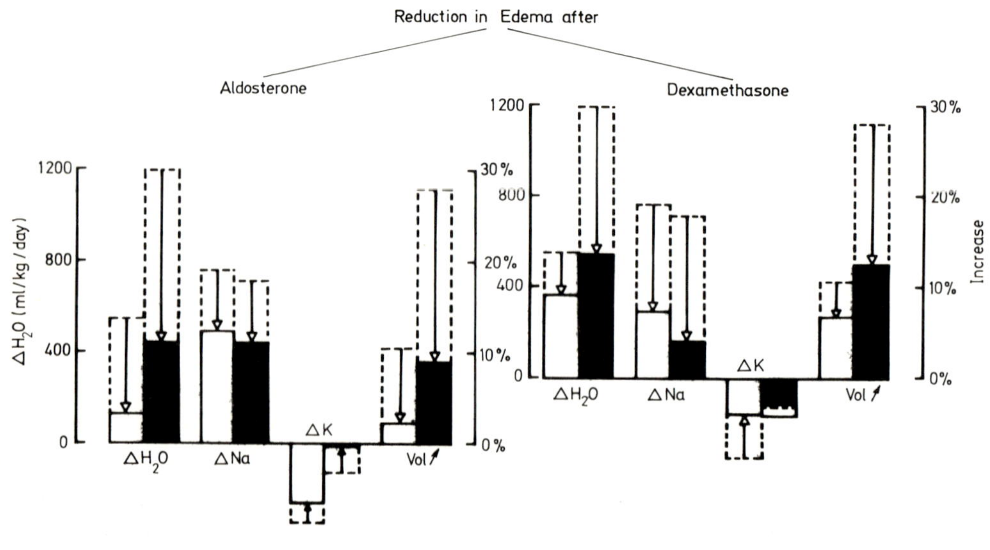

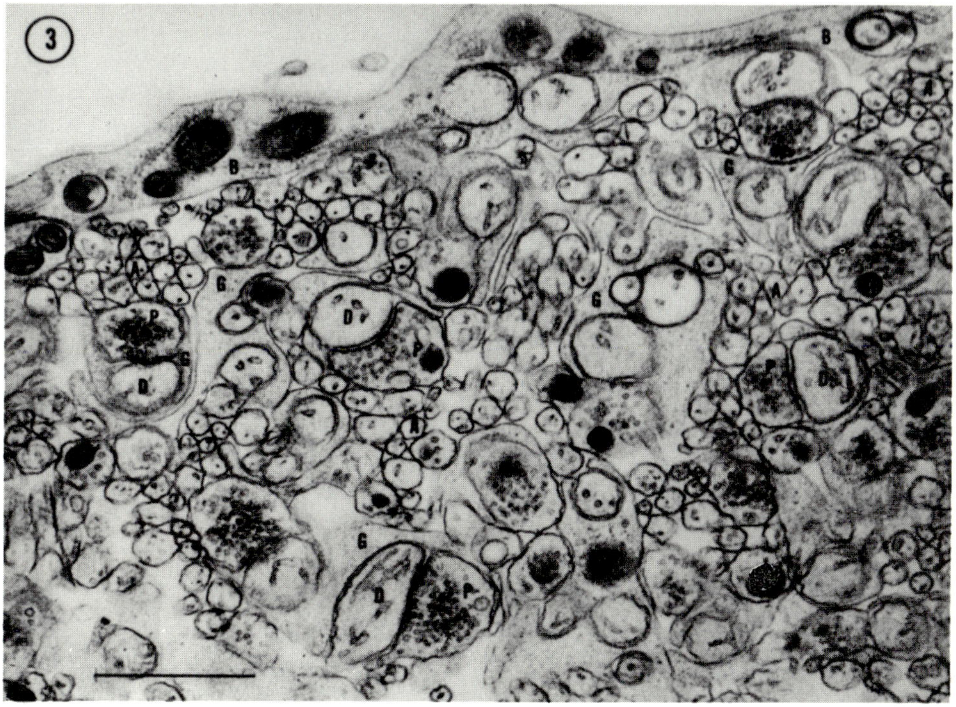

Fig. 7. Freeze-substituted molecular layer of the cerebellar vermis of a control ③ and after 6-aminonicotinamide (continued on p. 18)

◄

Fig. 6. The effect of treatment with aldosterone or dexamethasone (i.e. Ödemausschwemmung) on perifocal brain edema in man. Taking the edematous changes (ΔH_2O, ΔNa, ΔK) in perifocal areas, calculated from REULEN et al. (ref. Fig. 5) as a basis, the differences of the specifically pretreated and untreated groups of patients were subtracted (dotted lines). The solid columns (white = gray, black = white matter) symbolize the amount of edema remaining in the tissue

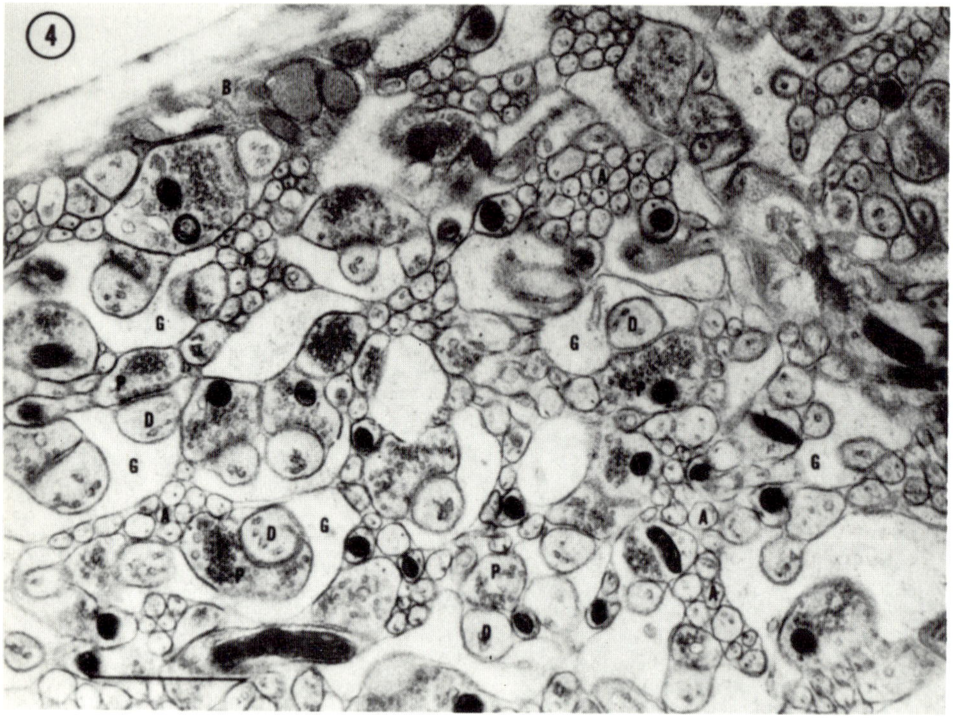

Fig.7. (continued) ④ showing non-myelinated nerve fibers, endfeet of BERGAMNN fibers, synaptic contacts and glial processes. The extracellular space is present under the pia-glia surface membrane, or in the axon fields. In ④the glial components are moreelectronstransparent than in the control preparation and have a swollen appearance, the extracellular space seems to be moderately reduced. The calibration line is 1 μ
(from: BAETHMANN, A. and A. van HARREVELD, [4])

Capillary Lesions and Hemorrhages in Brain Edema

F. MATAKAS, T. KLEMANN, and J. CERVÓS-NAVARRO

Intracranial hypertension is the most important consequence of brain edema. If the intracranial pressure exceeds a critical value it may reduce intracranial perfusion pressure and cerebral blood flow (CBF) (HEDGES, WEINSTEIN, KASSELL, STEIN, 1964; RISBERG, LUNDBERG, INGVAR, 1969; JOHNSTON, ROWAN, HARPER, JENNETT, 1972). Apart from the brain edema itself the immediate sequelae of intracranial hypertension are only of physiological nature. However, if they persist for some time they are soon followed by vascular lesions. The capillary lumen may be narrowed by endothelial swelling. Midbrain hemorrhages occur when brain edema develops to brain death. - The following experiments were undertaken to clarify the mechanism of both phenomena.

Material and methods

Six baboons and 11 cats were used for the experiments. All animals were anesthetised with pentobarbital sodium (40 mg/kg i.m.), relaxed with succinylbischol ine, and ventilated by means of a Starling pump via an endotracheal tube. Arterial pressure, ECG, EEG, body temperature, epidural pressure, and blood gases were constantly recorded. In 10 animals cerebral ischemia was produced by intracranial hypertension: An epidural balloon was inflated or mock CSF was injected into the intracranial space until the intracranial pressure equalled arterial pressure. In 7 cats the brachiocephalic trunk and the left subclavian artery were clamped. Cerebral ischemia lasted 20 minutes in all experiments. In those experiments which lasted for more than 1 hour sodium and potassium of the blood were controlled all 6 hours and balanced. Metabolic acidosis which developed after ischemia was compensated by Tris buffer, but not earlier than 2 to 3 hours after ischemia. Nine animals were sacrificed 1 hour, 2 animals 6 hours, and 6 animals 12 to 48 hours after cerebral ischemia. The animals which did not survive more than 1 hour were perfused with a carbon suspension before the end of the experiments. The rest of the animals were perfused with glutaraldehyde. Tissue samples of the brain were taken from all animals for electron microscopy.

Results

The technique for producing cerebral ischemia had no influence on the results. In all animals the EEG became isoelectric within 10 to 20 seconds after the beginning of cerebral ischemia. The mean arterial pressure after ischemia had to be raised by norepinephrine. It was maintained between 80 and 100 mm Hg. In all animals intracranial hypertension developed. One hour after cerebral ischemia the intracranial perfusion pressure was usually not greater than 30 mm Hg.

One hour after ischemia wide areas of the cerebrum were not perfused by the carbon suspension (Fig. 1). The nonperfused areas of the crebral cortex were predominantly located in the superior parts of the brain. The basal ganglia and brain stem showed only minor defects. Six hours after ischemia there was no perfusion of the cerebrum and large defects in the brain stem. After 12 hours the whole brain was not perfused. In most cases the defects were roughly symmetrical in both hemispheres.

In those areas where no perfusion had occurred the capillaries and venules showed severe lesions. The endothelium was thickened, the lumen was narrowed. In those animals which had survived more than 6 hours more than 80% of cerebral capillaries and venules were obstructed by endothelial swelling, blebs, or impacted erythrocytes (Fig. 2).

All animals had developed brain edema. The astrocytes, particularly in the perivascular region, were swollen and had a watery cytoplasm. Brain edema was moderate after 1 hour and extreme after 24 hours.

Six hours after cerebral ischemia small hemorrhages were found in the midbrain. They were most numerous in the medial parts of the midbrain, but extended in some cases into the posterior parts of the basal ganglia and medial parts of the occipital lobe (Fig. 3).

Discussion

Cerebral ischemia causes brain edema (REULEN, STEUDE, BRENDEL, HILBER, PRUSINER, 1970). Brain edema may cause intracranial hypertension and impairment of venous drainage (HEKMATPANAH 1970). As a consequence, the intracranial perfusion pressure is reduced and CBF diminishes. In our experiments the brain was subjected to a reduction of CBF by two mechanisms. Ischemia was first artificially produced for a limited time period. Afterwards brain edema and intracranial hypertension developed. Since in all animals the intracranial perfusion pressure fell to low values it seems justified to assume that the cerebral circulation was considerably reduced or even completely stopped. However, the results of our experiments show that another mechanism developed which must have contributed to disturbances of the cerebral circulation, viz. the lesions of capillaries and venules. Such lesions were first observed by HILLS, (1964) and CHIANG, KOWADA, AMES, WRIGHT, MAJNO (1968) immediately after cerebral ischemia. Only HILLS (1964) observed capillary obstruction after longer periods of recovery, but had applied a different technique. The results of our experiments demonstrate that the degree of capillary lesions increases in correspondence to the development of brain edema. In brain death all capillaries are affected (MATAKAS, CERVOS-NAVARRO, SCHNEIDER, 1973).

AMES, WRIGHT, KOWADA, THURSTON, MAJNO (1968) and GINSBERG, MYERS (1972) observed incomplete perfusion of the brain immediately after cerebral ischemia. Though in our experiments obstruction of capillaries was confined to such nonperfused areas we think that they were the result rather than the cause of the "no-reflow" phenomenon. The distribution of lesions makes it probable that first venous compression by brain edema caused a regional stop of the circulation, which was followed by lesions of the microvasculature.

Severe brain edema after cerebral ischemia or anoxia develops in two phases.

First intracranial hypertension is confined to the supratentorial space. Because of the "Axialverschiebung" (RIESSNER, ZÜLCH, 1939) hypertension in the infratentorial space may follow after an interval of some hours. This is proved by the fact that the no-reflow phenomenon was observed in the infratentorial space later than in the supratentorial space. The well-known fact that in brain death a stop of the intracranial circulation is first observed in the carotid artery and later in the vertebral artery is another support for this assumption. Thus brain edema beginning in the supratentorial space may reach a point of development where the veins draining the midbrain are compressed because they empty into the vein of Galen (HOLDORFF, CERVOS-NAVARRO 1971) while the arteries of this area are still supplied by the vertebral system. Obviously the midbrain hemorrhages develop in this phase. This explains why they are nearly always found in severe brain edema which started in the supratentorial space (KLINTWORTH, 1966) but usually only after an interval of some hours.

REFERENCES

1. AMES, A., R. L. WRIGHT, M. KOWADA, J. M. THURSTON and G. MAJNO: Cerebral ischemia. II. The no-reflow phenomenon. Am. J. Pathol. 52, 437-453 (1968)
2. CHIANG, J., M. KOWADA, A. AMES, R. L. WRIGHT and G. MAJNO: Cerebral ischemia. III. Vascular changes. Am. J. Pathol. 52, 455-476 (1968)
3. GINSBERG, M. and R. E. MYERS: The topography of impaired microvascular perfusion in the primate brain following total circulatory arrest. Neurology 22, 998-1011 (1972)
4. HEDGES, T.R., J.C. WEINSTEIN, N. KASSELL and S. STEIN: Cerebro-vascular responses to increased intracranial pressure. J. Neurosurg. 21, 292-297 (1964)
5. HEKMATPANAH, J.: Cerebral circulation and perfusion in experimental increased pressure. J. Neurosurg. 32, 21-29 (1970)
6. HILLS, C. P.: Ultrastructural changes in the capillary bed of the rat cerebral cortex in anoxic-ischemic brain lesions. Am. J. Pathol. 44, 531-551 (1964)
7. HOLDORFF, B. and J. CERVOS-NAVARRO: Die Pathologie der inneren ponto-mesencephalen Venen. Der Radiologe 11, 465-471 (1971)
8. JOHNSTON, I. H., J. O. ROWAN, A. M. HARPER and W. B. JENNETT: Raised intracranial pressure and cerebral blood flow. I. Cisterna magna infusion in primates. J. Neurol., Neurosurg., Psychiatr. 35, 285-296 (1972)
9. KLINTWORTH, G. K.: Evaluation of the role of neurosurgical procedures in the pathogenesis of secondary brain-stem hemorrhages. J. Neurol., Neurosurg., Psychiatr. 29, 423-425 (1966)
10. MATAKAS, F., J. CERVOS-NAVARRO and H. SCHNEIDER: Experimental brain death. I. Morphology and fine structure of the brain. Neurol., Neurosurg., Psychiatr. (in press)
11. REULEN, H. J., U. STEUDE, W. BRENDEL, C. HILBER and S. PRUSINER: Energetische Störung des Kationentransports als Ursache des intrazellulären Hirnödems. Acta. Neurochir. 22, 129-166 (1970)

12. RIESSNER, D. and K.J. ZÜLCH: Über die Formveränderungen des Hirns (Massenverschiebungen, Zisternenverquellungen) bei raumbeengenden Prozessen. Dtsch. Z. Chir. 253, 1-61 (1939)

13. RISBERG, J., N. LUNDBERG and D.H. INGVAR: Regional cerebral blood volume during acute transient rises of the intracranial pressure (plateau waves). J. Neurosurg. 31, 303-310 (1969)

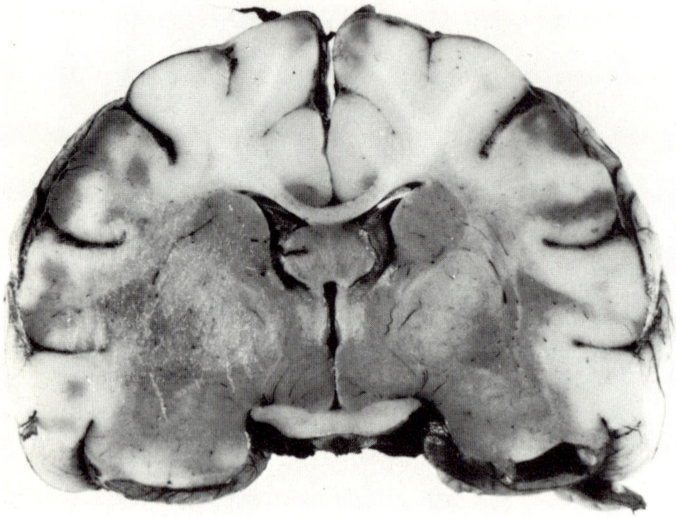

Fig. 1. Cat. coronal section. One hour after cerebral ischemia of 20 minutes. Large areas of the brain are not perfused

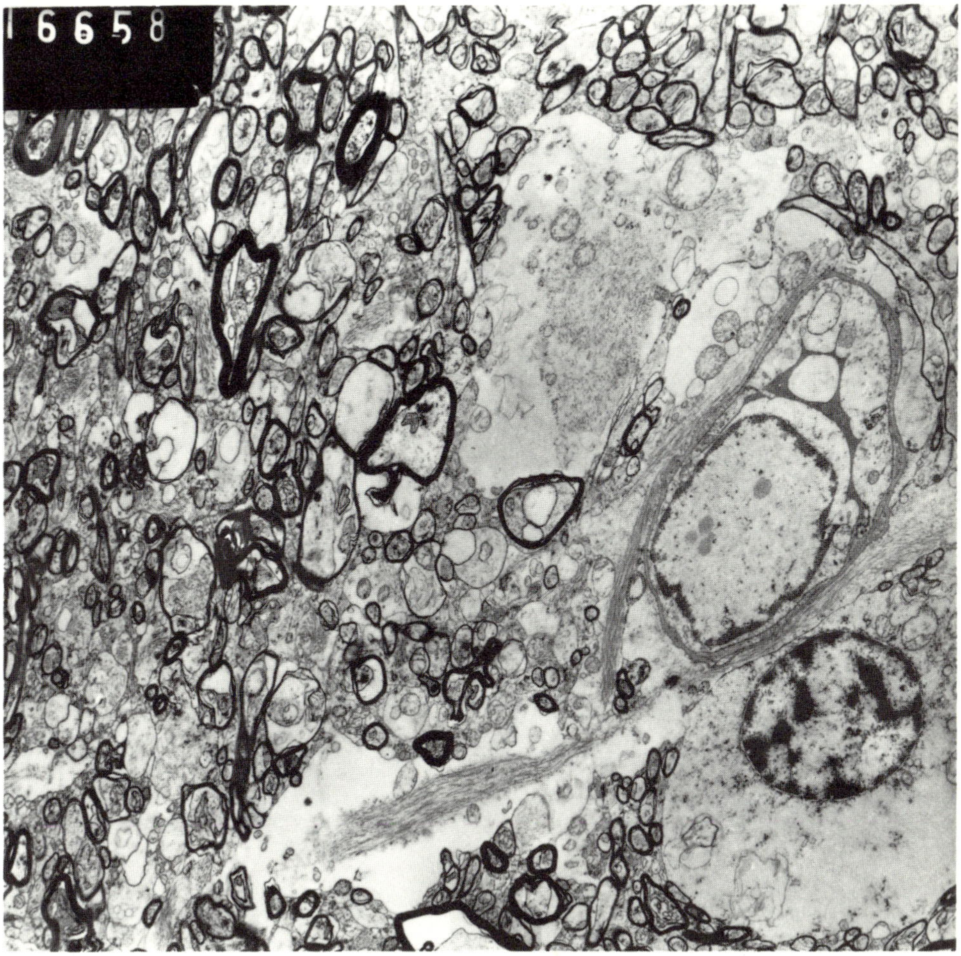

Fig. 2. Baboon. 12 hours after cerebral ischemia. Swelling of the capillary endothelium. x 4,500

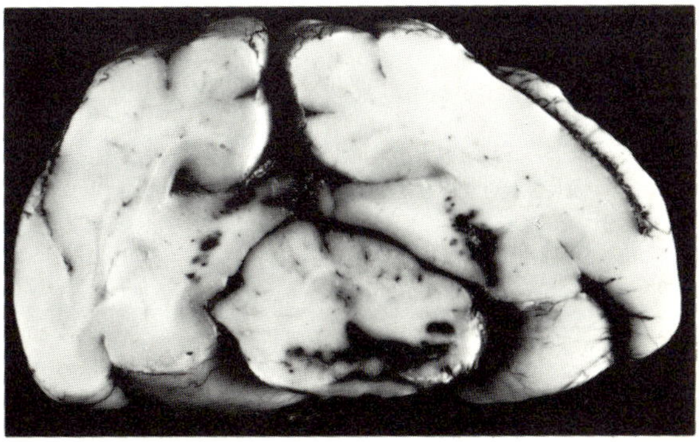

Fig. 3. Cat. six hours after cerebral ischemia. Hemorrhages in the midbrain and in medial parts of the occipital lobe

Blood Brain Barrier and Scintigraphy

L. PENNING and D. FRONT

A scintigraphic study of brain contusion confronted us again with the problem of the blood-brain barrier. It is generally accepted that damage of the blood-brain barrier is a cause of scintigraphic visualization of a brain lesion. However, the problem in brain tumors is quite different from that in brain contusion. It should be remembered that in tumors we are dealing with non-cerebral tissue. Their visualization in fact is dependent on the presence or absence of a blood-tumor barrier. Brain contusion serves as a pure model to study scintigraphically the damage of the blood-brain barrier itself.

Due to shortage of time we will have to limit ourselves to the demonstration of one illustrative case. It concerns a seven-year-old girl with a brain contusion after a car accident. There was a linear fracture of the left temporal bone. The scintigraphs made after 5 days (Fig. 1 a and b) demonstrate a diffuse lesion of the right hemisphere in the posterior view; in the lateral view only slight abnormalities in the temporo-occipital region are noticed. The scintigraphic investigation 3 weeks after the accident (Fig. 2 a and b) shows a quite different picture: a well-defined wedge-shaped lesion in the right occipital region. The rest of the right hemisphere has returned to normal. In a third study 4 months after the accident (Fig. 3 a and b) all abnormalities have disappeared.

What is the significance of those scintigraphic findings? The diffuse and vague shadow in the first investigation is often observed in the early stages of brain contusion. It has a tendency to disappear for the largest part rather quickly. In our opinion it represents the brain contusion with resultant brain edema. In the edematous region the brain tissue is not permanently damaged, which explains the quick disappearance of the largest part of the diffuse and vague scintigraphic shadow What we see in the second investigation closely resembles brain infarction due to primary vascular disease. Histological investigation of brain specimens after head injuries has shown that traumatic brain infarction is a common finding. Like non-traumatic infarction the lesion appears only after a certain interval of time. The last series of pictures shows that even large lesions may disappear completely at the end.

In conclusion we should like to stress that brain contusion serves as a suitable model to study in vivo traumatic lesions of the blood-brain barrier. Using sodium pertechnetate as a blood-brain barrier tracer we are now investigating in how far the observations in cold-injury animal experiments are correlating with our own in vivo scintigraphic findings.

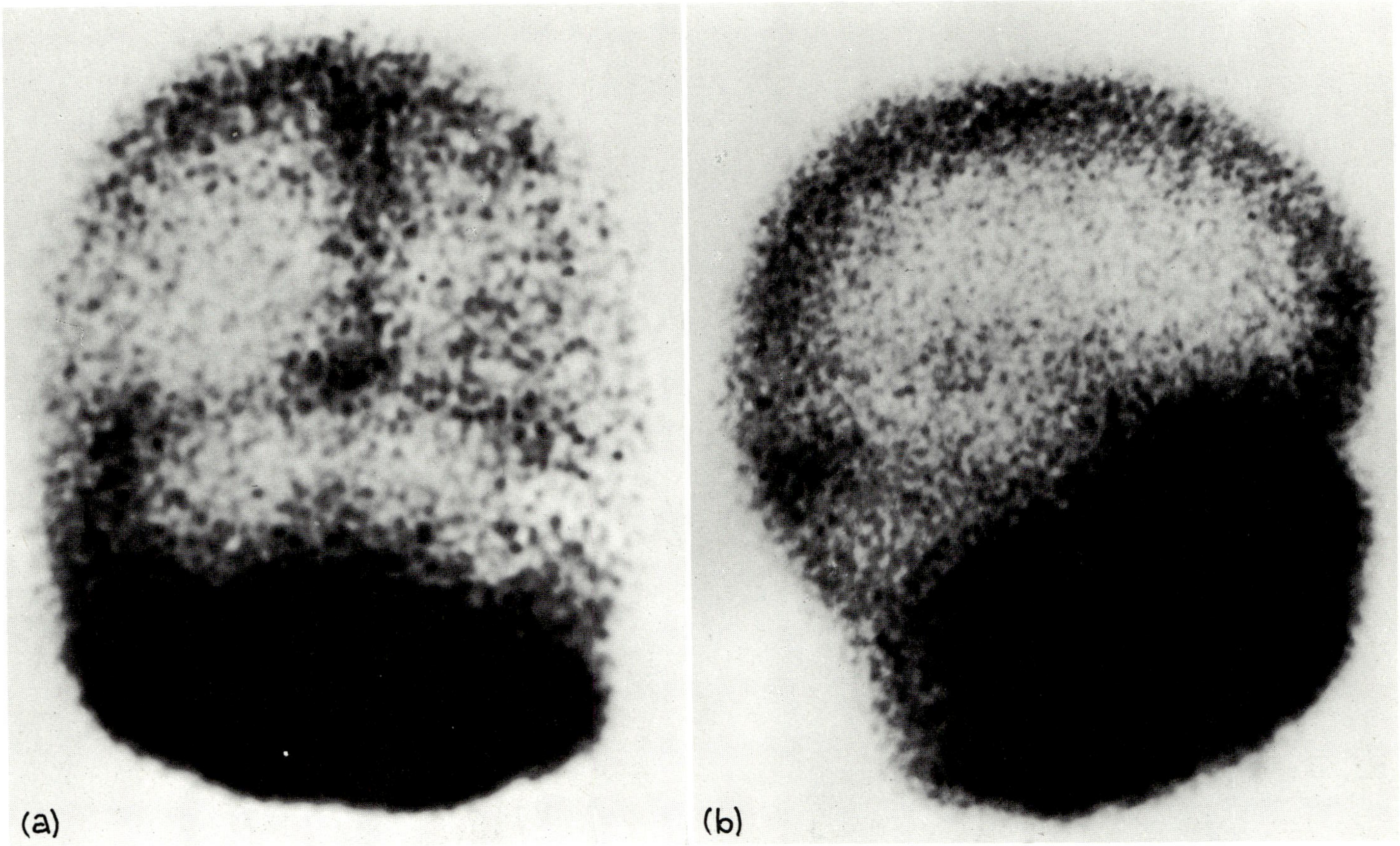

Fig. 1. Posterior and lateral scintiencephalographic views of a 7-year-old girl, hostpitalized because of brain contusion due to a car accident. X-ray pictures of the skull revealed a linear fracture of the left temporal bone. Extracerebral hematoma was ruled out by angiography. The EEG showed diffuse slow wave activity and local disturbances in the right posterior region. The scintigraphs (made 5 days after the injury) demonstrate a diffuse lesion of the right hemisphere in the posterior view (a). The lateral (b) view is normal

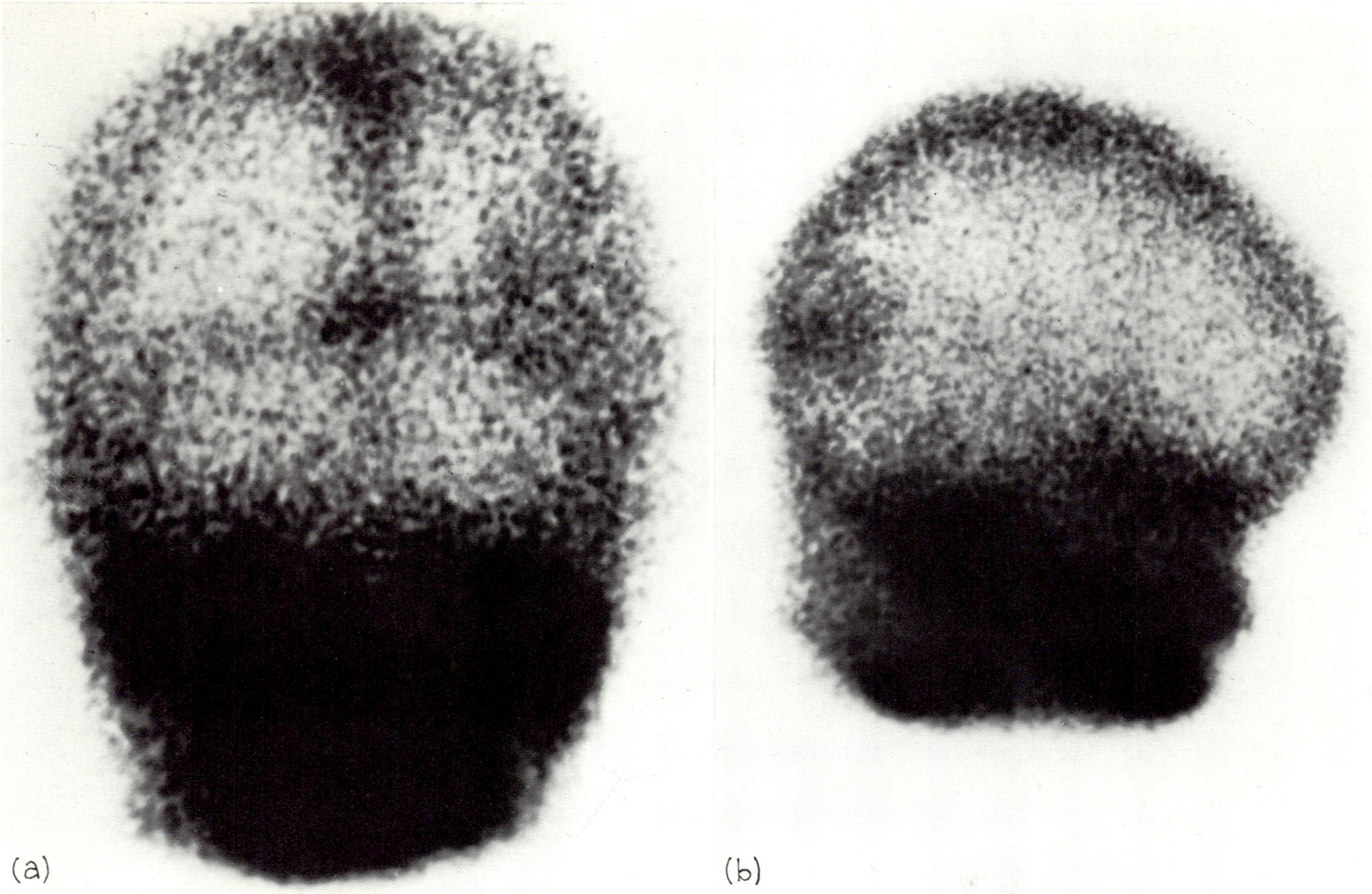

Fig. 2. Follow-up scintigraphy in the same patient 3 weeks after the injury. Well defined wedge-shaped lesion in the posterior view (a). On the lateral view (b) an abnormal accumulation of radioactivity with well-defined borders is visible in the occipital region

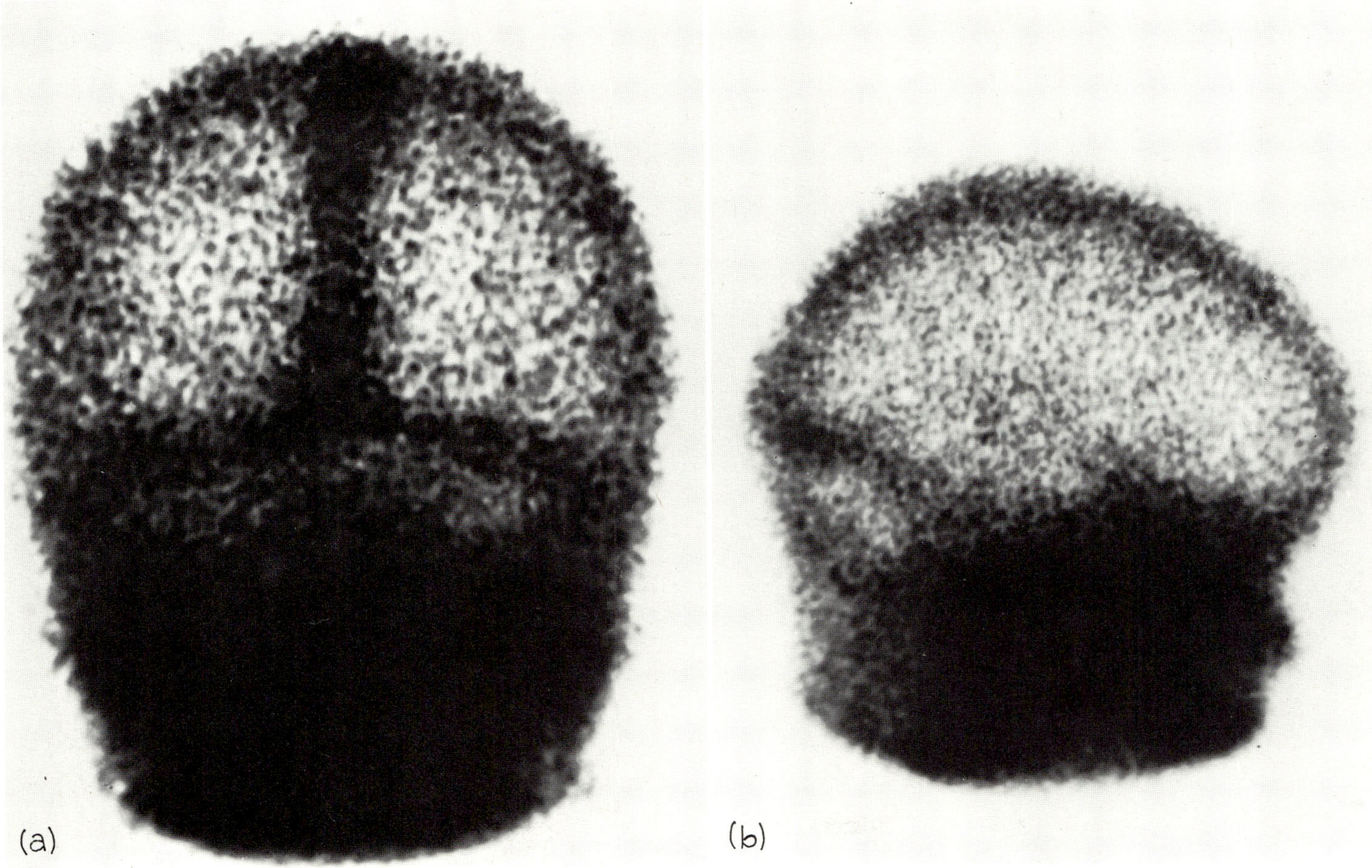

Fig. 3. Follow-up scintigraphy in the same patient 4 months after the injury. No abnormalities in the posterior (a) or lateral (b) view. When the girl left the hospital she had a mild spastic leftsided hemiparesis, and severe behaviour disturbances. No visual disturbances or visual field defects were found

Biochemical Disturbances in Experimental Brain Edema

A. GROMEK, D. CZAJKOWSKA, Z. CZERNICKI, J. JURKIEWICZ, and A. KUNICKI

The present studies were undertaken to examine the initial state of brain edema and the accompanying biochemical changes. We were especially interested in the reversible early changes.

An extradural balloon was used to induce brain edema in cats according to the method fo ISHII et al. (3). The duration of the experiment was 2 h (on the basis of our previous observation that the intracranial pressure starts rising after 2 h of brain compression).

Two groups of mongrel cats were used in the studies described: 19 animals with spontaneous respiration and 6 with artificial respiration. The control group consisted of 7 cats. From the group with spontaneous respiration we eliminated all cats with severe respiratory disturbances and other complications e.g. hemorrhage so that only 9 cats were left for final analysis. The animals were anesthetized with Nembutal (40 mg/kg body weight). A burr hole was made on the left occipital region and a bolt-screw with a latex balloon was screwed in. The balloon was inflated slowly at a rate of 0, 2 ml every ten minutes to reach the final volume of 0, 7 to 1, 1 ml in the group with spontaneous respiration and 0, 1 ml in the group with artificial respiration. The respiratory parameters were selected on the basis of gasometric measurements: pH, pO_2, pCO_2. After 2 h of brain compression with the final balloon volume brain tissue samples were taken from the left occipito-parietal region of animals still alive. The animals were then sacrificed.

The samples were examined in an electron microscope and biochemically under the three following aspects: oxidative phosphorylation, ATP-ases and free fatty acids (FFA). Oxidative phosphorylation was estimated by determining the respiration control index (RCI) and the index of oxidative phosphorylation ADP/O. Isolated mitochondria were examined according to the method of CHANCE. Mg and DNP-ATP-ase activity was calculated according to the method Fiske-Subbarow. Free fatty acids were determined using the colorimetric method of Itaya and Ui.

The results obtained are shown in the table I and the figures 1 and 2.

Table I concerns oxidative phosphorylation. There is a very slight reduction of RCI and ADP/O, which is higher in the group with spontaneous respiration. The ADP/O index decreased a little more than RCI, but there are values in both animal groups which correspond to the control group values. When albumin was added to the reacting solution in order to remove FFA, oxidative phosphorylation increased to values comparable with the control group. Thus oxidative phosphorylation is uncoupled very slightly, less for animals with artificial respiration (Fig. 1).

Table I. Oxidative phosphorylation in mitochondrial fraction from cat brain hemispheres

EXPERIMENTAL CONDITIONS	RCI - Albumin	RCI + Albumin+)	ADP/O - Albumin	ADP/O + Albumin
A. Control	$7,46 \pm 0,84$	$10,30 \pm 0,43$	$2,79 \pm 0,14$	$2,94 \pm 0,10$
B. Edema with natural respiration	$3,13 \pm 0,73$	$4,31 \pm 0,97$	$1,90 \pm 0,35$	$2,10 \pm 0,37$
C. Edema with artificial respiration	$4,50 \pm 0,48$	$7,88 \pm 0,68$	$2,41 \pm 0,16$	$2,71 \pm 0,20$

+) Albumin concentration -04%

The activity of Mg-ATP-ase, DNP-ATP-ase and Mg-DNP-ATP-ase is distinctly lowered. For Mg-ATP-ase this reduction is approximately 25% (Fig. 2).

The main biochemical changes concern the free fatty acid concentration. A significant rise of FFA was detected both in the homogenate (1, 5 times) and in the mitochondrial fraction (3 times). (Fig. 3)

The electron microscope examination showed changes in the structure of some mitochondria, an increase in size of the astrocytes surrounding the capillaries and an enlargement of endoplasmic reticulum. There was also a slight alternation of myelin. No signs of destruction were observed.

The results of the examinations performed indicate the great influence of respiratory disturbances on the course of the experiment. Thus, in experiments with brain edema only animals with artificial respiration should be used. One should also stress the great role of anesthesia.

Very interesting results were obtained in the albumin test. This test seems to indicate that free fatty acids participate in the uncoupling of oxidative phosphorylation. It is in agreement with the results of SATO et al. (5) and YAMAGUSHI et al. (6). In our experiments the observed disturbances of oxidative phosphorylation were reversible which correspond to the electron microscope picture - very slight alternations without any destruction.

It is well-known that FFA depress ATP-ase activities. However disturbances of ATP-ase activity have been found by many authors for example LIM et al. (4). Nevertheless such disturbances have not been investigated following only 2 h of brain compression.

The high rise of FFA concentration in our experiments corresponds to the results of BAZAN (1, 2). Thus free fatty acids are the main biochemical factors which facilitate edema development in our brain edema model.

Summary

Increased intracranial pressure was produced in cats by compressing the brain for two hours using an epidural balloon. A great increase in free fatty acid concentration was detected together with a distinct reduction of Mg and DNP-ATP-ase activities and slight uncoupling of oxidative phosphorylation.

The observed changes were reversible. The biochemical results were compared with the electron microscope picture.

REFERENCES

1. BAZAN, N.G.: Effects of ischemia and electroconvulsive shock on free fatty acid pool in the brain. Biochem. Biophys. Acta 218, 1-10 (1970)

2. BAZAN, N.G.: Free fatty acid production in cerebral white and grey matter of the squirrel monkey. Lipids 6, 211-212 (1971)

3. ISHII, S., R. HAYNER, W.A. KELLY and J.P. EVANS: Studies of cerebral swelling. II. Experimental cerebral swelling produced by supratentorial extradural compression. J. Neurosurg. 16, 152-166 (1959)

4. LIM, R., J.C. de la TORRE and S. MULLAN: Protein and enzyme alterations in experimental brain injury. Arch. Neurol 27, 314-322 (1972)

5. SATO, K., M. YAMAGUCHI, S. MULLAN: Brain edema: A study of biochemical and structural alternation. Arch. Neurol. 21, 413-424 (1969)

6. YAMAGUCHI, M., K. SATO, J.P. EVANS and S. ISHII: Experimental brain edema. The role of a factor in brain supernatant in the prevention of edema. Arch. Neurol. 22, 521-527 (1970)

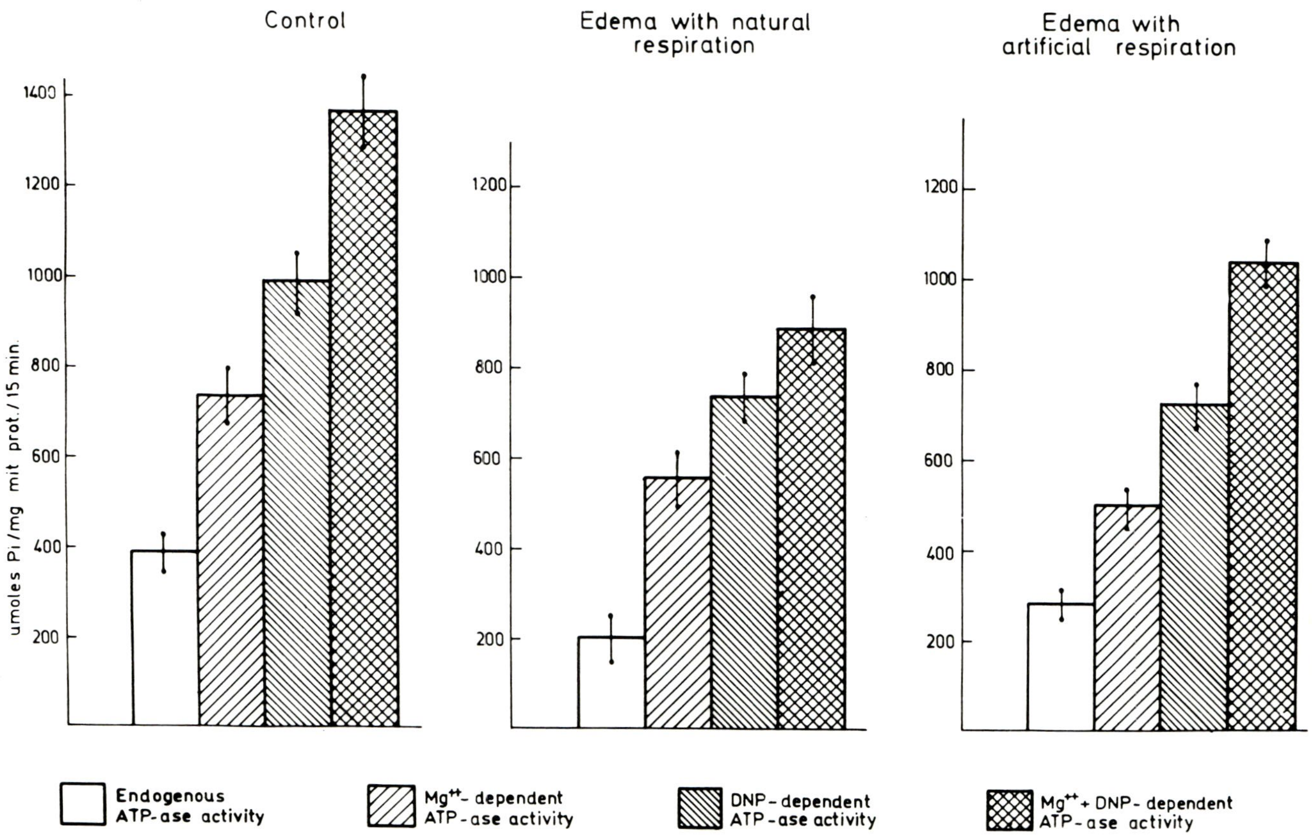

Fig. 1. ATP-ase activity of mitochondrial fraction from cat brain hemispheres

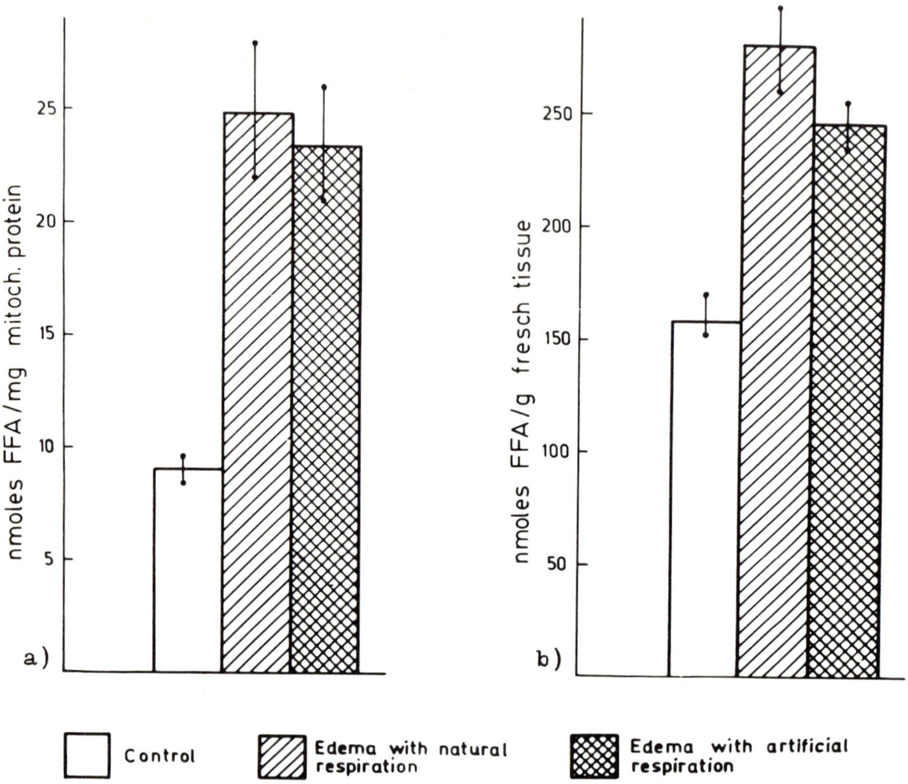

Fig. 2. a) Liberation of free fatty acids from mitochondrial fraction of cat brain; b) liberation of free fatty acids from hemogenates of cat brain

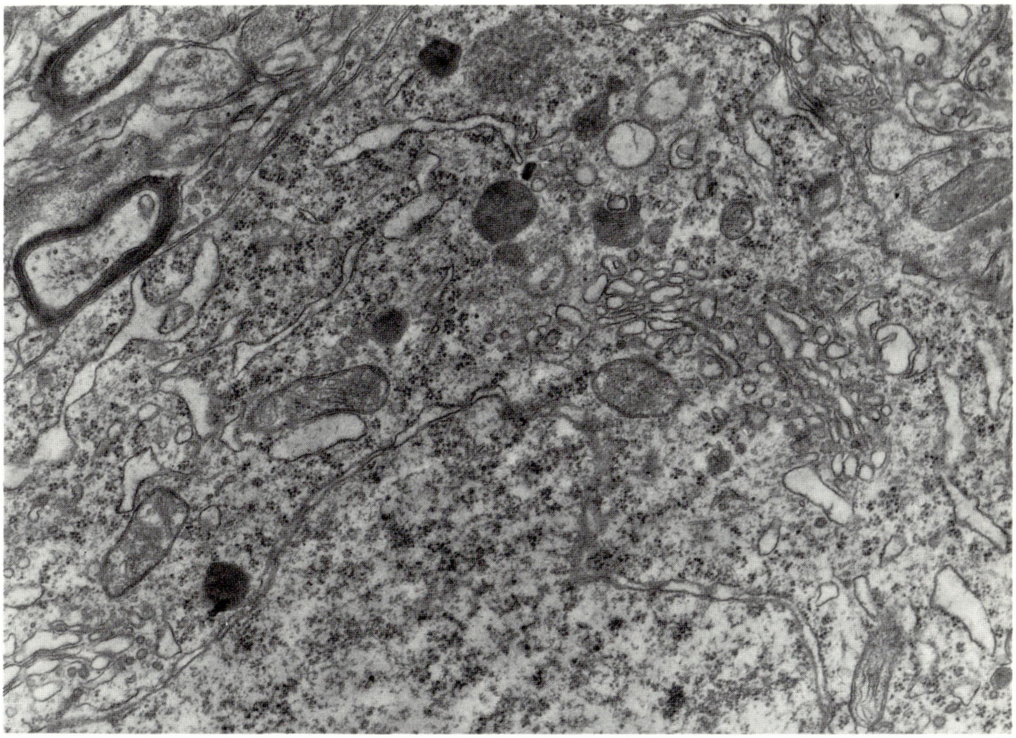

Fig. 3. Electron micrograph of the white - matter perivascular space in the cat after 2 hours of brain compression: enlargement of smooth and rough endoplasmic reticulum, lysosomes in the form of dense bodies and multivesicular bodies, partly damaged mitochondria (x 16500)

Alterations of Metabolism in Brain Edema Following Head Injury

I. HAUSDÖRFER, W. HELLER, P. OLDENKOTT, and C. STOLZ

Introduction

The systematic studies performed by our group in recent years had the purpose of demonstrating the changes in metabolism caused by head injuries and, if possible, of relating the degree of the lesion and its prognosis thereof (4).

The following metabolic parameters were evaluated under BMR conditions in the central venous blood of more than 100 patients with head injuries of different degree:

Pyruvate and lactate, to demonstrate disturbances of metabolism caused by shock and hypoxia with consecutive metabolic or mixed metabolic respiratory acidosis (6, 10, 11, 16, 20); ATP and 2, 3-DPG, to prove subsequent derangements in metabolism (8, 9, 12, 13). 2, 3-DPG is of particular importance in oxygen transport (1, 5) since, in connection with blood gas analysis, conclusions can be drawn on oxygen transport capacity. Furthermore, uric acid, CK, alpha-HBDH, transaminases and LDH were determined. ATP and CK analysis resulted in no statistically significant differences, therefore this matter will not be discussed. The results concerning the pathophysiology of the transaminase of LDH and its isoenzymes, of cholinesterase, acethylcholinesterase and MDH were reported elsewhere. The observed derangements will be considered here in context with the concomitant shock situation of most of the patients (18, 19).

Methods

The investigation comprised patients with signs of severe brain concussion as well as with brain contusion. Thirty-nine patients with brain concussion were compared to 68 patients with different clinical degrees of brain contusion. As regards the prognosis and the discussion of the metabolic parameters the total number of survivors was compared to the group of 34 deaths. The calculation of significance was performed according to student t-test. Lactate, pyruvate, ATP, CK and alpha-HBDH (isoenzyme 1 of LDH) were determined by methods as reported by BERGMEYER (3). 2, 3-DPG was evaluated according to BENESCH & BENESCH (2) as well as uric acid following a modification of SOBRINHO-SIMOES et al. (14).

Results

On day 1 and 2 as well as on day 5 after the injury the value of lactate (Fig. 1.) was found to be significantly greater in patients with brain contusion as compared to the values found in patients with brain concussion. The latter stayed clearly within normal range and differed from the very much elevated values discovered in patients with contusion at the time of admission to the hospital.

As expected from the change of lactate, pyruvate values turned out to be considerably higher at the time of admission in patients with brain contusion as compared to the values found in patients with brain concussion.

2, 3-DPG values proved to remain essentially eithin the normal range in both groups of patients, a significant difference could not be stated.

On the other hand, the determination of alpha-HBDH (Fig. 2) revealed a statistically significant difference on day 2 and 5 between patients with concussion and patients with contusion.

Differences in uric acid level were present in this group especially at the beginning, though they did not prove to be significant. Patients with brain contusion had uric acid levels slightly above normal range.

Lactate values were higher in patients with brain injury who survived as compared to those who died (Fig. 3), the difference being significant for several days. Fatally injured patients initially have very elevated values, by far exceeding the normal range. This is a distinct sign of unfavourable prognosis. In the course of further treatment (day 3 and 4), however, a stabilization sets in. The values of survivors and nonsurvivors remain within the normal range from then on. This range is never exceeded by the lactate values of the survivors. On day 7 after the accident, the corresponding value of fatally injured patients was again elevated beyond the normal limit and differed significantly from that of the control group.

Patients who did not survive the injury showed a distinct increase in pyruvate values (Fig. 4) as compared to those of the day of accident, and a considerable decrease thereafter. Their values were always increased over those of patients who survived, though they were at first distinctly elevated beyond normal range in both groups. In our opinion the pyruvate determination also bears prognostic significance in a very early stage.

The 2, 3-DPG values (Fig. 5) stayed within normal range in each group. A statistically significant difference was evident on day 1 after the accident.

Whereas the alpha-HBDH values (Fig. 6) exceeded the normal range in both groups of patients with head injuries, in the course of which the greater values were, as expected, found in patients who did not survive. Here the differences are significant on day 2, 4 and 5. The uric acid values (Fig. 7) proved to be a very important and reliable indicator for the further development of the lesions we are here interested in. In deadly injured patients they exceeded the normal range on the day of admission and on the following day and were significantly different from the control group.

Discussion

Comparing our results to those of other authors we could extend the interpretation of the reported lactate and pyruvate increase after head injury (7, 10, 16, 17) considering the prognostic evidence. 2, 3-DPG as a parameter of carbohydrate metabolism is distinctly affected which probably has to be seen in connection with the severe CNS damage. The specific effect fo organic phosphates, especially of

2, 3-diphosphorglycerate, is known in its importance for oxygen linkage to hemoglobin since CHANUTIN and CURNISH (1967) and BENESCH and BENESCH (1967) published their fundamental papers.

2, 3-DPG which has lost its relation to the Hemoglobin molecule results in a decreased tissue oxygen transport, since oxygen now holds on to hemoglobin via the Fe atoms.

Uric acid was determined with the notion to have in hands an important parameter of purin metabolism. With the disintegration of nucleated matter there has to be an increased formation of uric acid for a short time which may indicate a radical alteration of the nucleotid component of the damaged brain cell.

Alpha-HBDH expresses the decomposition of fat into ketogen substances which is preferably brought into action during adrenalin stress.

All mentioned parameters did correlate in their behavior with the changes of acid base conditions which were determined by bloodgas analysis, but in the scope of today's subject this may not be discussed.

From the results of our animal studies we expect further hints as to the possibility of correlating CNS damage to metabolic parameters measured in central venous blood.

Conclusion

The diagnostic and prognostic evaluation of recent head injuries poses great difficulties since the extent of the actual cellular damage remains unclear at first, and patients with a different degree of injury may show identical or very similar clinical pictures. A morphological evaluation is not possible under clinical conditions, but suitable metabolic studies which sufficiently reflect the cellular situation may offer an alternative.

By means of the above parameters we hope to arrive at an early prognostic statement sooner than by means of day-to-day clinical diagnostic evaluations.

REFERENCES

1. BENESCH, R. and R. E. BENESCH: The effect of organic phosphates from the human erythrocyte on the allosteric properties of hemoglobin. Biochem. biophys. Res. commun. 26, 162 (1967)

2. BENESCH, R. and R. E. BENESCH, Nature 221, 618 (1969)

3. BERGMEYER, H. U.: Methoden der enzymatischen Analyse, Weinheim 1970

4. BES, A., L. ARDUS, Y. LAZORTHES, M. ESCANDE, M. DELPLA and J. P. M. VERGNE: Hemodynamic and metabolic studies in "Coma Dépasse" a search for a biological test of the brain. In BROCK, M., C. FIESCHI, D. H. INGVAR, N. H. LASSEN and K. SCHÜRMANN: Cerebral Blood Flow, Springer, Berlin 1969

5. CHANUTIN, A. and R. R. CURNISH: Effect of organic and inorganic phosphates on the oxygen equilibrium of human erythrocyte. Arch. Biochem. 121, 96 (1967)

6. COHEN, P.J.: The metabolic function of oxygen and biochemical lesions of hypoxia. Anesthesiology 37, 160-163 (1972)

7. HURWITZ, B.S. and S.K. WOLFSON: Brain lactate in anoxia and hypothermia: relation to brain viability. Exp.Neurol. 23, 426-434 (1969)

8. KAASIK, A.E., L.NILSSON and B.K.SIESJÖ: The effect of asphyxia upon the lactate, pyruvate and bicarbonate concentrations of brain tissue and cisternal CSF and upon the tissue concentrations of phosphocreatinine and adenine nucleotides in anesthetized rats. Acta physiol. scand. 78, 433-447 (1970)

9. KAASIK, A.E., L.NILSSON and B.K.SIESJÖ: The effect of arterial hypotension upon the lactate, pyruvate and bicarbonate concentrations of brain tissue and cisternal CSF, and upon the tissue concentrations of phosphocreatinine and adenine nucleotides in anesthetized rats. Acta physiol. scand. 78, 448-458 (1970)

10. MEYER, J.S., A.KONDO, F.NEMURA, K.SAKAMOTO and T.TERAURA: Cerebral hemodynamics and metabolism following experimental head injury. J.Neurosurg. 32, 304 (1970)

11. SAMII, M., H.J.REULEN, A.FENSKE and U.HASE: Energy metabolism, lactate/pyruvate ratio and extracellular space in cortex and white matter adjacent and distant from a local freezing point. In: M.BROCK et al., Cerebral Blood Flow, Springer, Berlin 1969

12. SANDERS, A.P., R.S.KRAMER, B.WOODHALL et al.: Brain adenosin triphosphate, decreased concentration precedes convulsion. Science 169, 206-208 (1970)

13. SIESJÖ, B.K. and L.NILSSON: The influence of arterial hypoxemia upon labile phosphates and upon extracellular and intracellular lactate and pyruvate concentration in the rat brain. Scand.J.clin.Lab.Invest. 27, 83-96 (1971)

14. SOBRINHO-SIMOES, M. and M.J.PEREIRA, J.Lab.Clin.Med. 65, 665 (1965)

15. SPECTOR, R.G.: Content of lactic acid and adenosine mono-, diand triphosphate in anoxic-ischemic rat brain. J.Path.Bact. 90, 533-541 (1965)

16. STOECKEL, H. and S. HOYER: Hirndurchblutung und Hirnstoffwechsel nach schweren Hirntraumen. Prakt.Anästh. und Wiederbel. 6, 431 (1971)

17. SCHWEIZER, O. and W.S.HOWLAND: Prognostic Significance of High Lactate Levels. Anest.Analg. 47, 383-388 (1968)

18. VITEK, V. and R.A.COVLEY: Blood lactate in the prognosis of various forms of shock. Ann.Surg. 173, 308-313 (1971)

19. WEIL, M.H. and A.A. AFIFI: Experimental and clinical studies on lactate and pyruvate as indicators of the severity of acute circulatory failure (shock), Circulation 41, 989-1001 (1970)

20. ZUPPING, R.: Cerebral acid-base and gas metabolism in brain injury. J.Neurosurg. 33, 498-505 (1970)

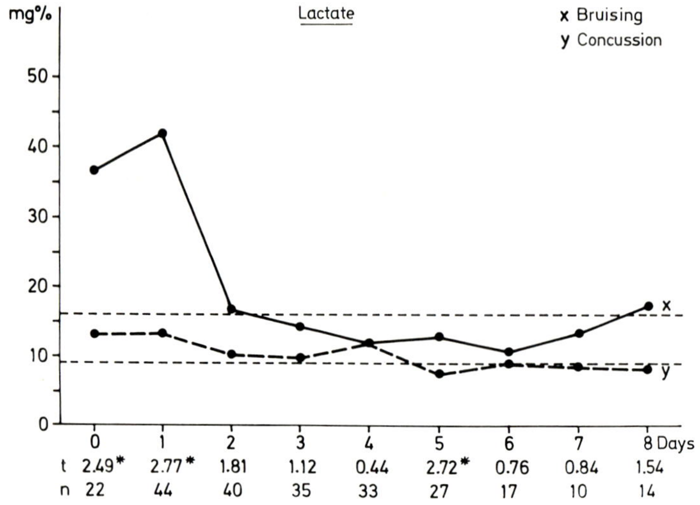
mg%
Lactate
x Bruising
y Concussion
50
40
30
20
10
0
0 1 2 3 4 5 6 7 8 Days
t 2.49* 2.77* 1.81 1.12 0.44 2.72* 0.76 0.84 1.54
n 22 44 40 35 33 27 17 10 14
x
y

Fig. 1

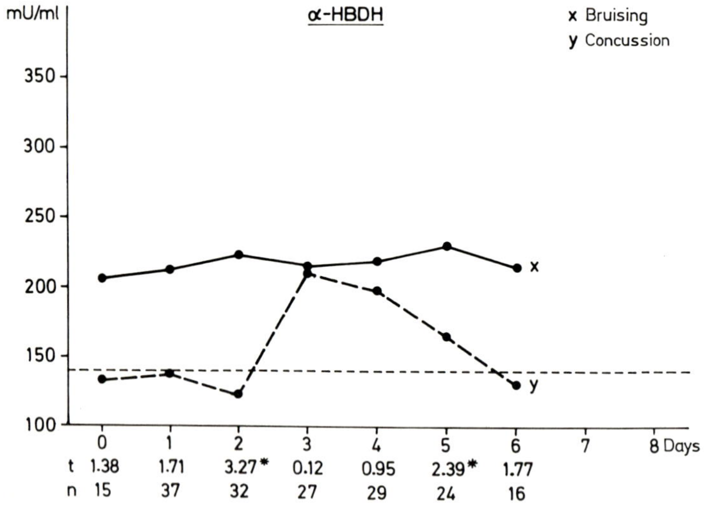
mU/ml
α-HBDH
x Bruising
y Concussion
350
300
250
200
150
100
0 1 2 3 4 5 6 7 8 Days
t 1.38 1.71 3.27* 0.12 0.95 2.39* 1.77
n 15 37 32 27 29 24 16
x
y

Fig. 2

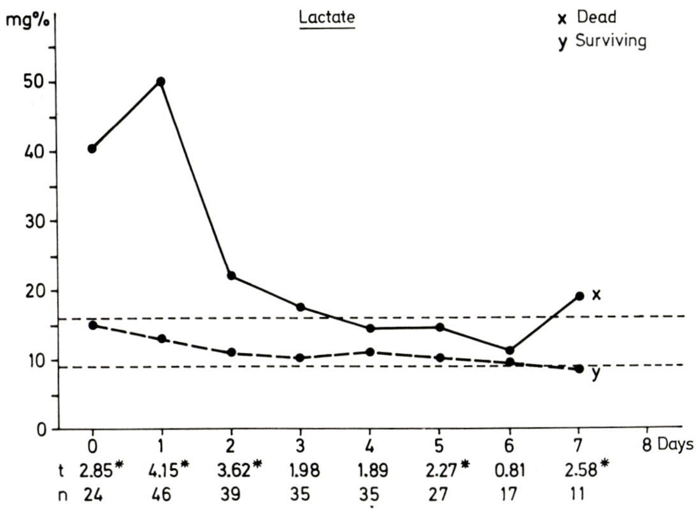

mg%
Lactate
x Dead
y Surviving
50
40
30
20
10
0
0 1 2 3 4 5 6 7 8 Days
t 2.85* 4.15* 3.62* 1.98 1.89 2.27* 0.81 2.58*
n 24 46 39 35 35 27 17 11

Fig. 3

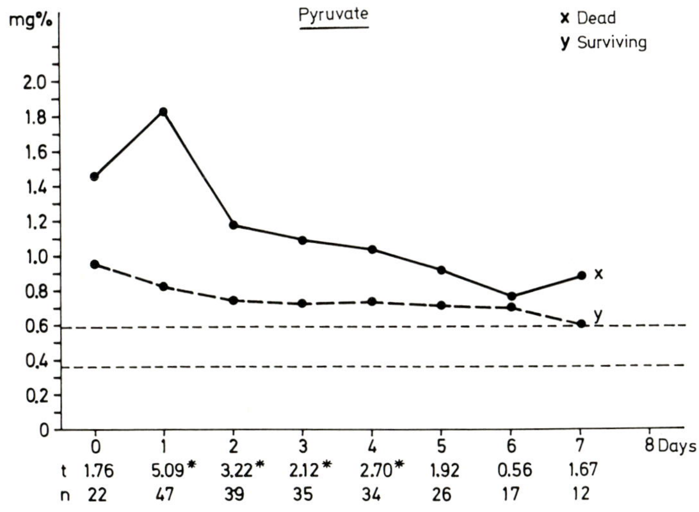

mg%
Pyruvate
x Dead
y Surviving
2.0
1.8
1.6
1.4
1.2
1.0
0.8
0.6
0.4
0.2
0
0 1 2 3 4 5 6 7 8 Days
t 1.76 5.09* 3.22* 2.12* 2.70* 1.92 0.56 1.67
n 22 47 39 35 34 26 17 12

Fig. 4

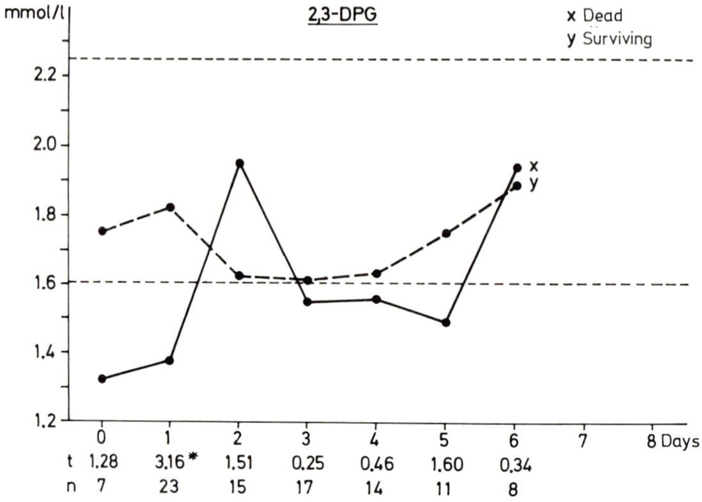
mmol/l
2,3-DPG
x Dead
y Surviving
2.2
2.0
1.8
1.6
1.4
1.2
0 1 2 3 4 5 6 7 8 Days
t 1.28 3.16* 1.51 0.25 0.46 1.60 0.34
n 7 23 15 17 14 11 8
x
y

Fig. 5

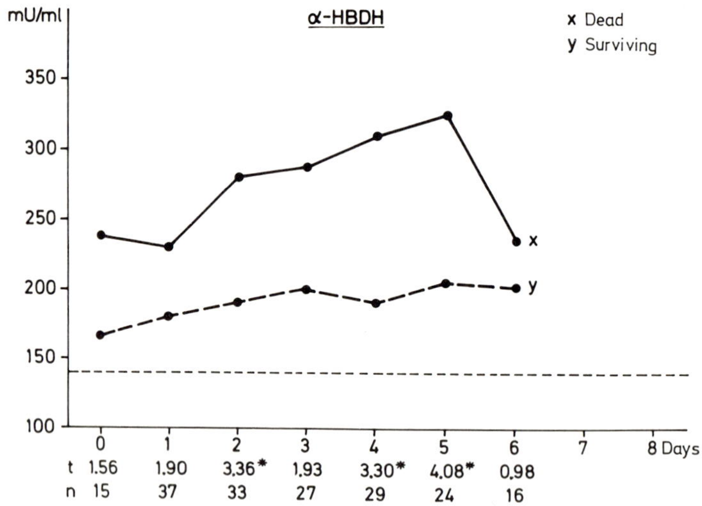
mU/ml
α-HBDH
x Dead
y Surviving
350
300
250
200
150
100
0 1 2 3 4 5 6 7 8 Days
t 1.56 1.90 3.36* 1.93 3.30* 4.08* 0.98
n 15 37 33 27 29 24 16
x
y

Fig. 6

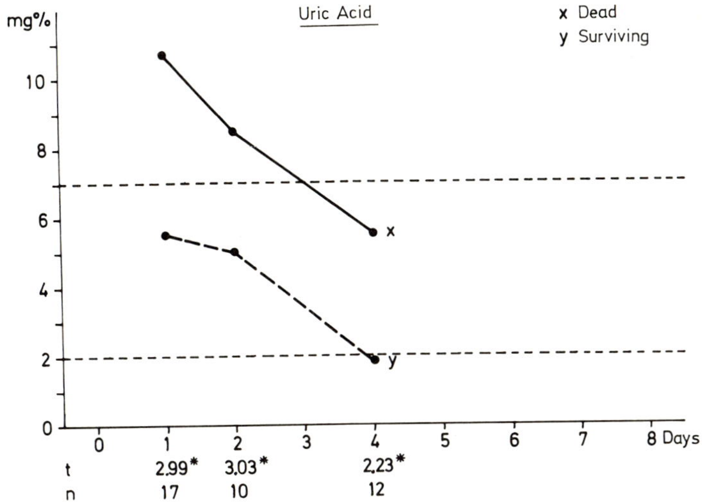
mg%
Uric Acid
x Dead
y Surviving
10
8
6
4
2
0
x
y
0
1
2
3
4
5
6
7
8 Days
t
2.99*
3.03*
2.23*
n
17
10
12

Fig. 7

Consequences of Cerebral Edema and Increased Intracranial Pressure

J. W. F. BEKS

Already in 1881, two German scientists, NAUNYN and SCHREIBER, reported that as result of increasing intracranial pressure, changes of vegetative functions may occur.

In 1902 these changes were described in detail by HARVEY CUSHING, pioneer of neurosurgery. He recorded:

increasing arterial pressure, changing of frequency of pulse and altering in the pattern of breathing.

Further investigation showed, that these reactions could not have been only induced by a space-occupying lesion, having led to increased intracranial pressure, but that these vegetative changes were also the result of compression of cerebral and vascular structures, caused by displacement of cerebral tissue.

The question could arise whether the term "increased intracranial" pressure is always correct. The expression has indeed only significance if the pressure inside the skull, viz. in various compartments is actually increased in the same degree. This pressure increase will indeed be equal everywhere as long as there is a liquid communication between various compartments (Pascal's Law). This is not the case anymore if this liquid communication is interrupted as may be observed under pathological conditions for instance herniation of cerebral tissue in the tentorial hiatus.

The mechanism of the displacement of cerebral tissue and the herniation of the brain stem and its resulting consequences have been described extensively by PIA (1957), LANGFITT (1964) and SEEGER (1968).

Herniation of cerebral tissue in caudal direction through the tentorial hiatus is considered to be a frequently occurring result of a supratentorially situated space-occupying lesion. If however in a closed system, subdivided into different communicating compartments the pressure remains equal in those different compartments, displacement of the contents cannot take place.

In animal experiments we tried to establish the degree of difference in pressure between various compartments necessary to effectuate a displacement of cerebral tissue.

In a number of anesthetized cats a needle was brought into the sella media of the right lateral ventricle by stereotactic means and also one into the great cistern in order to measure and register simultaneously the pressure in the ventricle system and in the great cistern. The average initial pressure amouted to 6-11

Table I. Summary of the changes of pressure in the intracranial compartments after a cold lesion

			mm Hg
Case No.	Initial Intraventricular Pressure	Initial Cisternal Pressure	Highest Cisternal Pressure
1	6	7	37
2	10	10	35
3	10	10	38
4	9	8	32
5	7	7	29
6	10	10	37
7	10	10	40
8	8	7	37
9	10	10	36
10	11	11	35
11	7	7	35
12	11	11	35
13	7	7	32
14	10	10	35
15	7	7	36
16	10	10	35
17	8	8	35
18	8	7	36
19	9	8	37
20	10	10	35

mm Hg infra- as well as supratentorially (Table I).

In order to be able to bring about a raise of intracranial pressure a cold induced lesion was applied to the cerebral cortex, in a way as has been described formerly by us in detail (BEKS c. s., 1965).

Consequently to the application of this lesion we observed a gradual increase in intraventricular pressure, as well as a rise of pressure in the great cistern. The increase of pressure in both instances was identical. This stands to reason because there is an open liquid communication between supra-and infratentorial spaces via the tentorial hiatus and the Sylvian aqueduct.

At a certain moment however a discrepancy appeared between the increase of pressure in both compartments and the pulsations in the infratentorial compartment disappeared.

This moment was determined by displacement of cerebral tissue as result of an increase of volume of a space-occupying lesion. At the moment we saw the appearance of the discrepancy in the rise of pressure in the supra-and infratentorial space, we injected an X-ray contrast medium into the ventricle system via a needle stuck into the right ventricle. It appeared that the Sylvian aqueduct did not show its normal course anymore, but snapped off at the level of the tentorium.

At the same time we could not transfer anymore to the infratentorial space, via the tentorial hiatus contrast medium injected into the subdural supratentorial space. Therefore we may assume that the liquid communication between both compartments had been interrupted.

After this we saw the pressure rise considerably in the supratentorial space whilst the pressure in the infratentorial space remained equal at first and finally still rose a little. This late rise of pressure can possibly be ascribed to an increase of volume of the infratentorial space by herniation of cerebral tissue via the tentorial hiatus.

The average pressure in the ventricle system, at the moment the pulsations in the great cistern disappeared, amounted to an average of 35 mm Hg (Table I).

At that moment no changes in vegetative functions could be observed. Namely no rise of arterial pressure was seen, nor a change in respiratory pattern. These symptoms did not appear until the supratentorial pressure had reached an average value of 90 mm Hg. This pressure equals about the arterial pressure offered to the brain (Table II).

This shows that a sharp rise of supratentorial pressure has consequences for the cerebral circulation.

Under normal conditions the pressure in the venous system of the brain varies according to GREENFIELD and TINDALL (1965) from 8-12 mm Hg.

These values are in accordance with the average pressure values in the cerebrospinal system LANGFITT (1972). If however the pressure in the supratentorial system rises, the venous system in the area where the pressure has increased, will be more or less compressed. The resistance in the venous system will increase by this narrowing, which will be of consequence for the cerebral circulation, because as a result the cerebral blood flow (CBF) will decrease. The circulation is a function of inflow- and outflow pressure, diameter of the vascular system and blood viscosity.

If the pressure rises in a certain area, the venous pressure in this area will have to remain at least equal to the pressure in the surroundings in order to maintain circulation. The maintenance of adequate cerebral circulation in varying conditions is called autoregulation.

In studying autoregulation various authors have examined different parameters of

Table II. Summary of the values of intraventricular pressure at different moments

			mm Hg
Case No.	Initial Intraventricular Pressure	Intraventricular Pressure at increase Bloodpressure	Intraventricular Pressure at Respiration Changes
1	6	70	109
2	10	95	118
3	10	96	117
4	9	95	124
5	7	96	110
6	10	88	112
7	10	91	110
8	8	95	117
9	10	93	115
10	11	97	112
11	7	93	111
12	11	93	110
13	7	92	110
14	10	96	115
15	7	90	112
16	10	91	113
17	8	93	110
18	8	93	113
19	9	88	115
20	10	95	118

importance to stable circulation. The main factors were blood pressure, PCO_2, PO_2, and PH.

The blood pressure, conducted to the cerebral vessels via the internal carotid artery amounts to an average 95 mm Hg. This pressure is further reduced by the arterioles and then reaches the capillaries.

If, for whatever reason, a reduction of arterial blood flow occurs, provided metabolism remains the same, the capillary PCO_2 will rise and the PO_2 decrease.

This will entail dilatation of the arterioles. Under normal conditions especially the arterioles are responsible for the resistance in the peripheral vascular system and therefore the blood pressure offered to the capillary system will rise. If the arterioles widen as a result of a rise of PCO_2 or else by a decrease of PO_2 the pressure offered to the capillary system will rise and indeed so much, that the difference between systemic arterial pressure (SAP) and jugular venous pressure (JVP) still increases more than under non-pathological conditions, because also the increased resistance, developed as result of the risen intracranial pressure, has to be levelled up to restore normal circulation.

If as a result of the increased intracranial pressure the resistance in the vascular system increases so much, that the normal blood pressure is not sufficient anymore to keep up normal circulation, the blood pressure will rise. In our experiments we arrived at the same conclusion.

If the intracranial pressure keeps rising further, the moment will come the arterial blood pressure cannot be adapted anymore to the disturbed circulation. This can be demonstrated with evidence in certain patients with sharply risen intracranial pressure in whom an attempt is made to perform angiography and in whom the contrast medium cannot be traced in subarachnoidal parts of the carotid or vertebral artery.

In his excellent monograph about "Zentrale Atemstörungen" FROWEIN (1963) stated that under certain conditions a vicious circle develops in which respiratory and circulatory disturbances mutually influence each other, leading that way to a stage in which it is difficult to judge what will be the concequences for the cerebral functions if either of these systems fails to work. This point of view is still valid.

In order though to gain some insight in the changes in respiratory pattern we observed in our experimental investigations, it is necessary that we first go further deeply into the problem of the nervous regulation of the respiration.

Though during the last ten years much research into the mechanisms which control respiration has been performed, there has not yet been found a generally accepted concept with respect to this problem.

Therefore it is impossible to summarize the information from the literature, because the data are often controversial.

The peripheral part of the nervous respiratory regulation mechanism contains much less fundamental uncertainties than does the central regulation system.

The central regulation is not determined by a limited group of neurons in a single respiratory centre, but the neurons, taking part in the central regulation, are situated in the cerebral hemispheres, the reticular formation in the medulla oblongata and in superficial parts of the brain stem and the lateral parts of the basis of the fourth ventricle.

Though these structures are diffusely spread, they are functionally closely mutually connected (LAMBERTSEN, 1968).

It is generally accepted that the group of neurons, initiating spontaneous rhythmic respiratory activities, is localized in the medulla oblongata, because animal experiments show remaining periodicity in case the medulla oblongate is isolated from her connection with higher situated centres.

This primary rhythmic a activity is based on alterating discharges of impulses by inspiratory and expiratory components and may be modificed in a complex way.

It is assumed. that in the reticular formation of the medulla oblongata two groups of neurons are localized, so-called inspiratory and expiratory neurons, forming together the primary respiratory centre.

This primary respiratory centre is. localized on both sides of the median line and it can be subdivided.

The dorso-lateral part is supposed to be involved mainly in the expiration whereas the medial part is responsible for the inspiration. The activities of these centres are supposed to control normal breathing.

The function of the primary respiratory centre may be modulated though by other neuronal complexes situated in various parts of the brain, i.a. pons, mesencephalon, diencephalon, and cerebral cortex. However the exact way of influencing by these cellgroups is not known.

Two centres, which can influence the respiratory centre in the medulla oblongata, are situated in the pons, viz. the so-called pneumotactic centre and a centre which can inhibit respiration, the so-called apnoestic centre.

The pneumotactic centre is localized in the cranial part of the tegmentum pontis. The apnoestic centre is situated in the middle and caudal part of the pons, namely in the extensive territory of the substantia reticularis lateralis.

Little is known yet about the influence the cerebral cortex has on the respiration.

According to FENN and RAHN (1965) stimulation of the ventral part of the frontal pole, the insula, the lateral part of the temporal pole and the frontal part of the cingular gyrus, induces inhibition of respiration. If, on the contrary, the motoric cortex the Sylvian gyrus and the median cingular gyrus are stimulated, the respiratory intensity increases.

Because the automatism of the respiration may be changed voluntarily, it is clear-that there will have to exist higher control mechanisms.

In the clinic no standardized lesions of the skull exist, which implicates, that it often is very difficult to analyse the symptoms and signs which occur. In animal experiments this is possible to a certain extent.

According to PLUM and BROWN (1963) there are among others, 3 basic forms of disturbed respiration:

1. Periodical breathing, or respiration according to Cheyne-Stokes.

   This respiration type may develop if influences of regulating mechanisms of supra-nuclear level are inactivated to a certain extent or inhibited, because the descending motoric tracks have been injured, causing a change in the influences on the primary respiratory centre in the brain stem. These tracks will become injured especially in cases of bilateral lesions, lying deeply in the cerebral hemisphere and in the basal ganglia and therefore damaging the intern capsule.

   The pathogenesis according to PLUM is based on a combination of an abnormally increased ventilation reaction on the CO_2 stimulus, resulting in hyperpnoea and an abnormally decreased ventilation stimulus from the cerebrum, causing the apnoea after hyperventilation.

   This form of respiration we observed in our experiments in case the supratentorial intraventricular pressure had reached an average value of 110 mm Hg, which is 10 times as high as the initial value (Table II).

2. The second fundamental form is the central neurogenic hyperventilation.

   This form of respiration consists of 24-36 respirations per minute, the inspiration lasting as long as the expiration and giving the impression that the expiration occurs more actively than passively.

   This form of respiration is supposed to develop in cases of lesions of the medial part of the rostral end of the pontine tegmentum, therefore between the lower midbrain and the lower 1/3 part of the pons.

   It develops in case of compression of the brain stem, occurring by transtentorial herniation, preventing regulating influences from higher situated centres to reach the primary respiratory centre, causing thereby autonomic functioning of this centre.

   It is not yet known whether these functional disorders are the result of mechanical compression of the tracks or either the result of anoxia, caused by vascular compression or obstruction.

   In our experiments we observed during the increase of the pressure difference between supra-and infratentorial compartment, periodical respiration change into central neurogenic hyperventilation.

   The appearance of central neurogenic hyperventilation after a period of Cheyne-Stokes breathing, may indicate a deterioration of the clinical condition.

   We also could make transfer experimentally a periodical form of respiration by raising the supratentorial pressure by means of an artificial increase of the PCO_2, by letting the test animal breath CO_2. As a result of the PCO_2 growth of the intracranial blood volume occurred, raising the pressure gradient between supra-and infratentorial compartment again making the incarceration of the brain stem still worse.

   The regulating influences of higher situated centres are excluded that way.

3. The third form is the atactical respiration, which is characterized by a strong irregularity in frequency and intensity of respiration with intermittent periods of apnoea lasting varying periods of time.

   This form of respiration occurs in cases of lesion of the essential centre, viz. the primary respiratiory centre in the medulla oblongata. There is in that case a dysregulation between activities of inspirational and expirational neuronal groups.

On the basis of our findings we would like to suggest to subdivide the process of transtentorial herniation in two phases, occurring in case a pressure gradient of a certain value has developed between supra-and infratentorial compartment, viz.:

1. the anatomical phase, in which communication between supra-and infratentorial phase via the tentorial hiatus has been interrupted by displacement of cerebral tissue.

2. the clinical phase, in which vegetative changes occur, viz. an increase of arterial pressure and changing of respiratory pattern.

The fact that the anatomical phase of transtentorial herniation is not accompanied by the appearance of clinical-vegetative signs, speaks for SCHEINKER's (1945) conception that herniation of the gyrus hippocampus on its own is not sufficient to cause neurovegetative changes.

The first perceived change in the clinical phase of the incarceration appeared at an average value of 90 mm Hg in the supratentorial area and 35 mm Hg in the infratentorial area and consisted of a rise of arterial bloodpressure. This increase of bloodpressure is, as appears from the above, necessary, in case the cerebral arterioles are maximally open already.

The respiratory changes in the animal experiments do not appear until a much larger pressure gradient has been reached, namely at an average value of intraventricular pressure of 110 mm Hg.

At this stage we observed the appearance of periodical breathing, which was transferred into central neurogenic hyperventilation at an intraventricular pressure of about 120 mm Hg.

REFERENCES

1. BEKS, J.E.F., C.A.TER WEEME, E.J.EBELS, W.G.WALTER and J.S. WASSENAAR: Increase in intraventricular pressure in cold induced cerebral edema. Acta physiol. Pharmacol. Neerl. 13, 317-329 (1965)
2. FENN, W.O. and H.RAHN: Handbook of physiology, Section III: Respiration. 1Ed. Washington, D.C.: American Physiological Society, p. 927 (1965)
3. FROWEIN, R.A.: Zentrale Atemstörungen bei Schädel-Hirnverletzungen und bei Hirntumoren. Springer Verlag, Berlin, 1963
4. GREENFIELD, J.C. and G.T.TINDALL: Effect of acute increase of intracranial pressure on blood flow in the internal carotid artery of man. J.Clin.Invest. 44, 1343-1351 (1965)
5. LAMBERTSEN, C.L.: Medical Physiology, ed. 12, Saint Louis: The C.V. Mosby Company, p. 613 (1968)
6. LANGFITT, T.W., J.D.WEINSTEIN, N.F.KASSELL and F.A.SIMEONE: Transmission of increased intracranial pressure. J.Neurosurg. 21, 989-997 (1964)
7. LANGFITT, T.W.: Pathophysiology of increased ICP. In: Intracranial Pressure, edited by BROCK and DIETZ. Springer Verlag, 361-364 (1972)
8. NAUNYN, B. and J.SCHREIBER: Über Gehirndruck. Naunyn-Schmiedeberg's Arch. exp. Path. Pharmak. 14, 1 (1881)
9. PIA, H.W.: Die Schädigung des Hirnstammes bei raumfordernden Prozessen des Gehirns. Acta Neurochir. (Wien) Suppl. 4 (1957)
10. PLUM, F. and H.W.BROWN: The effect on respiration of central nervous system disease. Am.N.J.Acad.Sci. 109, 915 (1963)
11. SCHEINKER, M.: Transtentorial herniation of the brain stem. Arch.Neurol. Psychiat. 53, 289 (1945)
12. SEEGER, W.: Atemstörungen bei intrakraniellen Massenverschiebungen. Acta Neurochir. (Wien) Suppl. 17 (1968)

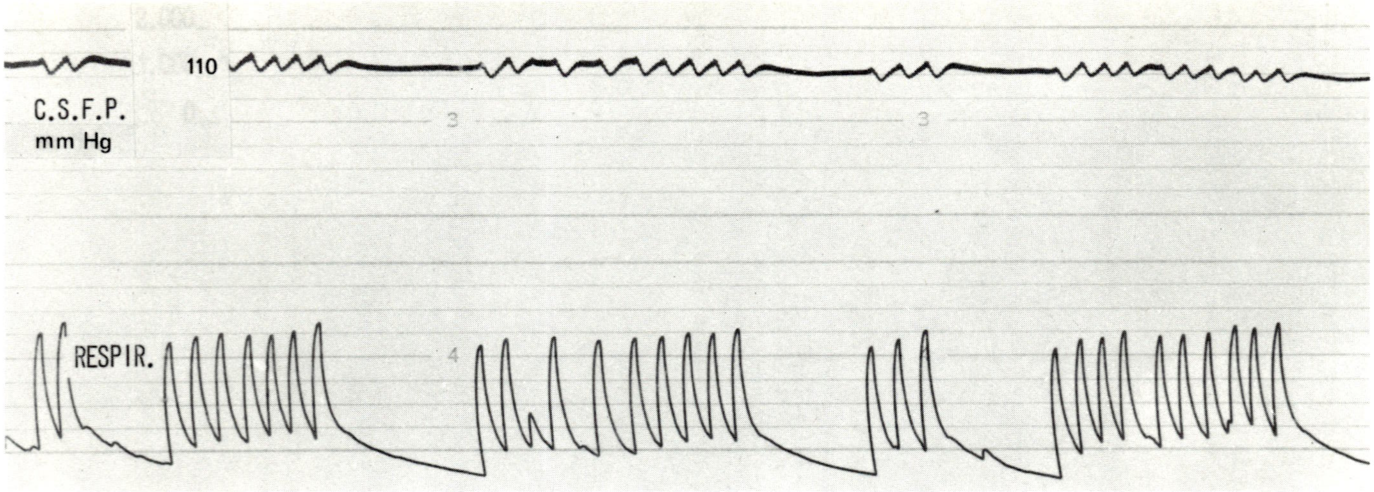

Fig. 1. Recording of the respirationpattern of periodic respiration

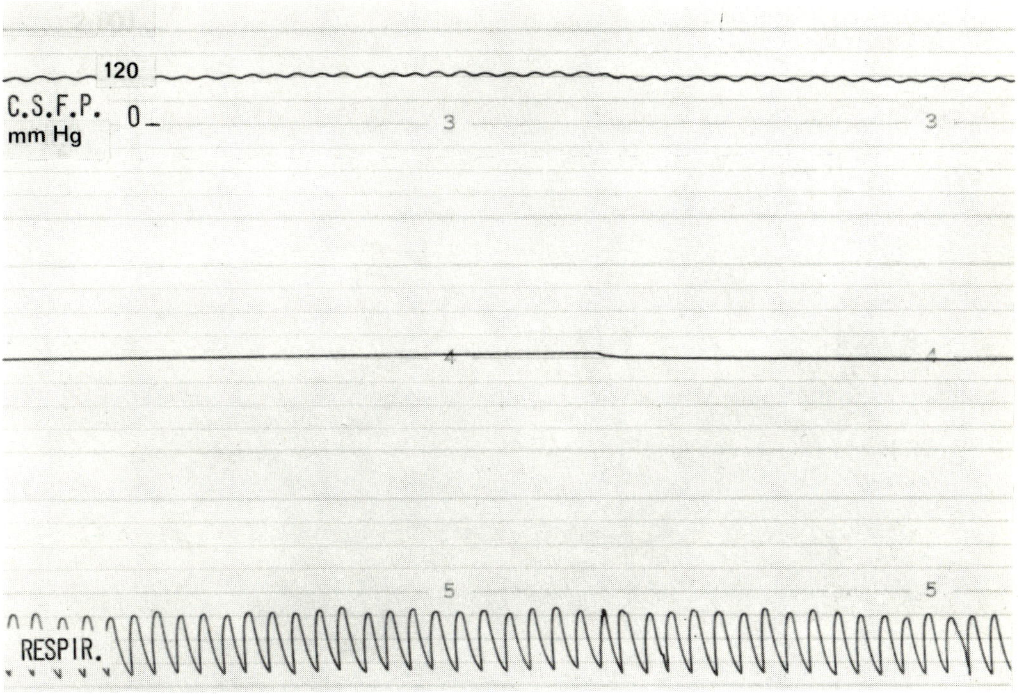

Fig. 2. Recording of the central neurogenic hyperventilation

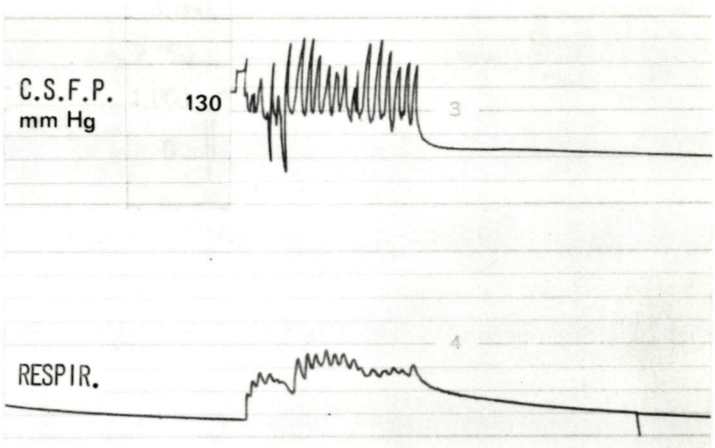

Fig. 3. Recording of atactical respiration

Intracranial Pressure Measurements in Clinical Practice

B. JENNETT

Introduction

Raised intracranial pressure (ICP) is the mechanism whereby many clinical conditions eventually threaten brain function and life itself. Neurosurgeons are therefore frequently concerned to recognise whether ICP is raised, and if so to try to reduce the level of pressure. Continuous clinical monitoring of pressure was shown to be feasible by GUILLAUME and JANNY in France in 1951, and a large series of neurosurgical cases was reported from Sweden in 1960 by LUNDBERG. Their observations showed that the level of pressure is often variable so that single estimations of pressure may be misleading; the clinical state of the patient has likewise been shown to be an unreliable guide to ICP. In these circumstances widespread adoption of continuous monitoring of ICP might have been expected, but last year's conference in Hannover revealed that it has become routine in comparatively few centres. In the Glasgow Institute some 300 patients have now been monitored by the LUNDBERG method, a plastic catheter being introduced into the ventricle via a frontal burr hole and linked through a fluid-filled system to a bedside transducer and chart recorder. Monitoring is continued for 2-5 days as a rule but only one patient has developed intracranial infection and he recovered, which confirms a recent report of an extremely low incidence of infection (0.5%) with LUNDBERG's method in almost 1,000 cases (SUNDBÄRG et al, 1972).

Many management decisions are made easier by the availability of reliable information about the level of ICP. These include decisions about diagnosis, either of the nature of the disease process as a whole, or of changes in that state; decisions about treatment, by indicating whether reduction of pressure is necessary and then whether measures taken have been effective; and decisions about prognosis, particularly after severe head injury.

Diagnosis

It may at first seem curious that the most useful single application in clinical circumstances has been the recognition that ICP is not unduly high in patients whose clinical picture was suggestive of raised pressure. After severe head injury, for example, patients frequently show signs of brain stem dysfunction which may be ascribed either to primary stem injury, or to brain shift due to focal haematoma or to more generalised brain edema. Particularly in the first 24 hours after injury it is sometimes difficult to be certain whether this clinical state has been present from the onset or has developed secondarily; in some centres there is a tendency to treat all such patients indiscriminately with measures designed to reduce ICP - such as hypertonic solutions or even hyperventilation, on the unproved assumption that there is likely to be "cerebral edema". Our investigations have shown that many such patients have a consistently normal pressure; the subsequent course of such patients usually indicates that the damage sustained has been either a diffuse white matter lesion, or a primary brain stem injury, or sometimes both. In another group of patients, in whom angiography shows evidence of a focal expanding lesion, the ICP may prove to be only moderately raised or even normal; if volume/pressure measurements (vide infra) show that intracranial compliance is normal then it is probably safe to assume that we are dealing with a well-compensated situation; we believe that we have avoided unnecessary surgery in a number of such patients with temporal lobe swelling, who had suffered swollen contusions rather than haematomas but whom we would previously have felt obliged to explore surgically on the basis of the angiographic findings. In patients who deteriorate clinically at a later stage after injury increasing pressure may be suspected; but again monitoring may show that ICP is not rising, and another explanation must be sought for their changing clinical condition. Apart from head injuries, a similar situation may arise <u>after intracranial surgery</u> of any kind, when anxiety about the possible development of an intracranial haematoma may be allayed by ICP monitoring, and the patient may be spared further neuroradiological investigation, or an unnecessary second operation. In a different situation again, are patients <u>with a ventricular shunt</u> in position in whom deterioration is assumed to indicate shunt blockage and subsequent ICP; in a number of such instances we have found normal ICP, there being some alternative explanation for the patient's deterioration, such as spread of tumor. Different yet again are patients suspected of <u>pseudo-tumor,</u> (benign intracranial hypertension). In 5 of 24 such patients monitoring revealed normal ICP and the final diagnosis of pseudo-papilledema was confirmed in 4 by fluorescein angiography (JOHNSTON and PATERSON, 1972).

Only in patients undergoing routine ICP monitoring (in our clinic severe head injuries and post-operative craniotomies) could we expect to discover raised ICP when it was not suspected clinically. This occurred only occasionally in our experience. But the availability of monitoring gave us considerably increased confidence in the management of the small number of patients in a neurosurgical unit for whom controlled ventilation is recommended - usually for a combination of chest injury and head injury. Such a regime deprives the neurosurgeon of many of the clinical signs on which he normally relies to detect intracranial complications associated with raised ICP, and we have detected intracranial haematomas in such patients.

Treatment

In regard to <u>treatment</u>, monitoring may indicate whether or not measures need be instituted to control ICP, and will also show how effective these are in the individual patient. Change in clinical state is a poor guide as to whether or not pressure has been effectively reduced; lack of improvement may indicate either that the pressure is still high, or that there is such severe underlying brain damage that in spite of reducing ICP brain function does not recover. When monitoring shows one method of lowering ICP to be ineffective an alternative can be tried. For example when intravenous mannitol fails to control ICP the aspiration of a small amount of ventricular CSF through the recording catheter will often lower the pressure for several hours; indeed the possibility of doing this is an advantage of the intraventricular method of pressure monitoring.

Prognosis

The relationship between the level of ventricular fluid pressure and the outcome from severe head injury has been reported from Scandinavia by LUNDBERG et al (1965) and more recently by VAPALAHTI and TROUPP (1971). Whilst our own studies confirm that high pressure has serious significance they do not support the corollary that normal pressure is usually favorable. Indeed we would regard the discovery of normal pressure (<20 mmHg) in a patient with bilateral extensor rigidity, together with other signs of brain stem dysfunction, soon after injury, as indicating severe primary white matter damage of the kind which, although it may be survived for a time, is likely to give rise to a persistent vegetative state. The ability to predict such an outcome soon after injury is of considerable importance in allocating treatment resources to patients with a more favorable outlook.

Intracranial pressure and cerebral vascular dynamics

Not only are ICP measurements helpful in the very practical situations just described, but they have also advanced our understanding of the dynamic relationship between ICP and cerebral flow (CBF). Such relationships are of considerable clinical significance because it is probably by its effect on CBF that ICP (as distinct from brain shift) is harmful. The crucial parameter is the oxygen supply to the brain which depends not only on oxygen content and blood flow, as does available oxygen in any tissue in the body, but also upon ICP - which may be sufficiently high to compete with the arterial pressure; what matters is the relationship between the two, the cerebral perfusion pressure, defined as the difference between mean arterial pressure and mean ICP.

The intracranial contents are made up of different volumes of brain tissue, of intravascular blood and of CSF, with a small amount of extracellular fluid. As each of these components is virtually incompressible, an increase in the volume of any one of these should cause an increase in ICP, unless (or until) compensation occurs by a reduction in the volume of one of the other intracranial components - such as by the extrusion from the intracranial cavity of venous blood or of CSF. Intracranial blood volume is the only component which can change rapidly, such as when vasodilatation is induced by hypercapnia or hypoxia. These are by no means uncommon occurrences in clinical practice, particularly in unconscious patients. We have shown that the volatile anaesthetic agents in common use (halothane, trichlorethylene and methoxyflurane) also have a vasodilatory effect on cerebral vessels, and ipso facto cause a rise in ICP (JENNETT et al, 1969). Whilst prior induction of hypocapnia by hyperventilation will reduce this rise of pressure it cannot be relied on to abolish it; in any event the resultant cerebral vasoconstriction in such a critical situation may in itself be harmful, because the reduction in flow is greater than the reduction in volume.

This rise also varies according to the compensatory capacity of the intracranial cavity - in patients without space-occupying lesions the rise is trivial, but in those with a mass it can be dramatic; such a rise can occur even when the ICP is not markedly raised prior to the introduction of the volatile agent. This suggests that the effect which an increase in the volume of the intracranial contents has on ICP will depend on which part of the volume/pressure curve applies at the time. My colleague Douglas MILLER has therefore proposed that the compensatory capacity of the intracranial cavity should be tested by observing the effect on ICP of induced changes in CSF volume by the infusion or the withdrawal of 1 ml through the ventricular cannula. In over 40 patients he has found a good correlation between the sensitivity of the volume/pressure response and the resting level of ICP (MILLER et al, 1973). At any given pressure level, however, considerable variation is found in the volume/pressure response, but this sensitivity is greatly reduced by the removal of a mass lesion even when this does not greatly alter the resting pressure level. In a series of 16 patients with head injury a better correlation was found between angiographic shift and volume/pressure sensitivity than between shift and resting ICP (MILLER and PICKARD, 1973). This test, which indicates how dangerous high pressure is, and whether normal pressure is safe, adds another dimension to ICP monitoring which therefore becomes an even more sensitive guide to the true state of intracranial dynamics, and in turn a more reliable guide to management. Moreover these findings provide an explanation of our earlier observations on volatile anesthetic agents, in which we found such a variable response of ICP to the same dose of agent. It also explains some other clinical situations familiar to neurosurgeons; these include the ease with which certain other events may precipitate a crisis in a patient with a space-occupying lesion - e. g. ventriculography, an epileptic fit or the administration of analgesic drugs which also cause respiratory depression. Each of these events may induce a small increase in the volume of the intracranial contents and if the patient is already on the steep (vertical) part of the volume/pressure curve, then a serious rise of ICP may result.

Neuropathological correlations of raised ICP

Evidence for the importance of intracranial dynamics does not rest only on theoretical considerations or on clinical evidence. Detailed neuropathological examination of the brains of patients who have died after severe head injury in this Institute provides clear evidence of extensive ischaemic damage in over half the cases (GRAHAM and ADAMS, 1971). Although much of this damage is of a type typical of perfusion failure, it was more common in patients under the age of 40 and could not therefore be ascribed to degenerative arterial disease; nor could the findings be ascribed to agonal changes. No close correlation was found between recorded ICP and ischaemic brain damage, but other factors affecting substrate delivery to the brain may have been important - variations in arterial blood pressure and in the oxygen content of the blood. Professor ADAMS' laboratory has, however, shown a close correlation between pathological signs of brain shift and herniation and increased pressure levels recorded during continuous monitoring (ADAMS and GRAHAM, 1972).

Conclusions

We are no longer in doubt that continuous ICP monitoring provides information which is of direct use to the clinician managing severely ill neurosurgical patients. Quite apart from that, we believe it is a useful research tool, both in the clinical and experimental situation. Much remains to be learned, both in regard to the most effective and safest way to monitor ICP, and in explaining the various phenomena which continuous monitoring reveals. It is too soon to declare that every neurosurgeon should be undertaking such measurements because both the setting up and maintenance of the system and its interpretation call for considerable effort and attention to detail. Nonetheless it seems likely that in a few years it will seem as primitive to try to manage acute neurosurgical problems without ICP measurements as it would be to practise cardiology without electrocardiography or neurosurgery without angiography.

REFERENCES

1. ADAMS, H. and D. I. GRAHAM: The relationship between ventricular fluid pressure and the neuropathology of raised intracranial pressure. In: M. BROCK and H. DIETZ (eds.): Intracranial Pressure. Springer-Verlag, Berlin-Heidelberg-New York 1972, 250-253

2. GRAHAM, D. I. and J. H. ADAMS: Ischaemic brain damage in fatal head injuries. Lancet 1, 265-266 (1971)

3. GUILLAUME, J. and P. JANNY: Manometrie intra-cranienne. Intérêt physiopathologique et clinique de la méthode. Presse méd. 59, 953-955 (1951)

4. JENNETT, W. B., J. BARKER, W. FITCH and D. G. McDOWALL: Effect of anaesthesia on intracranial pressure in patients with space-occupying lesions. Lancet 1, 61-64 (1969)

5. JOHNSTON, I. H. and A. PATERSON: Benign intracranial hypertension: Aspects of diagnosis and treatment in "The Optic Nerve" Proceedings of the Second William Mackenzie Memorial Symposium, ed. J. S. Cant, 1972, Henry Kimpton, London

6. LUNDBERG, N.: Continuous recording and control of ventricular fluid pressure in neurosurgical practice. Acta psychiat. scand. (Suppl. 149), 36 (1960)

7. LUNDBERG, N. H. TROUPP and H. LORIN: Continuous recording of the ventricular fluid pressure in patients with severe acute traumatic brain injury. J. Neurosurg. 22 581-590 (1965)

8. MILLER, J. D., J. GARIBI and J. D. PICKARD: Induced changes of cerebrospinal fluid volume during continuous monitoring of ventricular fluid pressure. Arch. Neurol., 28 265-269 (1973)

9. MILLER, J. D. and J. D. PICKARD: Intracranial volume/pressure studies in patients with head injury. (in press) 1973

10. SUNDBÄRG, G., A. KJÄLLQUIST, N. LUNDBERG and U. PONTEN: Complications due to prolonged ventricular fluid pressure recording in clinical practice. In: M. BROCK and H. DIETZ (eds.): Intracranial Pressure. Springer-Verlag, Berlin-Heidelberg-New York 1972, 348-352

11. VAPALAHTI, M. and H. TROUPP: Prognosis for patients with severe brain injuries. Brit. med. J., 3 404-407 (1971)

Nature and Significance of the CUSHING Reflex

J. CERVÓS-NAVARRO, F. MATAKAS, and E. FUCHS

NAUNYN and SCHREIBER in 1881 first described the arterial pressure response (APR) during intracranial hypertension subsequently called CUSHING (1902) response. Two questions remained controversial since then: the adequate stimulus for the APR (WEINSTEIN, LANGFITT, CASSELL, 1964) and the significance of the APR in intracranial hypertension. It was described by SCHUTTA, KASSELL, LANGFITT (1968) and others that arterial hypertension may enhance the development of brain edema. Thus it seems possible that the APR is of disadvantage for the patient in conditions of brain edema.

Material and Methods

All animals were anesthetised with pentobarbital sodium (40 mg/kg) relaxed with succinylbischolin and artificially respirated by a Starling pump. Mean arterial pressure (MAP), cysternal pressure, epidural pressure, EEC, ECG, and body temperature were constantly recorded. In 44 cats the intracranial pressure (ICP) was elevated by injecting mock CSF (DAVSON, 1967) into the subarachnoid space for time periods of 2 to 5 minutes. In 14 animals (monkeys and cats) ICP was elevated by inflating an epidural balloon.

Results

Whenever the ICP was elevated an APR occurred. The increase of the MAP equalled the ICP when the latter was low. Thus the intracranial perfusion pressure (= MAP - ICP) was remained constant (Fig. 1). However, when the ICP became greater than 50 to 70 mm Hg the APR did not compensate the ICP and the intracranial perfusion pressure became smaller.

If blood was withdrawn from an animal during an APR and injected into a second animal no pressure response was observed in the animal receiving the blood. Blocking of peripheral alpha-receptors with phentolamine (10-15 mg/kg) abolished the APR. About 30 sec. after the beginning of intracranial hypertension the MAP fell by 5 to 10 mm Hg. Blocking of peripheral beta-receptors with propanolol (1.7 - 2.5 mg/kg) produced an up and down movement of the MAP on a level lower than normal during intracranial hypertension (Fig. 2).

After a sudden relief of the intracranial space the MAP fell always to subnormal values.

When the ICP approached the MAP alterations of the ECG were observed, particularly ventricular extrasystoles and a decrease of the ST-interval. After application of atropine heart rate and blood pressure amplitude changed parallel to the MAP. When the arterial pressure increased heart rate and arterial pressure amplitude showed a slight increase,too.

When intracranial hypertension was produced by an epidural balloon the ICP was dependent on the MAP. Thus the ICP became greater when the MAP increased and vice versa. However, the relationship between MAP and ICP was not so vigorous as to prevent the intracranial perfusion pressure to increase during arterial hypertension (Fig. 3). Thus in all 14 animals the intracranial perfusion pressure could be increased by 10 to 50 mm Hg by artificial arterial hypertension although the ICP was considerably elevated.

Discussion

The experimental data lead to the hypothesis that an increased intracranial pressure stimulates sympathetic fibers reaching the alpha-receptors of peripheral vessels in an early alpha-phase within 30-35 seconds and fibers predominantly reaching the beta-receptors of the myocardium and peripheral vessels in a second phase.

When the beta-receptors were blocked only alpha-adrenergic fibers had an effect on their target organs (predominantly the peripheral vessels). Consequently only that component of the APR that is caused by vasoconstriction, viz. the early rapid increase of the blood pressure was observed. The consecutive fall of the blood pressure may be explained by an inhibition of central vasomotor centers (HOFF, REIS 1970). These centers are stimulated by beta-adrenergic fibers but are not subjected to the blocking effect of propanolol. This hypothesis is supported by the fact that the blood pressure decrease appeared after a time interval identical to that which usually preceeds the second phase in the normal APR, i. e. the blood pressure plateau.

When the alpha-receptors were blocked, we found an inversion of the MAP 30 sec. after the beginning of intracranial hypertension. Vasodilatation by stimulation of beta-receptors and a resulting reduction of the venous return obviously could not be compensated for by an increased cardiac output. That a reduced venous return diminishes the APR is proven by the findings of MEYER and WINTER (1970) who observed an attenuated APR in hypovolemia.

There has been a long discussion as to whether the adequate stimulus of the APR is distortion of the brain stem, intracranial pressure, cerebral hypoxia or reduction of the cerebral blood flow (WEINSTEIN, LANGFITT, KASSELL, 1964; JOHNSTON, ROWAN, HARPER, JENNETT, 1972). The results of SAGAWA, ROSS and GUYTON (1961) and MATAKAS, LEIPERT, FRANKE (1971) showed that the degree of the arterial pressure increase is dependent on the degree of the reduction of the CBF or intracranial perfusion pressure. Since chemoreceptors usually have a latent period of 30 - 42 sec. (Korner, 1971), which corresponds well with the starting time of the second phase of the APR, it seems reasonable to assume that beta-adrenergic fibers in the APR are activated by arterial chemoreceptors. The early increase of the arterial pressure on the other hand appears so early that it may well be provoked by baroreceptors.

The fact that slight and moderate intracranial hypertension is compensated by the APR indicates that the latter is a compensating mechanism for preventing reduction of the CBF. This was established with more certainty by measuring the intracranial perfusion pressure during arterial hypertension in conditions of intracranial hypertension. The relationship between ICP and APR is of complex nature. Once the intracranial pressure is elevated the mean arterial pressure contributes to its height. However, the perfusion pressure may still be increased by arterial hypertension. Thus in intracranial hypertension the mechanism may be as following: By increased ICP the intracranial perfusion pressure is reduced. This provokes an APR. By elevation of the MAP the ICP is further increased but not as much as the arterial pressure itself. Consequently the intracranial perfusion pressure is raised and cerebral blood flow may be improved.

REFERENCES

1. CUSHING, H.: Some experimental and clinical observations concerning states of increased intracranial tension. Am.J. med. sci. 124, 375-400 (1902)

2. HOFF, J.T. and D.J. REIS: Localisation of regions mediating the CUSHING response in CNS of cat. Arch. Neurol. 23, 228-240 (1970)

3. JOHNSTON, I.H., J.O. ROWAN, A.M. HARPER, W.B. JENNETT: Raised intracranial pressure and cerebral blood flow. I. Cisterna Magna infusion in primates. J. Neurol., Neurosog., Psychiatr. 35, 285-296 (1972)

4. KORNER, P.I.: Integrative neural cardiovascular control. Physiol. Rev. 51, 312-367 (1971)

5. MATAKAS, F., M. LEIPERT and J. FRANKE: Cerebral blood flow during increased subarachnoid pressure. Act. Neurochir. 25, 19-36 (1971)

6. NAUNYN, B. and I. SCHREIBER: Ueber Gehirndruck. Arch. Exp. Pathol. Pharmakol. 14, 1-73 (1881)

7. MEYER, G.A. and D.L. WINTER: Spinal cord participation in the CUSHING reflex in the dog. J. Neurosurg. 33, 662-675 (1970)

8. SAGAWA, H., J.M. ROSS and A.C. GUYTON: Quantitation of cerebral ischemic pressure response in dogs. Am. J. Physiol. 200, 1164-1168 (1961)

9. SCHUTTA, H.S., N.F. KASSELL and T.W. LANGFITT: Brain swelling, produced by injury and aggravated by arterial hypertension. A light and electron microscopic study. Brain 91, 281-294 (1968)

10. WEINSTEIN, J.D., C.W. LANGFITT and N.F. KASSELL: Vasopressor response to increased intracranial pressure. Neurology 14, 1118-1132 (1964)

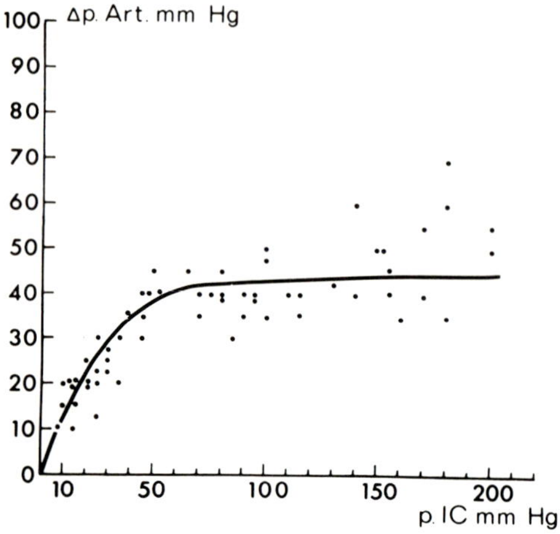

Fig. 1. Relationship between intracranial pressure (ICP) and arterial pressure increase (Δ p Art.). Increase of intracranial pressure is compensated by APR as long as the first does not exceed 50-70 mm Hg

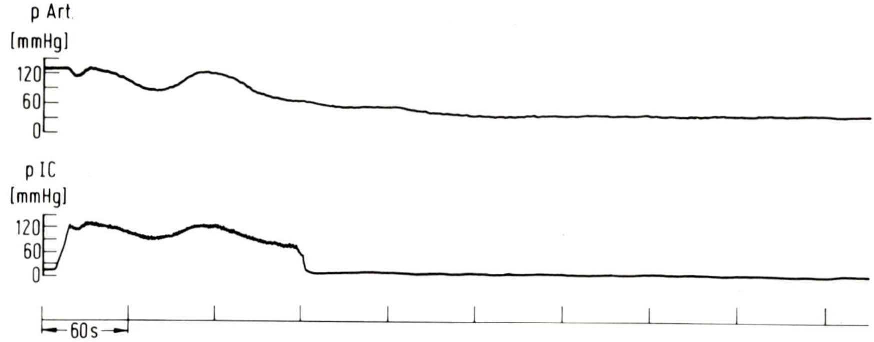

Fig. 2. Arterial pressure during artificial intracranial hypertension in a cat. 15 minutes after application of propanolol. The first short downward movement of the arterial pressure is greater than in the "normal" APR. The arterial pressure moves up and down. These changes are transferred onto the intracranial pressure. After relief of the intracranial space the arterial pressure falls below the initial value

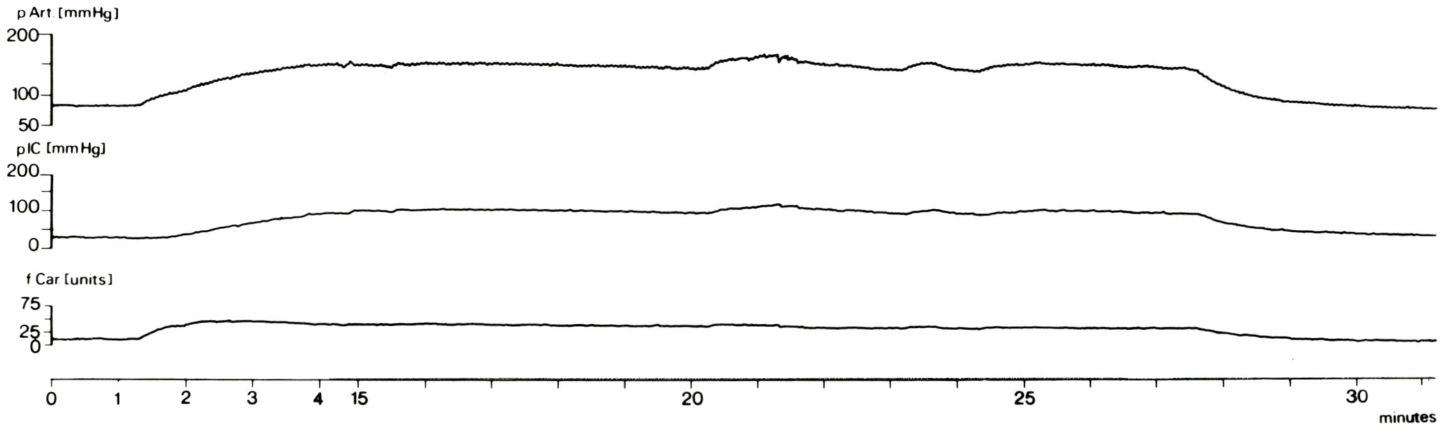

Fig. 3. Rhesus-monkey. By inflating an epidural balloon a moderate intracranial hypertension was produced. By application of norepinephrine the arterial pressure is elevated. There is a parallel movement of both pressures. Measurement of the carotid flow (f car.) after ligation of the external carotid artery demonstrates improvement of carotid flow because of increased intracranial perfusion pressure

Ventricular Fluid Pressure in Children with Severe Brain Injuries

H. TROUPP and M. VAPALAHTI

On April 26th, 1964, a 6-year-old girl was admitted unconscious to the Neurosurgical Clinic of the Helsinki University Central Hospital. A left posterior temporal extradural haematoma was removed. As she did not regain consciousness a check angiogram was done, and this showed some haematoma remaining. To help us decide whether a second operation was necessary, a ventricular fluid pressure recording was started on April 28th. It showed a basic pressure of some 15-20 mmHg, with minor plateau waves reaching 30-40 mmHg; the pressure was later classified as being in the 30-60 mmHg range (see methods). The remaining haematoma was left untouched, and the patient regained consciousness on May 2nd, when the recording was stopped.

This case - the first patient on whom a ventricular fluid pressure recording was done in our department - shows a rather rare indication for doing such a pressure recording in children: to judge whether a small haematoma is worth removing. The indications for ventricular fluid pressure recording in brain injuries can be classified as follows:

1. assessing the severity of the brain injury, establishing a prognosis, and monitoring the patient;
2. gauging the effect of treatment - or lack of such effect;
3. ventricular drainage;
4. as an aid to doubtful decisions.

This paper analyzes our experience with continuous ventricular fluid pressure (VFP) recording in brain-injured children. Children, unlike adults, do not as a rule remain vegetative wrecks even after a severe brain injury; if they survive, they show an amazing power of recuperation and compensation, and VFP recording can be particularly helpful in the handling of severe brain injuries in children.

Methods

For the ventricular pressure recording, LUNDBERG's (1) method was used. A HOLTER ventricular catheter was inserted into one lateral ventricle through a burr hole and securely anchored in the hole with the aid of a rubber plug. The catheter was connected to a Statham P23AA pressure transducer through a 3-metre piece of plastic tubing. The signal from the transducer was amplified, and recorded either with an ink-writer or with a point recorder making a mark on the record every 1-2 seconds. The latter proved better for prolonged use: there was far less paper to look through, and there were fewer mechanical failures.

In two instances the arterial blood pressure (Fig. 1) with a nylon catheter in the superficial temporal artery.

For assessment of the recordings the following criteria were used:

1. Range under 30 mmHg: mean pressure well below 30 mmHg, with, at most, occasional rises slightly above this level.
2. Range 30-60 mmHg: mean pressure might be below 30 mmHg, but with frequent rises above 30 mmHg, sometimes plateau waves to 50-60 mmHg. Fig. 1 provides an example of this type.
3. Range above 60 mmHg: either a pressure keeping steadily above 60 mmHg or a mean pressure below 60 mmHg but with plateau waves reaching far above this level. Fig. 2 provides an example of the latter type.

There were no complications from the VFP recording in this series of 25 patients.

The VFP recordings were started on average 25 hours after the accident, and lasted for an average of 4 days. Fifteen recordings were started within 24 hours after the injury, and five later than 48 hours after the accident.

In 12 instances the pH_{csf} was determined soon after the start of the VFP recording; mean pH_{csf} was 7.30, with no apparent correlation to outcome in this series.

The Patients

In the years 1964-1972 twenty-five children under 15 years of age with severe acute brain injuries were monitored with continuous ventricular fluid pressure (VFP) recordings. This series represents the most severe brain injuries among the children admitted over this period; at first our use of VFP recording was rather tentative, until we gained confidence enough in the method to use it regularly with severely brain-injured children.

Mean age at the time of injury for the 25 children in the series was 7.3 years. Mean follow-up time for the survivors was 4 years (Table I).

All 25 children had at least one carotid angiogram; a haematoma was removed in four patients; in five more patients a small mass lesion was found at angiography but was not considered large enough to necessitate an operation.

Eleven children had significant extracranial injuries; significant here means that the extracranial injury necessitated some procedure in the acute stage. Five of these children died. In three instances the extracranial injuries could be considered mainly responsible for the child's death; in these it did not seem to be the brain injury which caused the child's deterioration, and the VFP stayed continuously below 30 mmHg.

Thirteen children had extensor spasms; four of these died; this sign would suggest an almost hopeless prognosis in adults (5). Two children developed

Table I

25 CHILDREN UNDER 15 WITH SEVERE BRAIN INJURIES			
Ventricular fluid pressure	Outcome		Total
	Survivors	Dead	
Under 30 mm Hg	9	1	10
30 - 60 mm Hg	4	3	7
Above 60 mm Hg	2	6	8
	15	10	25

hyperthermia very quickly although there was no apparent infection and pulmonary ventilation was adequate; they both died. P_aCO_2 over the first two days did not correlate with outcome.

Fifteen children survived; ten died, on an average 5. 5 days after the injury, median 4 days. See Table I for the correlation between VFP and outcome. Those that survived were unconscious for an average period of 22 days, median 9 days. One 8-year-old boy was unconscious for four months; he has recovered enough to take care of himself and go to school, but is not likely to become self-supporting; he was one of the two patients who survived in spite of a VFP in the above 60 range. Of the fifteen survivors, eight have a chance of becoming self-supporting; of these, one was unconscious for 19 days and one for 37 days. The two children who seemed to have no residua at follow up had been unconscious for 4 and 7 days. For this analysis, unconsciousness was defined as not obeying simple commands like "open your eyes", "squeeze my hand", let go my hand".

Treatment

Twenty-four children were intubated at some stage; only the youngest one (8 months) was not, as he seemed to maintain a free airway on his own. Six children had a tracheotomy at some stage, of whom one, a girl of 7 had considerable difficulties with tracheal stenosis later.

Seven children received massive doses of corticosteroids; there were no apparent complications, and the one child who died from a perforated gastric ulcer had not received corticosteroids at all, as his VFP was well controlled with hyperventilation and ventricular drainage.

Ten children were hyperventilated in a respirator; seven of these belonged to the pressure range above 60 mmHg, two to the 30-60 mmHg range, and one had a VFP classified as below 30 mmHg. The latter patient had aspirated both blood and gastric contents. Six of these ten children died; of the other four deaths, without hyperventilation, three children died of their extracranial injuries, and in the remaining child the VFP was so high in comparison to blood pressure that the brain was probably dying before the start of the recording, and VFP was recorded for three hours only.

Seven children had ventricular drainage; four of these died. Ventricular drainage was often used as a last resort, as were also dehydrating agents; but it may well be that drainage should be used more often and at an earlier stage. It has the drawback that it may render the VFP recording unreliable. Dehydrating agents were used mainly in an acute emergency; previous experience had led to considerable caution in this report (2, 3).

Discussion

We would recommend the following measures for the child with a severe brain injury: acute resuscitation as usual, i.e. clearance and maintenance of airways, treatment of shock if any, carotid angiography to establish or disprove significant haematomas; then a ventricular fluid pressure (VFP) recording; hyperventilation if the patient had an elevated P_aCO_2 on arrival or if the VFP shows at least long excursions into the 30-60 mmHg range. The effect of hyperventilation is easy to see, though adults must be distinguished from children in this respect. Judging from our experience with adults (4, 5) none with pressures above 60 mmHg survived as anything but a vegetative wreck, and those that hyperventilated most on their own fared worst (5).

Corticosteroids should perhaps also be started early; in three dead children the macroscopic brain damage was surprisingly slight, but there was severe edema of the brain. If the VFP constantly rises above 30 mmHg in spite of hyperventilation and corticosteroids, ventricular drainage may be tried. Dehydrating agents we would reserve for sudden and severe rises in VFP, in particular immediately before and during the removal of a haematoma (cf. Fig. 2).

We cannot prove that the recording of ventricular fluid pressure was a decisive advantage in the handling of these brain-injured children; we have no exactly comparable series without VFP recording. However, we know that VFP is correlated to outcome (Table I; 4) so that the physician can direct his energies purposefully, and unnecessary interference is avoided, as in the case report which opens this paper. This is important precisely because children, if they survive the acute stage, have such recuperative powers. The case of the 8-month-old baby, whom we did not hyperventilate because it was not then our practice to do so, is very instructive as to the resilience of children. His pressure was the highest in the 30-60 mmHg group but his recovery was good after 6 days of unconsciousness. It is possible that his fontanel functioned to some extent as a safety valve.

Summary

The records of 25 children - under 15 years of age - with severe brain injuries were analyzed. These were all the children who had had ventricular fluid pressure (VFP) recordings in the acute stage after a severe brain injury in the years 1964-1972 in the Neurosurgical Clinic of the Helsinki University Central Hospital.

Ten of the children died, , seven from their brain injury, three mainly from their extracranial injuries; fifteen survived, and of these eight are likely to become self-supporting. None became a vegetative wreck.

The VFP recording was started on average 25 hours after the injury, and lasted for an average of 4 days. Ten children, of whom nine survived, had a pressure classified as under 30 mmHg. Seven children, of whom four survived, had a pressure over 60 mmHg. These two survivors were considerably crippled .

Basic treatment was the same for all: adequate airway maintenance, diagnosis of intracranial haematomas by carotid angiography, and adequate fluid therapy and replacement of lost blood as well as immobilization of injured limbs. Ten children were treated by hyperventilation in a respirator; seven received massive doses of corticosteroids; and seven were treated by ventricular drainage. Treatment was very much guided by the VFP recording.

Ventricular fluid pressure recording is useful for assessing the brain injury, establishing a prognosis, guiding therapy and monitoring the effect of treatment. A ventricular catheter also makes it possible to withdraw samples of cerebrospinal fluid; and ventricular drainage probably contributed to the survival of three children.

REFERENCES

1. LUNDBERG, N.: Continuous recording and control of ventricular fluid pressure in neurosurgical practice. Acta psychiat. neurol. scand. 36, Suppl. 149 (1960)

2. TROUPP, H.: Intraventricular pressure in patients with severe brain injuries. J. Trauma 5, 373-378 (1965)

3. TROUPP, H.: Intraventricular pressure in patients with severe brain injuries. J. Trauma 7 , 875-883 (1967)

4. VAPALAHTI, M.: Intracranial pressure, acid-base status of blood and cerebrospinal fluid, and pulmonary function in the prognosis of severe brain injury. Thesis, University of Helsinki, 1970

5. VAPALAHTI, M. and H. TROUPP: Prognosis for patients with severe brain injuries. Brit. med. J. 3, 404-407 (1971)

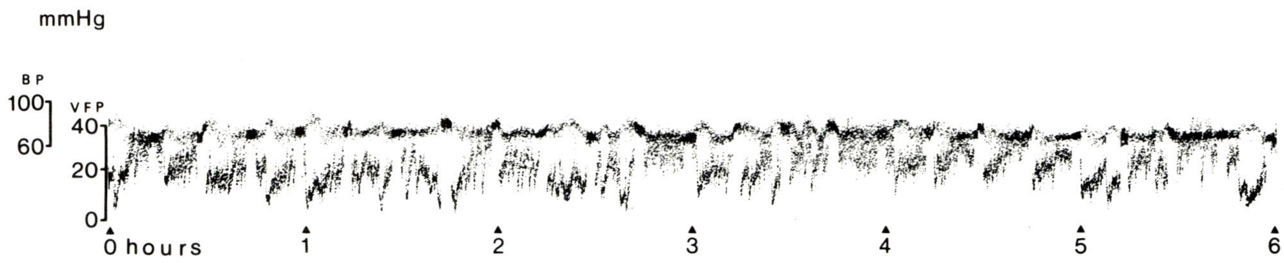

Fig. 1. Boy, 4. This recording was obtained 4 days after the injury. As there were frequent rises above 30 mm Hg, the recording was classified in the 30-60 mm Hg range. No hyperventilation, no corticosteroids. The boy recovered consciousness the day after this recording was obtained, and made a good recovery

Note that the blood pressure (upper trace) remains very steady in spite of the sudden swings in ventricular fluid pressure (lower trace, sometimes overlapping the blood pressure trace); sometimes there is a drop in blood pressure coinciding with a rise in ventricular fluid pressure, and vice versa. Note also how the point recorder compresses a 6-hour recording into a small space; our present point recorders produce only 122 cms. of recording per day

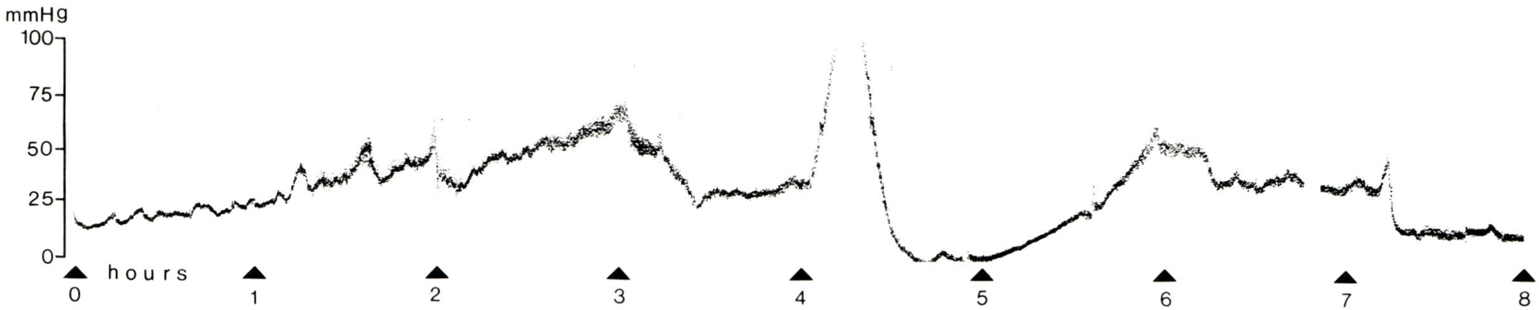

Fig. 2. Boy, 5. This recording was obtained 6 days after the injury. Mean pressure is definitely below 60 mm Hg, but there are rises to 60 mm Hg at 3 and at 6 hours; and at 4 hours there is a plateau wave rising above 100 mm Hg; this recording was consequently classified in the above 60 mm Hg range. This recording was obtained just before the decision to evacuate a temporal lobe hematoma; after the operation the ventricular fluid pressure settled to between 20 and 30 mm Hg. The VFP recording was stopped 12 days after the injury, and the child's condition seemed to have stabilized well when he suffered a cardiac arrest 17 days after the injury. At autopsy no reason for his sudden death could be found

Intracranial Pressure, Hemodynamics and Metabolic Disorders in Patients with Severe Head Injury

W. GOBIET, W. J. BOCK, J. LIESEGANG, and W. GROTE

Experimental studies have shown that cerebral perfusion pressure, i.e. the difference between mean arterial and intracranial pressure, can be lowered to about 40-60 mm Hg without marked cerebral hemodynamic or metabolic disorders (1, 2, 3). Below this limit significant decrease of cerebral blood flow and increase of cerebral tissue and jugular vein lactate concentration was noticed (4, 5, 6, 7, 8). In the above experiments low cerebral perfusion pressures were produced either by decreasing the arterial or by increasing the intracranial pressure.

The purpose of this investigation was, to study the effect of lowered cerebral perfusion pressure on cerebral blood flow and metabolism in man.

Method

In 15 patients with severe head injury the intracranial pressure (ICP), mean arterial blood pressure (MAP), cerebral blood flow (CBF) as well as pO_2, pCO_2, pH and lactate concentration in arterial and jugular venous blood were measured.

To obtain better information about the interaction between ICP, MAP and CBF these values were continuously recorded.

ICP was measured with a miniature pressure transducer in the epidural space as described in an earlier paper (8). We used the new Sensotec BW 7 transducer, which can be calibrated in situ. As an index for CBF we determined the flow in the internal carotis with an electromagnetic blood flow probe Statham 2202. This standard method in experimental medicine had been used in man only for a short time during Carotis surgery (11, 12). This Statham 2202 model allows long time monitoring because zero point reference can be obtained without occluding the artery.

Before implantation the pressure transducer and the flow probe were sterilized with Detergicide solution. The implantation period lasted between 1 and 11 days. No local disturbances due to the insertion of the probes could be observed.

Blood pressure was measured in the femoral artery with an external Statham transducer P 23 db and a Siemens Elektromanometer. ICP, MAP and CBF were recorded on a Siemens Meditape 12. pO_2, pCO_2 and pH were determined with an AVL Gascheck Analyzer, lactate concentration with the Boehringer enzymatic method.

Results

The relationship between CBF and CPP is shown in Fig. 1. Normal perfusion pressure from 70-120 mm Hg is associated with cerebral blood flow above 200 ml/min. (mean 270 ml/min.). Lowering perfusion pressure (CPP) by increasing ICP is accompanied by a reduction of CBF. In most cases CBF is uphold in normal range until CPP is reduced under 50 mm Hg. Then a marked decrease of CBF can be noticed.

In our study no relationship between CPP and arterial or jugular venous pO_2 and pCO_2 could be found.

Fig. 2 shows the values of jugular venous pH plotted against CPP. The area between dotted lines indicates normal values.

Down to perfusion pressures of 50-60 mm Hg pH remains in normal range. Further diminishing of CPP accompanied by reduced CBF leads to cerebral tissue acidosis indicated by a sharp fall of jugular venous pH to values between 7,1 and 7,2.

The increasing anerobic glycolysis causes a rise of jugular venous lactate concentration as shown in Fig. 3. Lactate levels increase with decreasing CPP. Excessively high lactate values over 40 mU were noticed when CPP was below 40 mm Hg.

As an example, the recording of a patient with increased ICP (Fig. 4) shows the interaction between ICP, CBF and blood pressure (BP). An initially normal CPP is upheld by a slight elevation of BP, although ICP is increased to about 40 mm Hg. Loss of autoregulation in the final stage causes a fall in BP accompanied by a significant reduction in CBF down to 10-15 ml/min. ICP rose up to 60 mm Hg. The lactate concentration above 72 mU and the pH of 7,05 indicate the complete metabolic imbalance.

Discussion

We found that also in man lowered CPP either by increasing ICP and / or falling MAP causes a reduction of CBF. When CPP is lowered below 50 mm Hg CBF is reduced below 1/4 of normal values in most patients.

At the same time, the increase of lactate concentration accompanied by a decreasing pH in jugular venous blood reflects the progressive brain tissue acidosis (3, 5, 6, 7).

These results are in good accordance with previous experimental studies (4, 5, 11).

In our opinion simultaneous continuous monitoring of cerebral blood flow, intracranial pressure, and blood pressure will provide better information on cerebral hemodynamics in the presence of brain edema.

REFERENCES

1. KJÄLLQUIST, A., B.K. SIESJÖ and N. ZWETNOW: Effects of increased intracranial pressure on cerebral venous PO_2, PCO_2, PH lactate and pyruvate in dogs. Acta physiol. scand. 75, 267-275 (1969)

2. GRANHOLM, L. and B.K. SIESJÖ: The effects of hypercapnia upon the cerebrospinal fluid lactate and pyruvate concentrations and upon the lactate, pyruvate, ATP, ADP, phosphocreatine concentrations of cat brain tissue. Acta physiol. scand. 75, 257-266 (1969)

3. SIESJÖ, B.K. and N.N. ZWETNOW: Effects of increased CSF pressure upon adenine nucleotides and upon lactate and pyruvate in rat brain tissue. Acta neurol. Scandinav. 46, 187-202 (1970)

4. MATAKAS, F., M. LEIPERT and J. FRANKE: Cerebral blood flow during increased subarachnoid pressure. Acta Neurochirurgica 25, 19-36 (1971)

5. MEINIG, G., H.J. REULEN, C. MAGAVLY, U. HASE and O. HEY: Changes of cerebral hemodynamics and energy metabolism during increased CSF pressure and brain edema. Intracranial pressure. Springer-Verlag Heidelberg 79-84 (1972)

6. ZWETNOW, N.N.: Effects of increased CSF pressure on the blood flow and on energy metabolism of brain. Acta physiol. Scandinav. suppl. 339 1-31 (1970)

7. ZIMMERMANN, W.E.: Hypoxie und Gewebsstoffwechsel. Der Anaesthesist 13,4 122-127

8. HUCKABEE, W.E.: Excess Lactate and anaerobiosis. Pharmacol. Rev. 17, 247-252 (1965)

9. GOBIET, W., W.J. BOCK, J. LIESEGANG and W. GROTE : Long-time monitoring of epidural pressure in man. Intracranial pressure. Springer Verlag Heidelberg, 14-17 (1972)

10. LOWELL, H.M. and B.M. BLOOR: The effect of increased intracranial pressure on cerebrovascular hemodynamics. J. Neurosurg. 34 760-769 (1971)

11. GREENFIELD, J.C. and G.T. TINDALL: The effect of acute increase in intracranial pressure on blood flow in the internal carotid artery in man. J. clin. Invest. 44, 1343-1351 (1965)

12. NORNES, N.: Recurrent hemorrhage and hemostasis in patients with ruptured intracranial saccular aneurysm. Intracranial Pressure. Springer Verlag Heidelberg 244-249 (1972)

►

Fig. 1. Internal carotid flow plotted against cerebral perfusion pressure (CPP). Blood flow is markedly reduced at a CPP below 50 mm Hg

►

Fig. 2. pH values in jugular venous blood. Reduction of CPP below 50-60 mm Hg is accompanied by increasing acidosis. (Interrupted lines=normal values)

Fig. 1

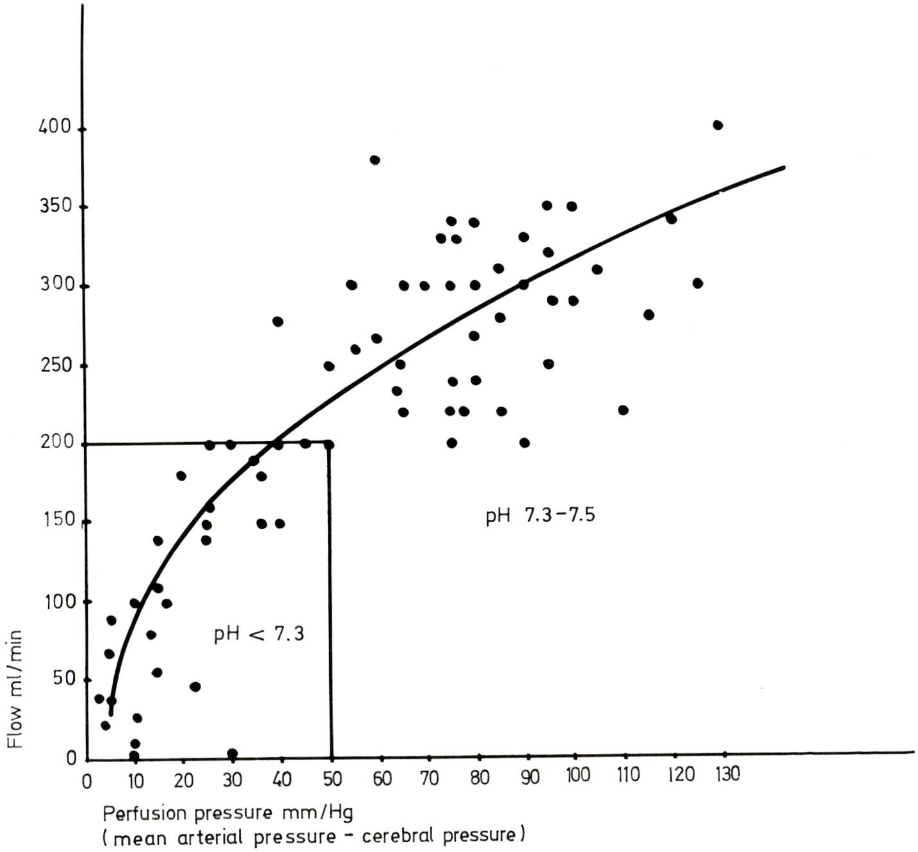
400
350
300
250
200
150
100
50
0
Flow ml/min
pH 7.3-7.5
pH < 7.3
0 10 20 30 40 50 60 70 80 90 100 110 120 130
Perfusion pressure mm/Hg
(mean arterial pressure - cerebral pressure)

Fig. 2

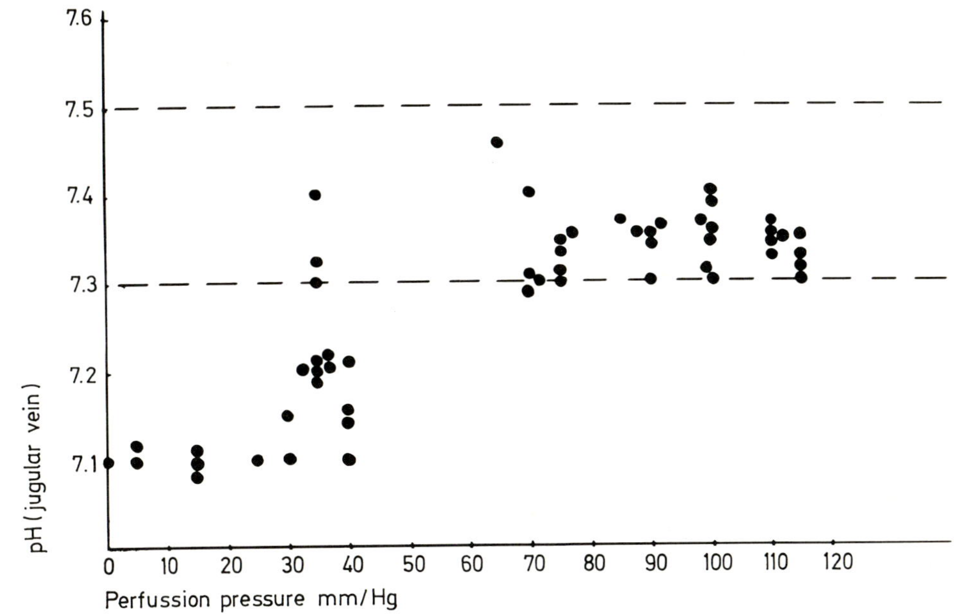
7.6
7.5
7.4
7.3
7.2
7.1
pH (jugular vein)
0 10 20 30 40 50 60 70 80 90 100 110 120
Perfussion pressure mm/Hg

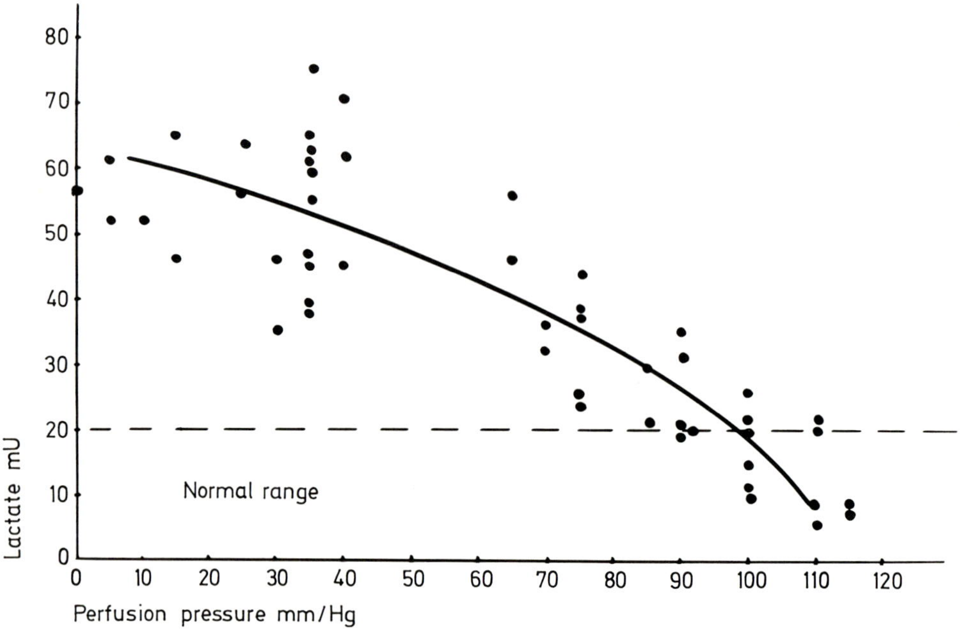

Fig. 3. Lactate concentration in jugular venous blood. Decreasing CPP causes elevated lactate levels

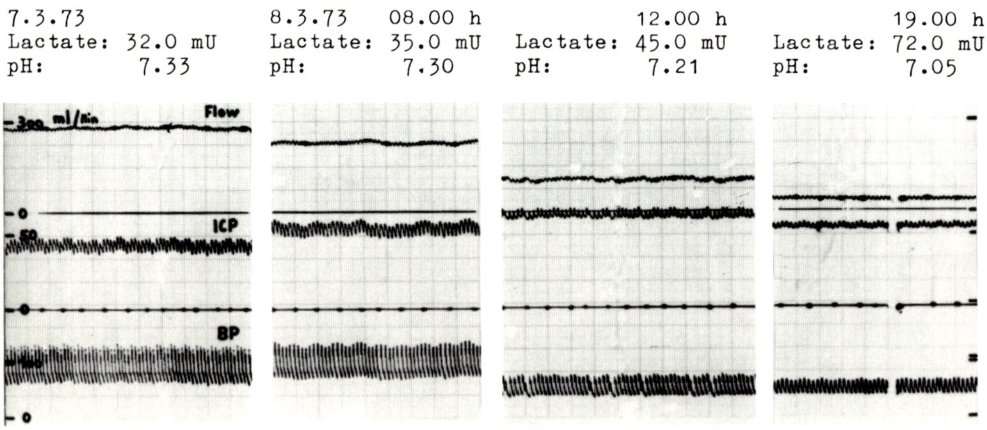

Fig. 4. Sections from an original recording. Loss of autoregulation in the terminal stage leads to a marked decrease of BP and blood flow. ICP remains high. (BP= Blood pressure, Flow= Blood flow in the art. Carotis interna, ICP= intracranial pressure)

Chapter II.

Clinical Therapy of Brain Edema

Hypertonic Solutions and Diuretics in the Treatment of Brain Edema

H. BRENNER

Generally known decongestant and diuretic therapies are often applied according to established treatment schedules, schedules which are changed as soon as a new presumably more potent drug is discovered. Since decades this is the general practice, a practice molded by clinical observations and experimental results as well as theoretical concepts, analogies and traditions.

Hypertonic and diuretic therapies have been widely discussed in the literature with little agreement of the various authors as to its value. The "Handbuch der Neurochirurgie" dedicates a single page to the subject: it could mean that the author attributes no importance to the problem or suggest that all has been said and further proof is no longer required. Some authors, such as KLINGLER, discussed the subject with resignation, others - such as W. E. DANDY - with indisguised objection.

A variety of therapeutic modalities has been attempted with the purpose of combatting the dreaded clinical manifestations of focal brain edema. In such attempts the effects of decongestant and diuretic therapies may be quite variable in different cases. Both beneficial clinical effects have been observed as well as unchanged conditions side by side with situations which suggest a detrimental action. Beyond that, the clinical treatment of edema as generally practiced, particularly the application of decongestants, fails to duplicate various experimental results. It has therefore been criticized both on theoretical grounds and on clinical evidence.

In pertinent experiments the intracranial pressure and more precisely the cerebrospinal fluid pressure are generally considered as evidence of, and measure for, any pathophysiologic and therapeutic changes. In view of the quite complex relationships between edema, displacement and compression of brain structures, localization of the underlying process and its course in terms of progression, adaptability and C. S. F. pressure, this approach appears to be somewhat questionable. But experimental investigations to shed light on the clinical and therapeutic implications of the edematous process proper present considerable difficulties and have consequently been limited in number. The difficulties encountered in such investigations do not relate primarily to inherent differences between man and animal - this is a problem faced in variable degrees in any experimental situation -; they rather relate to the following factors:

Any experimental method to study brain edema from a surgical point of view must satisfy the following conditions:

1. The edema must originate from a focus, such as in cases of cerebral tumor, abscess, contusion, etc.

2. The edema must be uniformly reproducible and should not be exposed to unpredictable alterations by secondary vascular factors, e.g. arterial compression, herniation and phlebothrombosis. (This condition is unfortunately not satisfied by methods which rely on inflatable balloons to serve as artificial space-occupying bodies).

3. The edema must be evaluated in its entirety, i.e. in quantitative terms, for analyses of tissue samples are known to vary with the distance from the focal lesion, from which the edema originates.

Comparative investigations require a standardized "edema model" which, in addition, should simulate human conditions. Among the parameters with which edematous processes of the brain, their course as well as the effects of therapy can be traced satisfactorily, albumin occupies a prominent place. It is a highly sensitive indicator. Its rise is 100 to 400 times higher than that of water and minerals and precedes variations of other substances. Moreover, its accumulation in the extravascular spaces, i.e., in the brain parenchyma, can be traced more effectively with radioactive labelling than is possible with fluorescein coupling and blue staining.

A visible and palpable reduction of intracranial pressure in a patient with cerebral prolapse who has been given potent diuretic treatment prompts the assumption that the excreted urinary volume has at least temporarily reduced the peritumorous edema. This can also be demonstrated experimentally on the closed skull reducing the intracranial pressure.

The assumption that the edema volume is reduced, is supported by analyses of bioptic brain tissue carried out by the group of Mainz. These analyses indicated that water, sodium and chloride levels were lower after 4 days of diuretic treatment than in the untreated controls. But then, REULEN, SAMII and SCHÜRMANN suggest that dysfunction of the renal tubuli may play a role in the development of brain edema.

However, there is no derth of experimental observations which make the efficacy of this approach questionable. Three years ago GO and coworkers, i.e. BEKS' group in Groningen, demonstrated that the osmotic and oncotic barrier action required an intact blood brain barrier. While ^{14}C and ^{3}H-labelled diuretics did not enter normal brain tissue, they penetrated into edematous tissue areas. And after a short lapse of time a balance was found to establish. Hence even the most potent diuretics including urea did not possess any anti-edematous effect; they rather acted in terms of expanding the plasma volume.

These findings are in good agreement with the results of SCHMIDT (previously Freiburg) and WISE (San Francisco), who hold that the decongestant effect of any drug is lost once the BBB is no longer intact.

If in a test animal with unilateral cold induced edema RISA is injected, enormous quantities of albumin are found to accumulate in the edematous area in albumin turnover.

	Albumin	Globulin
Normal white matter	1.3%	98.7%
Edematous white matter (total protein increase of 70%)	22.4%	77.6%
Therefore:		
Proteins of edemat. transudation	52.0%	48.0%

Edematous white matter has some 70% more protein, with the albumin share increasing from 1.3% to 22.4%. By means of a simple calculation, the edematous transudate can be seen to consist of equal shares of albumin and globulin. Moreover, the albumin in edematous white matter can be seen to be 96% "pathologic" (edema specific) and only 4% "normal" (pre-existent).

Albumin in edematous white regions:

Pre-existent	3.5%
From edema	96.5%

When killing the test animal, perfusing its brain and removing the hypothermally induced necrotic areas, the activities of the intact and the edematous hemisphere can be compared and related to blood activities (Table I).

These findings as well as the previously mentioned results indicating an inadequate effect on the edema proper on the one hand and the uncontestable reduction of intracranial pressure observed clinically under diuretic medication on the other hand are not contradictory. For what seems to be contradictory is explained by the fact that the diuresis primarily affects the intact brain parenchyma with its balanced BBB, while it fails to counteract the pathologic forces of the edematous process proper. The edema surrounding a furuncle on the back of the hand equally fails to subside after the passage of 2 to 4 liters of urine! The results presented also explain why, of all edematous processes, the diffuse low-grade brain edemas respond best to diuretic medication - here we are confronted with a situation that differs widely from that encountered by neurologists and internists. Beyond that, the results serve to explain why circumscribed edematous areas may expand after general diuresis: the reduction of brain volume produced by general dehydration permits further expansion of the hemisphere involved, thus promoting mass-shifting. Focal edema requires decompression and expansion towards the surface and not towards the midline of the brain.

Experimental investigations also indicated that damage of the vascular walls constituted the portal of the development of edema. This mechanism suggests the prophylactic administration of anti-inflammatory agents to seal the vascular walls and thus curb the expansion and slow down the rate of edema development. Vitamins C and P, calcium, steroids, butazolidine and chestnut derivatives are indicated prior to the onset of edema formation.

What are now the indications for hypertonic diuretic treatment?

Prior to surgery the surgeon will only rarely be faced with this problem, as

Table I. RIHSA accumulation in experimental brain edema (149 cats and rabbits)

n	RIHSA dosis	RIHSA application time	survival time	antiedematous medication	Q	I
5 controls	1 µC	10 min	24 hours		0,96	0,000022
12	1 µC	10 min after cold	24 hours		6,25	0,134
5	1 µC	10 min after cold	48 hours		2,2	0,048
3	1 µC	30 min before sacrification	24 hours		1,34	0,022
7	50 µC	30 min before sacrification	- " -		1,62	0,029
15	1 µC	10 min after cold	- " -		6,7	0,132
5	1 µC	60-90 min after cold	- " -		4,8	0,129
5	1 µC	10 min before cold	- " -		6,5	0,137
5	5 µC	10 min after cold	- " -		6,6	0,148
25	50 µC	10 min after cold	- " -		6,3	0,145
3	50 µC	10 min before cold	- " -		7,3	0,162
8	50 µC	10 min after cold	- " -	human albumin	7,5	0,212
8	50 µC	10 min after cold	- " -	urea	5,4	0,155
8	50 µC	10 min after cold	- " -	vitamin C	6,0	0,114
8	50 µC	10 min after cold	- " -	acetocolamide	7,4	0,167
8	50 µC	10 min after cold	- " -	rutin	5,9	0,148
8	50 µC	10 min after cold	- " -	extr. chestnut	5,4	0,138
8	50 µC	10 min after cold	- " -	calcium	6,9	0,167
8	50 µC	10 min after cold	- " -	fursemid	8,1	0,136

Q = rates of counts: involved hemisphere / intact hemisphere

$$I = \text{rates of counts: } \frac{\text{involved hemisphere - intact hemisphere}}{\text{1 ml blood}}$$

causal therapy or at least a palliative procedure for short-term relief will be prominent.

During surgery there are much more potent and much better controllable methods to reduce intracranial pressure. In the last 6,000 craniotomies we performed mannitol and sorbitol solutions had to be given only in those rare instances where anesthesia emergencies occurred.

After surgery diuretic osmotherapy to combat potential edema development is equally indicated in conditions following respiratory or general circulatory hypoxemia. If, in exceptional cases, trepanation was done in completely inoperable cases and attempts at decompression failed, these procedures will have to be tried. This also applied to children with craniosynostoses, who show a tendency to develop severe, often fatal diffuse brain edema.

In those cases where temporary or persistent occlusion of a cerebral artery or vein can be expected to produce regional hemispheral edema - these include the majority of our post-operative problem-patients - extensive decompression of the surgical field and a priori application of high doses of drugs with a vascular seal effect appear to be more appropriate. This approach is more promising than an attempt at diuresis with the skull closed, which would risk progressive mass displacement on account of volume reductions of the intact brain structures.

After surgery on particularly delicate neural structures where a local but not mass-shifting edema should be prevented, the above arguments against osmotherapy lose their relevance. In these cases the initial given vascular sealing medication should be completed on the 2nd and 3rd day with osmotic and hyperoncotic therapy. The latter is designed to become effective at the time of maximum edema expansion. Timing the therapy to coincide with the postoperative edema peak and limiting it to no more than approximately 48 hours have been chosen for

		Vasc. seals	Hypert. sol. diuretics
Pre-operative		where required	
Intra-operative	in anesth. emergencies		++
Postoperative	after anesth. emergencies	+	+++
	in cranio-synostoses	+	+++
	in inoperable non-decompressed cases		++
	lesion of cerebral artery or vein	+++	
	after surgery on delicate neural structures	+++	++ (on 2nd and 3rd day)

the reason that the drugs are known to gradually lose their efficacy and that a possible rebound effect will be better tolerated after the edema peak.

When selecting the medication it should be borne in mind that all of the pertinent agents are capable of penetrating the broken-down blood brain barrier and accumulating in the tissue. If blood concentrations drop rapidly, the extra intravascular gradient will soon be balanced or even inverted. This applies particularly to glucose in cases where an insulin response causes hypoglycemia.

Beyond that, it should be remembered that the administration of hypertonic solutions is limited quantitatively by plasma osmolarity. BECKER and VRIES found a control osmolarity in excess of 310 mosm/l to be fatal in all their cases. Whether intra-carotid mannite application offers essential advantages we can not say, as we do not have any pertinent experience.

If hypertonic solutions are used for their circulatory effects, high-molecular substances, e. g., albumins and dextrane, should be given preference.

At the Vienna Neurosurgery Clinic diuretic treatment was not performed in more than 1 % of all trepanations.

The Influence of High and Low Dosages of Mannitol 25% in the Therapy of Cerebral Edema

Comparative Study with Monitoring of Intraventricular Pressure

A. KÜHNER, B. ROQUEFEUIL, E. VIGUIE, PH. FREREBEAU, E. PERAZ-DOMINGUEZ, M. BAZIN, J. M. PRIVAT, and C. GROS

Cerebral edema has been treated by hypertonic solutions for many years. Urea and mannitol are the solutions most often used.

Since the introduction of intracranial pressure monitoring the usefullness of hypertonic solutions has been analyzed and confirmed by many authors. The efficacity of a hypertonic solution on cerebral edema is a function of the speed of injection and of amount used (22). The doses used vary from 1 to 4 g/kg for different authors. The intravenous route is used most often; to our knowledge only one author has studied the effect of mannitol by the intra-carotid route (21). This author noted a greater effect on CBF and ICP by this route but he also noted certain dangers such as: the risks inherent to intraarterial perfusion itself and a rebound phenomenon with decrease of CBF if the perfusion is stopped suddenly.

Since mannitol is not metabolized (26, 27, 28) the quantity used should be reduced to a minimum because, in acute traumatic cerebral edema, there are major metabolic disorders (water and sodium retention with a breakdown of free-water clearance) necessitating quantitatively limited reanimation. Since the effectiveness is relatively shortlasting (1 to 6 hours according to the dose) repeated perfusions are necessary to obtain an action lasting 24 hours. Therefore with doses of 1 to 4 g/kg the total for 24 hours dose surpasses reasonable limits.

Because of this, we looked for smaller doses which were still effective; so we analyzed the action of mannitol at the reduced doses of 0, 30 and 0, 15 g/kg in intravenous injections.

Methods

We analyzed the action of 25 % mannitol on a series of 30 patients with severe traumatic cerebral edema. All of these patients were comatous, intubated or tracheotomized and under artificial respiration. The gazometric and manometric conditions were the same in each case, thus eliminating the influences of respiratory parameters on ICP. ICP was measured by our intraventricular catheter and a Statham-type pressure-cell connected to a variable speed polygraph which permitted the study of both the immediate and long term effects. Concurrently we recorded central venous pressure, tracheal pressure, blood pressure and EKG on the same recorder.

Two different doses were used for rapid intravenous injection (less than 1 minute): 0, 15 and 0, 30 g/kg that is 50 cc and 100 cc respectively on an average. 4 to 6 injections are given per 24 hours. We chose the intraventricular pressure as our parameter because there is less chance of error than with extradural pressure (5). Both pressures are in direct linear correlation with the extradural pressure being generally higher (13, 24). Before studying the variations of ICP following administration of mannitol we considered it necessary to record ICP for at least 1 hour prior to injection so as to know the exact mean ICP, since it is absolutely necessary to take into account the physiologic variations, especially the plateau-waves which can last from 5 to 20 minutes.

Results

In 82 % of the cases we obtained a constant response after each injection. In 18 % there was no action on ICP. A rebound phenomenon was observed in 6, 6 % (2 patients), and, finally, we often noticed a decreased effectiveness starting with the 4th or 6th injection. Each time there was no action on ICP there was also no osmotic diuresis and a hyponatriemia with severe hemodilution. The effectiveness of mannitol seems to be dependant on the initial plasma osmolarity and on renal function.

For each dose several parameters were studied.

A. Initial decompressive action (Fig. 1 and 2):

We observed, for each of the two doses, an immediate lowering of ICP. This action is progressive with a maximum lowering after 10 to 15 minutes and exceptionally after 30 to 40 minutes. The rapidity of the initial decompressive action is identical for the two doses. The curves in figures 1 and 2 show this immediate action for the 100 and the 50 cc doses. We can also notice at the same time a slight elevation of the blood pressure by the parallel volemic effect.

B. Duration of the decompressive effect:

While the plateau of maximum lowering is relatively short we constantly noticed a long enough period of time during which the ICP is less than the initial value; the curve progressively approaches the initial level.

For the 100 cc dose, the mean time of action on 30 patients was two hours (Fig. 3) while for the 50 cc dose it was never longer than one hour (Fig. 4).

On all the recordings we are able to notice a regular flattening of the hemodynamic interferences (cerebral pulse) during the time of the mannitol effect.

C. Degree of the decompressive action:

The fall of the ICP is immediate and progressive with a maximum in approximately 15 minutes. The ICP progressively returns to its initial value. For the 100 cc dose we obtained a mean lowering in ICP of 60 to 80 % while with the 50 cc dose the lowering was in the range of 20 to 50 %. Fig. 5 summarizes the different action profiles of the two doses of mannitol.

D. The rebound phenomenon:

This was observed in two cases (Fig. 6). This phenomenon is explained by an intracellular passage of mannitol (7, 20) which inverts the osmotic disequilibrium previously created by the mannitol injection. The rebound phenomenon has been known to exist for a long time and has been reported for various hypertonic solutions: 19 % RINGER's solution (6), hypertonic saline and glucose solutions (2, 3, 4, 8), urea (16) and mannitol (16, 22, 12). But this phenomenon has been greatly disputed; for example, it has not been observed in certain cases with urea (11, 23, 14) and mannitol (4, 26, 27, 28).

JAVID and Coll. (11) studied this particular problem in detail and concluded that the rebound phenomenon is very rare and that many cases reported in the literature are often doubtful; they defined this effect as an increase in ICP above the initial values shortly after the injection. An increase in ICP 12 or even 18 hours after injection is, according to these authors, too late to be called a true rebound for only a substance which rapidly enters into the cell is able to cause this phenomenon.

Studies with C14-urea (19) have shown that the equilibration of the levels of blood urea and intra-cellular urea necessitates 12 hours but already 6 hours after the injection 50 % of the urea has been eliminated.

We are convinced that if there is a rebound it is most likely to appear if there is no osmotic diuresis after mannitol injection. In fact, in the case shown in Fig. 6 there was no osmotic diuresis. This may explain the relatively small decompression (10 mm Hg) and the rebound.

Discussion

The efficacity of mannitol on cerebral edema is admitted by most authors, but the doses used are very variable. Some use the dose of 1, 5 g/kg and obtain a decompressive effect lasting 4 hours (16, 25). Others (22) used a dose of 1 g/kg with a decompressive effect lasting 3 hours. A comparative study (26, 27, 28) of doses of 2 g/kg and 4, 5 g/kg gave identical results for the two doses with an effect lasting 6 hours, the lowering of ICP was in the range of 50 to 90 %. Repeated i. v. injections of 30 g of mannitol (12) gave a lowering 20 to 25 % in ICP.

The results of WISE and CHARTER (26, 27, 28) showing the equal effectiveness of 2 g/kg and 4, 5 g/kg doses encouraged our study especially since the doses used seemed too large for a 24 hour time span. For example at a dose of 2 g/kg 2400 cc would be necessary and at 4, 5 g/kg 4400 cc are necessary. The infusion of 2400 cc or even 4400 cc to obtain a prolonged decompression is certainly unthinkable. From this point of view, the results which we have obtained are extremely interesting. The degree of lowering obtained with the 0, 30 g/kg dose (100 cc) is, at 60 to 80 %, practically identical with that obtained by much larger doses. The duration of the action is shorter, approximately two hours, but the quantity theoretically necessary for 24 hours (Fig. 7) much less (1200 cc). It goes without saying that there should be regular controls of the serum osmolarity. We feel that the osmolarity should not go above 320 milliosmoles.

Conclusion

Repeated injections of 25 % mannitol at a dose of 0, 30 g/kg are sufficient for the treatment of cerebral edema and prevent the appearance of hemodynamic overloads with all their risks, without any loss of efficiency of the decompressive effect.

The 50 cc dose, 0, 15 g/kg, was shown not to be effective enough in severe cases, but may be adequate in cases of moderate intracranial hypertension. The continuous monitoring of ICP is not only necessary to control the effectiveness of the treatment but it also permits adapting the treatment in function with the ICP level.

Summary

The efficiency of hypertonic solutions in the therapy of brain edema, especially post-traumatic, depends not only on the dosage but also on the velocity of injection.

The frequent metabolic disturbances observed in such cases (water and sodium retention, breackdown of free-water clearance) demand a restriction of liquid intake. Solutions not metabolized, such as mannitol, must be restricted as much as possible because at high dosages they expose the patient to several risks such as hemodynamic overload, osmotic nephrosis, hyponatriemia by dilution or hypernatriemia by dehydration.

Because of these different reasons the authors have studied the action of mannitol (25 %) at low dosages on intracranial pressure. The dosages employed were 0, 15 g/kg and 0, 30 g/kg (50 ml and 100 ml respectively on the average) in rapid intravenous injection. The lowering of intraventricular pressure obtained depends on the dosage: lowering of 20 % with 50 ml and 80 % with 100 ml average dose. The lowering rate for the 100 ml average dose is exactly the same obtained by others with an average dose of 1100 ml (4 g/kg).

The action is almost immediate with a maximum effect 15 minutes after injection followed by a progressive decrease of action. The effect lasts for about one hour at the 50 ml dosage and for about two hours with 100 ml. While the rate at which pressure is lowered is the same with low and high dosage the effect of the high dose (4 g/kg - 1100 ml) is much longer, it lasts about six hours. But the quantity theoretically necessary to cover 24 hours is much less at the low dosage utilized by the present authors: 1200 ml/24h with the average dose of 0, 30 g/kg (100 ml/injection) against 4400 ml/24h with the average dose of 4g/kg (1100 ml perfusion in 1 hour).

Thus, the low dosage permits avoiding the dangers of mannitol therapy mentioned above without any loss of efficiency of its action on intracranial pressure. Finally, this technique has another advantage: the possibility of preventing a sudden rise of pressure with continuing need for injections.

REFERENCES

1. AVIRAM, A., A. PFAU, J.N. CZACZKES and I. D. ULMAN: Hyperosmolarity with hyponatriemia caused by inappropriate administration of mannitol. Amer. J. Med. 42, 648-650 (1967)

2. BRAGDON, F.H.: Alterations observed in cranio-cerebral injuries following the use of dehydrating agents. Res. Publ. Ass. Nerv. Ment. Dis. 24, 545-561 (1945)

3. BROWDER, J.: Dangers in the use of hypertonic solutions in the treatment of brain injuries. Amer. J. Surg. 8, 1213-1217 (1930)

4. BULLOCK, L.T., M.I.GREGERSEN and R.KINNEY: The use of hypertonic sucrose intravenously to reduce CSF pressure without a secondary rise. Amer.J.Physiol. 112, 82-96 (1935)

5. CORONEOS, N.J., J.M.TURNER et Coll.: Comparison of extradural with intraventricular pressure in patients after head injury. In: M.BROCK and H.DIETZ (eds.): "Intracranial pressure" Springer Verlag Berlin-Heidelberg-New-York 1973, 51-58

6. EBAUGH, F.G. and G.S.STEVENSON: The measurements of intracranial pressure changes in epileptic and its experimental variations. John.Hopk.Hosp. Bull. 31, 440-447 (1920)

7. ELKINTON, J.R.: The volume of distribution of mannitol as a measure of the volume of extracellular fluid, with a study of the mannitol method. J.Clin.Invest. 26, 1088-1097 (1947)

8. HUGHES, J. and L.LAPLACE: The effect of hypertonic solutions of sodium arabinate on the CSF pressure. J.Pharmacol. 38, 363-383 (1930)

9. JAVIER, W. and SETTLAGE: Effects of urea on CSF pressure in human subjects. J.A.M.A. 160, 943-949 (1956)

10. JAVID, M.: Urea new use of an old agent. Reduction of intracranial and intraocular pressure. Surg.Clin.N.Amer. August 1958, 907-928

11. JAVID, M., D.GILBOE and Th.CESARIO: The rebound phenomenon and hypertonic solutions. J.neurosurg. 12, 1059-1066 (1964)

12. JOHNSTON, I.H., A.PATERSON, A.M.HARPER and W.B.JENNET: The effect of mannitol on intracranial pressure and CBF. In: M.BROCK and H.DIETZ: "Intracranial pressure". Springer Verlag Berlin-Heidelberg-New-York 1972, 176-180

13. JORGENSEN, P.B. and J. RIISHEDE: Comparative clinical studies of epidural and ventricular pressure. Idem. pp. 41-45

14. KEEGAN, H.R. and J.P.EVANS: Studies on cerebral swelling III. Long term recordings of CSF pressure before and following parenteral urea. Acta neurochir. 10, 466-472 (1962)

15. MASSERMAN, J.H.: Effects of intravenous administration of hypertonic solutions of dextrose, with special reference to the CSF pressure. J.A.M.A. 102, 2084-2086 (1934)

16. McQUEEN, J.D. and L.D.JEANES: Dehydratation and redehydratation of the brain with hypertonic urea and mannitol. J.Neurosurg. 21, 118-128 (1964)

17. MILLES, G. and P. HURNITZ: The effect of hypertonic solutions on CSF pressure with special reference to secondary rise and toxicity. Arch.Surg. Chic. 24, 591-601 (1932)

18. ROSOMOFF, H.L.: Distribution of intracranial contents after hypertonic urea. J.neurosurg. 19, 859-864 (1962)

19. SCHOOLAR, J.C., C.F.BARLOW and L.G.ROTH: The penetration of carbon-14 urea into the CSF and various areas of the cat brain. J.Neuropath.Exp. Neurol. 19, 216-227 (1960)

20. SCHWARTZ, J.L., E.S.BREED and M.H.MAXWELL: Comparison of the volume of distribution, venal and extravenal clearances of insulin and mannitol in man. J.Clin.Invest. 29, 517-520 (1950)

21. SHALIT, M.N.: The effects of intra-carotid artery administration of mannitol on the CSF and intracranial pressure in experimental brain edema. In: M.BROCK and H.DIETZ: "Intracranial pressure". Springer Verlag Berlin-Heidelberg-New-York 1972, 171-175

22. SHENKIN, H.A., B.GOLUBOFF and H.HAFT: The use of mannitol for the reduction of intracranial pressure in intracranial surgery. J.Neurosurg. 19, 897-901 (1962)

23. STUBBS, J. and J.PENNYBAKER: Reduction of intracranial pressure with hypertonic urea. Lancet 1, 1094-1097 (1960)

24. SUNDBERG, G. and H. NORNES: Simultaneous recording of the epidural and ventricular fluid pressure. Idem 46-50 (Référence n°12)

25. WALKER, W.D. and D.THOMSON: Reduction of intracranial pressure in dogs with mannitol and fructose-mannitol solutions. Brit.J.Anesth. 43, 445-448 (1971)

26. WISE, B.L. and N.CHATER: Use of hypertonic mannitol solutions to lower CSF pressure and decrease brain bulk in man. Surg.Forum 12, 398-399 (1961)

27. WISE, B.L. and N.CHATER: Effect of mannitol on CSF pressure. The actions of hypertonic mannitol solutions and of urea compared. Arch.Neurol. Chic. 4, 200-202 (1961)

28. WISE, B.L. and N.CHATER: The value of hypertonic mannitol solution in decreasing brain mass and lowering CSF pressure. J.Neurosurg. 12, 1038-1043 (1962)

Fig. 2. Initial decompressive action of 50 cc PA = systemic blood pressure ▶

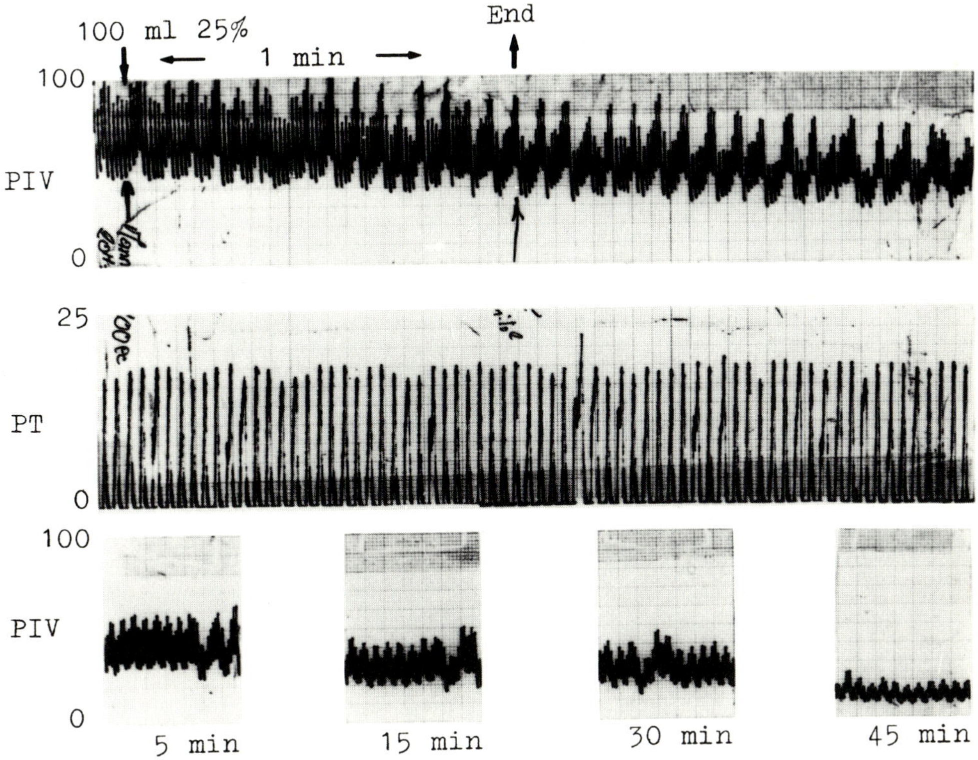

Fig. 1. Initial decompressive action of 100 cc PIV = PCSF, PT = tracheal pressure

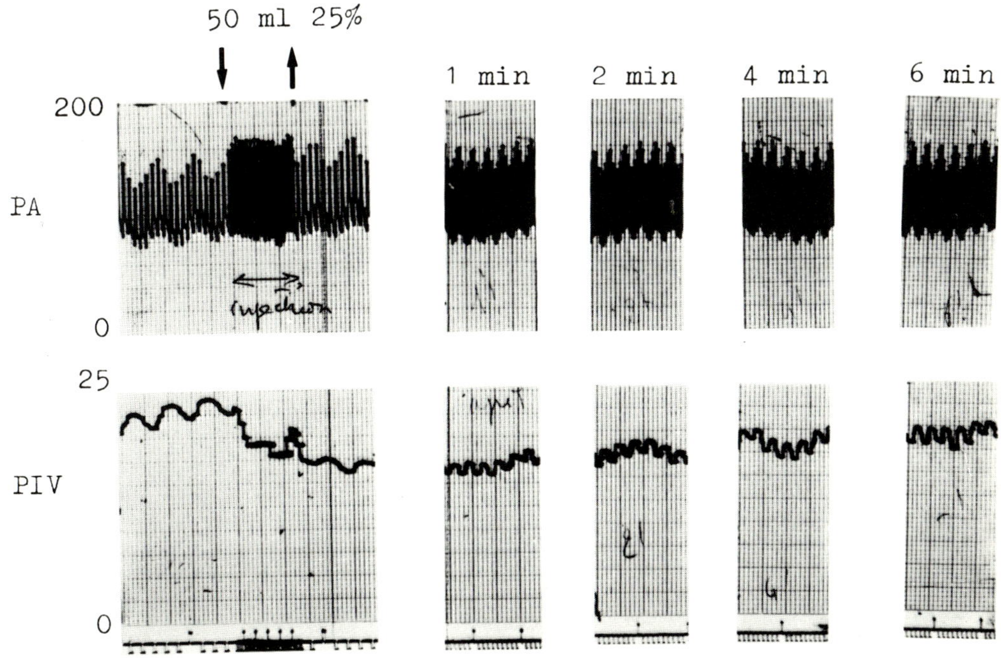

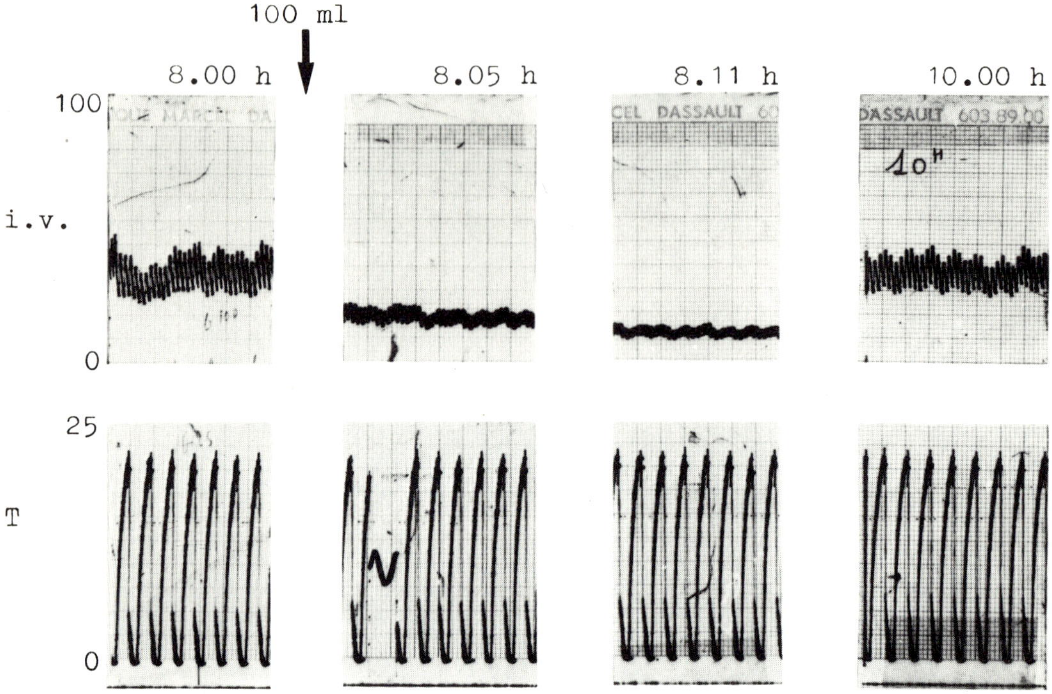

Fig. 3. Duration of the decompressive effect of 100 cc: 2 hours. Note the flattening of the cerebral pulse during all the time of mannitol-action

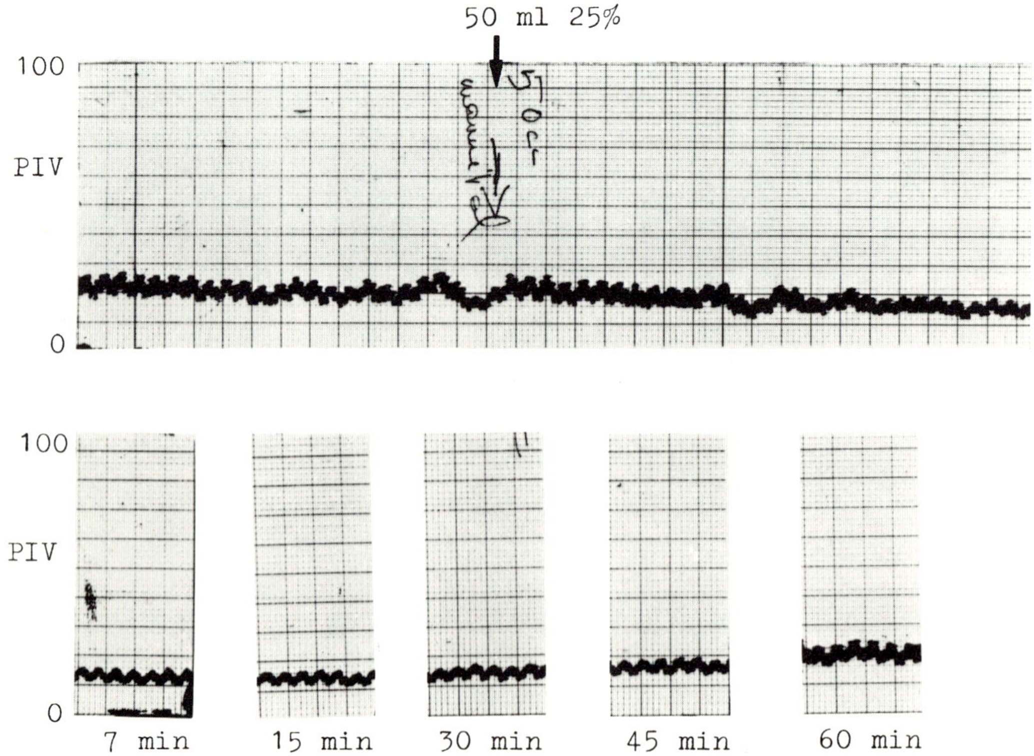

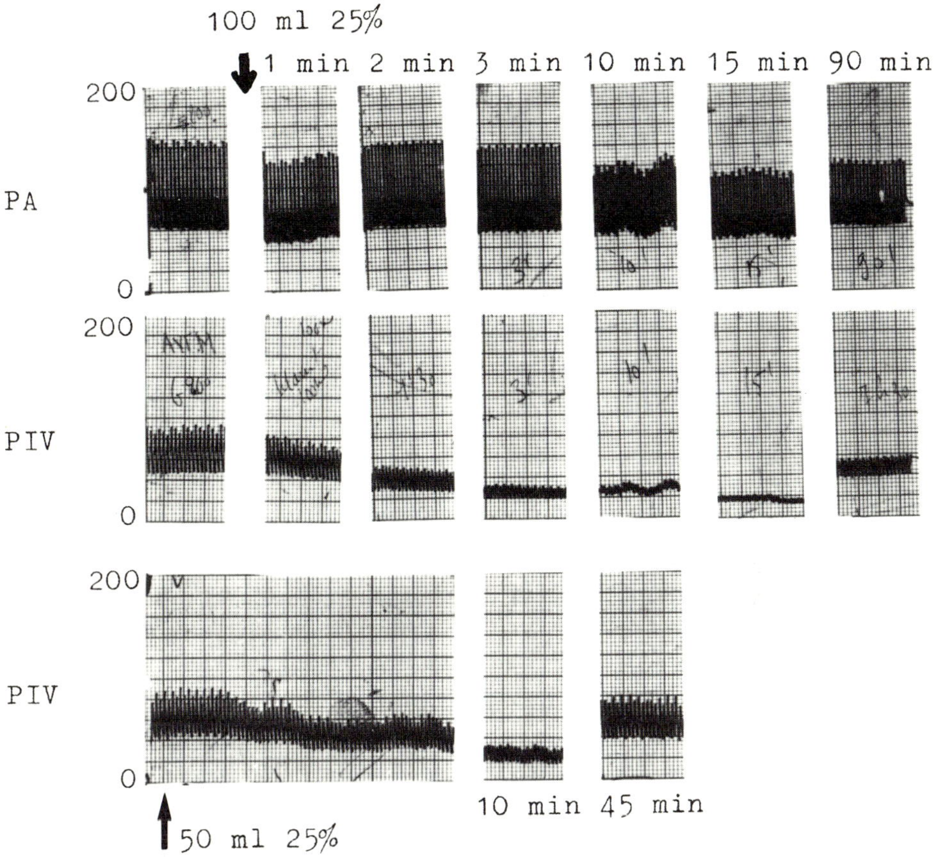

Fig. 5. The different actions of the 100 cc and the 50 cc doses. Duration of 90 minutes for 100 cc and only 45 minutes for the 50 cc dose in the same patient

◀ Fig. 4. Duration of the decompressive effect of 50 cc: 1 hour

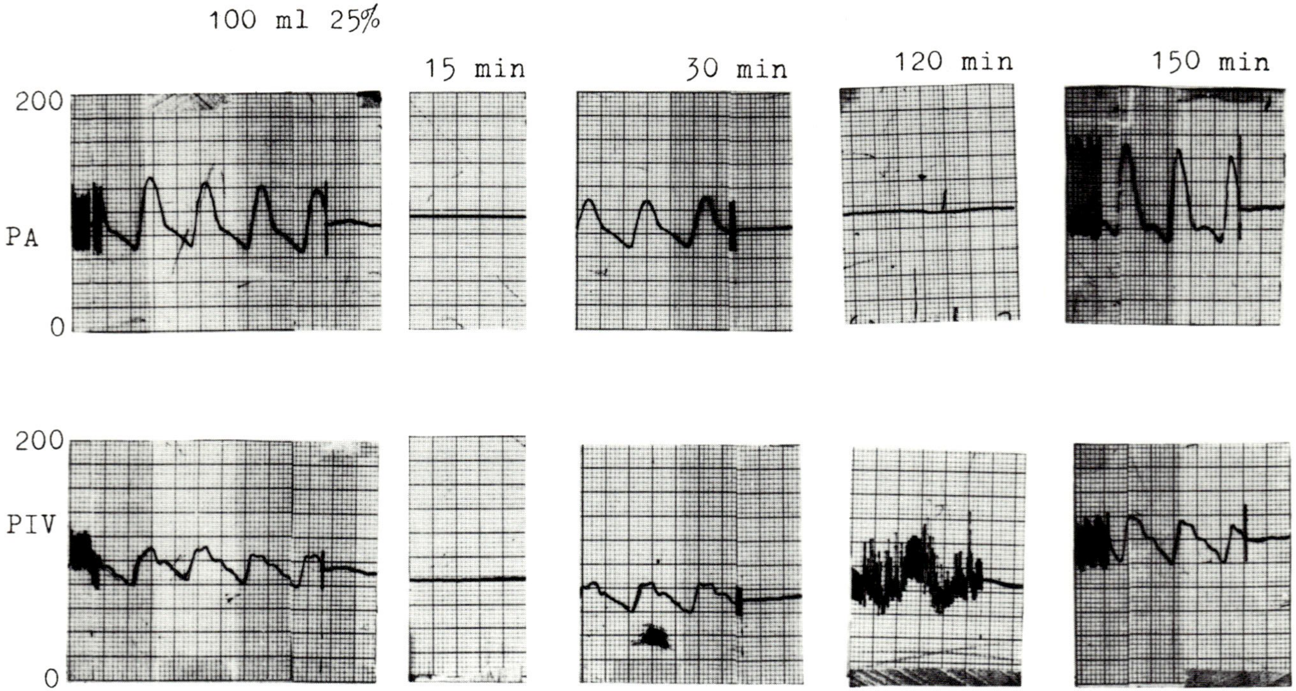

Fig. 6. Rebound-phenomenon and little decompressive effect

Dosage Mannitol 25 %	Rate of Injection	Decrease in IVP(%)	Duration of action	Theoretical quantity necessary for an adult (70 kg) in 24 hours
50 ml 0, 15 g/kg	Flash	10 to 20	1 hr	1. 200 ml 300 g
100 ml 0, 30 g/kg	Flash	50 to 80	2 hrs	1. 200 ml 300 g
300 ml 1 g/kg	in 15'	30 to 60	3 hrs	2. 400 ml 600 g
600 ml 2 g/kg	in 15'	60 to 90	6 hrs	2. 400 ml 600 g
1. 100 ml 4 g/kg	in 60'	60 to 90	6 hrs	4. 400 ml 1. 120 g

Fig. 7. The effectiveness of mannitol at different doses

Steroids in the Treatment of Brain Edema

H. J. REULEN, A. HADJIDIMOS, and U. HASE

Increasing experimental and clinical evidence has been accumulated on the efficacy of steroids in the treatment of brain edema since the first reports of GALICICH and FRENCH in 1961. Based on a large clinical study, this group showed that dexamethasone often resulted in the rapid and dramatic relief of symptoms and signs of increased intracranial pressure and neurological dysfunction associated with cerebral edema (11, 12, 20). Since this enthusiastic report, subsequent workers were able to demonstrate the correctness of most of these statements, using more refined techniques. The present report is an attempt to summarize these recent findings and to evaluate critically this mode of treatment of brain edema.

Brain edema in man

KLATZO (17) and BAETHMANN (2) at this meeting discussed the morphological and chemical characteristics of brain edema mainly as based on experimental findings in animals. Fig. 1 summarizes schematically the respective chemical results of human brain edema. The figure shows the alterations in water content of different brain areas in patients with brain tumors (7, 8, 28, 31). According to these data edema effects mostly the deep white matter of the tumor-bearing hemisphere, which is compatible with gross morphological findings. Water content of the deep white matter may increase from 70 % to about 82 %, which represents a local increase in tissue volume of about 70 - 90 %. In the cortex only small changes can be noted. Obviously, other brain areas such as the arcuate white matter, corpus callosum, internal capsule, putamen and thalamus remain unaffected in this type of edema. Changes in water content of the edematous white matter are closely correlated with changes in both sodium and potassium content and are of the magnitude expected if the edema fluid is derived from the plasma (28).

It should be stressed, however, that the accumulation of edema fluid in brain tissue is only the first step in the pathophysiological sequence of events (Fig. 2). Tissue volume enlarges and intracranial pressure rises as a consequence. A diminution of regional cerebral blood flow (rCBF) occurs (4, 13, 24) which is closely correlated with the local accumulation of edema fluid (26). The reduction in perfusion of the edematous areas may result in a critical underoxygenation of tissue and a rise in tissue lactate as well as CSF lactate levels (9). Brain lactacidosis may impair local regulation of blood flow and induce a state of vasoparalysis with loss of autoregulation and CO_2-regulation (18).

Therefore, when trying to assess the effect of a drug on brain edema, we rather should examine the various links of this pathological chain than concentrating only on one aspect of the phenomenon.

Effect of dexamethasone on human brain edema

a) Brain water and electrolyte content: Brain edema is a pathological increase of fluid in the brain tissue. Acceptence of such a definition implies that one criterion for the effectiveness of steroids on brain edema is the demonstration of a reduction in pathological increased tissue water content. Fig. 3 represents the findings of an investigation in patients with brain tumors or brain lesion. 16 patients undergoing craniotomy were pretreated with dexamethasone (4 mg every 6 hours intramuscularly) during 4 to 6 days. 18 patients were not pretreated and served as control. At the time of craniotomy tissue samples of gray and white matter were obtained from areas adjacent to the tumor which had to be operatively removed (26).

The changes found in the perifocal brain tissue (Fig. 3) in untreated patients consisted in a marked increase of the water and the sodium content of the white matter as compared to values obtained from morphologically normal areas (28) during lobectomy or from normal human brain at autopsy (7, 8). In patients treated with dexamethasone 4-6 days prior to the craniotomy, the water and sodium content of the perifocal white matter was significantly reduced by about 3.5 %. However, this value is still higher than the value of normal white matter which was reported as 69 - 71 % (7, 8, 31). In the cortex a moderate decrease in sodium content was observed. These results are thus in agreement with electron microscopical findings of LONG et al. (19), who provided evidence of significant reduction of ultrastructural characteristics of peritumoral brain edema following dexamethasone administration.

SCHMIEDEK et al. (29) recently showed a similar effect on human brain edema by aldosterone, a mineralo-corticoid. This group has started a double-blind-study to compare dexamethasone with aldosterone, both clinically and chemically. This, in fact is of great importance since aldosterone, even in the large doses used in this study, proved to have only small side-effects.

b) Cerebral blood flow: Following the introduction of methods for measuring regional cerebral blood flow (rCBF), it was shown by several groups, that the blood flow of the tumor-bearing hemisphere is significantly diminished (4, 13, 24). The most significant reduction, however, is found in the perifocal brain tissue. Regions corresponding to the tumor location may be hyperemic or ischemic. According to recent studies this drop in rCBF is primarily induced by an increased tissue pressure due to brain edema (27) and to a smaller extent only by an increased intracranial pressure (ICP) (22).

Consequently, if dexamethasone reduced the amount of brain edema, an increase in rCBF should be expected. 14 patients with a brain tumor or a space-occupying lesion were submitted to rCBF measurement before and after 5-7 days of dexamethasone treatment (24 mg daily). rCBF measurement was performed with a 16 channel scintillation probe equipment using the intraarterial ^{133}xenon clearance technique. Blood flow was recorded at rest, during induced hyperventilation and during induced arterial hypertension (14, 26). Before treatment patients showed a significant reduction of mean hemispheric blood flow as compared to normal values (about 50 - 55 ml/100 g min). Induction of arterial hypertension disclosed an increase in CBF indicating a defective autoregulation. Hyperventilation showed an impairment of CO_2 regulation of CBF (Fig. 4). Following dexamethasone treatment, a marked and significant increase in mean hemispheric blood flow occurred in these patients, mostly concomitant with a clinical improvement.

Functional tests revealed that the cerebrovascular response to blood pressure changes as well as to hyperventilation was improved or restored.

For clinical purposes the regional pattern of these changes shall be illustrated by the report of one of the cases. Carotid angiography in this 60-year-old male patient showed a left side temporal tumor, which later was histologically verified as an astrocytoma. Brain scan was negative. The position of the probes for regional recording of CBF is shown schematically in fig. 5. Before steroid administration blood flow of the focus corresponding to the tumor as well as the perifocal edematous areas amounted to about 10 ml/100 g./min as compared to the blood flow of the residual hemisphere of about 25 ml/100 g/min. Following this rCBF measurement the patient received dexamethasone (3 x 8 mg daily i.m.) during 6 days and thereafter the study was repeated. The most striking observation was an increase of the flow rate of the focus to 27 ml/100 g/min while the flow of the residual hemisphere was increased to 29 ml/100 g/min (Fig. 6a). Study of the autoregulatory capacity disclosed a focal disturbance of about 34 % while the surrounding brain tissue showed a normal autoregulation. This focal autoregulatory defect became obviously improved following dexamethasone. Similarly, the defective focal CO_2-response seemed partially restored following the steroid therapy (Fig. 6b). Thus, the results indicate that dexamethasone exerts a favorable effect on CBF in patients with brain tumors and improves the focal or global vasomotor paralysis present in edematous areas. We believe, that the reduction of brain edema may account for the restoration of circulation.

c) Intracranial pressure: If steroids reduce brain edema respectively brain volume, an increased ICP should also decline. KULLBERG (16) previously reported on continuous intraventricular pressure recordings in patients with brain tumors, which clearly indicated a fall of an increased ICP following steroids. Most striking was the finding that the first change occurring during steroid therapy was a reduction of the "high pressure episodes", while the basal pressure decreased only later. According to KULLBERG, a raised intraventricular pressure following severe head injuries generally responds less to steroids, especially in patients with continuous elevation of ICP to a high level.

In conclusion, steroids efficiently reduce brain edema and exert a favorable effect on the pathological situation of the edematous brain tissue. This is of utmost importance since the extent of this focal pathology is closely related with the final outcome of patients.

Clinical response of brain edema to steroids

The second part of this report is concerned with the available clinical data as related to the steroid therapy. According to experiences existing so far, the response to dexamethasone differs considerably in the various cerebral diseases associated with brain edema (Fig. 7). The best and most rapid response is seen in patients with brain tumors, especially with cerebral metastasis and with glioblastomas. The response in meningiomas and astrocytomas ranges behind these malignancies (20). It is interesting to mention that the same range has been reported in the tendency of these tumors to develop perifocal brain edema (33).

In an attempt to assess the clinical improvement more quantitatively, MAXWELL et al. (20) examined various symptoms and neurological disturbances in 815 patients with brain tumors. They found that a raised ICP, a hemiparesis and a dysphasia revealed a positive response in about 75-85 % of the patients, in whom they occurred.

Clinical signs of an increased ICP such as headache, nausea, vomiting and depression of sensorium improved or were completely alleviated within 12 - 36 hours. A poor response of a hemiparesis to dexamethasone was usually associated with a low grade astrocytoma or was due to a destructive lesion of the motor area. Resolution of papilledema was seen only in about 30 % incidence, probably due to the fact, that this process reacts with a relatively long delay.

Supportive evidence for the efficacy of steroids in patients with brain tumors was obtained by a retrospective study. In this study we examined the lethality following operation and removal of supratentorial brain tumors in adults. 100 patients receiving dexamethasone at least 3 days before craniotomy and post-treated in the manner, described below, were compared with 65 patients whithout steroids (Fig. 8). (Pituitary adenomas are not included in this study). Lethality in the group not receiving dexamethasone amounted 23 % as compared to 10 % in the dexamethasone treated group. We believe, that this important decrease in lethality from 23 % to 10 % is mostly related to dexamethasone, although additional improvement in basic treatment and anesthesia during this period (about 2 1/2 years) may have contributed. It is interesting however, that other groups also observed a drastic drop in operative mortality. BUCY and IEELSMA (5) found a reduction from 21 % to 3 % in 186 glioblastomas and MÜCKE (23) a fall from 19 % to 11 % following administration of steroids.

Except for brain tumors the best response to dexamethasone is seen in brain edema associated with brain abscesses. We started to treat patients with brain abscesses and increased intracranial pressure with dexamethasone only recently, when other groups reported on their positive experience (20, 25). In agreement with these reports we found that treatment with dexamethasone and systemic antibiotics enabled a better control of brain swelling and increased ICP. Operation which often had to be performed under poor condition of the patient could be better planned with edema under control, and at some occasions it had even to be postponed until encapsulation. This could be demonstrated by repeated brain scan or / and carotid angiography. With all simultaneous administration of systemic antibiotics we have not seen an exacerbation of the local brain inflammation.

The response to steroids is far less apparent in severe closed head injuries than in brain tumors or abscesses. The often dramatic clinical response to steroids in patients with brain tumors is uncommon following severe head injury. Several investigators observed an increased survival rate in acute head injury patients treated with steroids, but these reports did not contain controls (30). A double blind study has been conducted by RANSOHOFF, RAND and WOOD (25) in critically ill acute closed head injury patients without angiographic shift or significant clots, but with documented increase in ICP. Patients received methylprednisolone, 125 mg every 6 hours for 4 days. The results showed that although there was a distinct trend to a better survival rate in the steroid treated group, (48 %) as compared to the placebo group (28 %), this was not statistically significant, since the number of patients was too small. The quality of survival also appeared better in the treated patients, but did not reach significance.

Laboratory studies using a model of a brain lesion showed that the timing of steroid administration may be a major factor. Pretreatment resulted in a smaller edema territory than treatment at the time of lesion production or when steroid treatment was delayed (15, 21). An additional factor may be the dosis and administration of the steroid. Undoubtedly, a properly conceived double blind study with a sufficiently larger number of patients would be most important to make a clinical conclusion.

Dosage and duration of steroid therapy

Plasma half-lives of 140 - 370 min. have been reported for dexamethasone in blood (32). Thus, the repeated administration of dexamethasone every 6 hours seems pharmacologically reasonable. Whether the empirical choice of 16 mg / day (11,12) is an optimal dosage for all types of brain edema is not known, since no dose-effect studies have been done.

In patients undergoing brain surgery, most authors use a pretreatment of 2 - 4 days. Therapy is started with a loading dose of 1o mg of dexamethasone i. v. followed by 4 mg every 6 hours i. m., as recommended by GALICICH and FRENCH (11, 12). This schedule is continued following operation for 3-4 days, then the steroid is tapered over a 4-7 days period, depending on the patient's condition.

Dexamethasone may become a most important adjunct in therapy in the group of patients with inoperable gliomas, recurrencies or multiple cerebral metastasis. Relief of symptoms, improvement of the sensorium can be often achieved after 2 - 3 days of the usual high steroid dosis (16 mg/day). The doses can then be reduced individually until symptoms will reoccur. Patients can often be maintained in good condition and live at home for weeks with this individually adjusted dose and an orally administered form of dexamethasone. We consider this as a very important aspect of this therapy.

Steroid dependent brain

Several groups have encountered patients with brain tumors who had been placed on high-dose long term steroid therapy before referring to the hospital. Reducing the steroid in the usual manner following the operation in these patients, through the 5 - 7 days taper, results in an often acute deterioration, depression in sensorium and sometimes in coma. Continuous intraventricular pressure recordings in some of these patients showed a rapid elevation if ICP when steroid therapy was discontinued and a pressure decrease when steroid administration was restarted (16). These patients require a careful and gradual taper of the steroid over several weeks. It should be stressed, that the steroid dependency of the brain has never been observed in the usual short term pre- and posttreatment of patients undergoing brain surgery. Whether this phenomenon is related to some alterations of CNS membrane function or/and depression of adrenal cortical function is still a matter of discussion (1).

Side-effects of steroids in the treatment of brain edema

Complications attributed to the steroid therapy were not very frequent in most reports (3, 6, 10, 11, 12, 20, 23, 25). This may well be due to a screening of all patients for any history concerning gastric ulcers or diabetes. In addition, all patients were covered with an antiacid during steroid administration. Finally, the high dose steroid treatment should not be continued longer than 10 - 12 days.

With these restrictions, gastro-intestinal hemorrhage was observed by different groups (3, 6, 20) in 3 - 10 % of the patients. Since this complication is seen more frequently in comatous patients with severe head injuries, the complication rate may depend on the proportion of head injuries in the respective series.

Delayed wound healing or an increased incidence in wound infection of pulmonary infection was not observed by most groups (3, 20, 25) and this is in line with our own experiences. Other side effects, such as mild electrolyte disturbances or hyperglycemia, sometimes occurring in the immediate postoperative course, could be managed without difficulties and they disappear after discontinuing the steroid.

REFERENCES

1. BAETHMANN, A., A. van HARREVELD: Physiolgical and biochemical findings in the central nervous system of adrenalectomized rats and mice. In: Steroids and Brain Edema, pp 195-202, Berlin-Heidelberg-New York, Springer 1972
2. BAETHMANN, A.: Pathophysiology of cerebral edema, chemical aspects. Vortrag Kongress Deutsche Gesellschaft für Neurochirurgie in Mainz, April/Mai 1973
3. BEKS, J. W. F., H. DOORENBOS, G. J. M. WALSTRA: Clinical experiences with steroids in neurosurgical patients. In: Steroids and Brain Edema, pp 233-238, Berlin-Heidelberg-New York, Springer 1972
4. BROCK, M., A. HADJIDIMOS, J. P. DERUAZ, and K. SCHÜRMANN: Regional cerebral blood flow and vascular reactivity in cases of brain tumor. In: Brain and Blood Flow, oo 281-284, London, Pittman Medical and Scientific Publishing & Co. 1971
5. BUCY, T. C. and P. K. IELSMA: The treatment of glioblastoma multiforme. Excerpta Med. Int. Congr. Series, No. 193 (1969)
6. CANTU, R. U., H. AMIR-AHMADI and A. PRIETO: Evaluation of the increased risk of gastro-intestinal bleeding following intracranial surgery in patients receiving high steroid dosages in the immediate post-operative period. Int. Surg. Dig. 50, 325-335 (1968)
7. FEIGIN, I., and M. ADACHI: Cerebral oedema and the water content of normal white matter. J. Neurol. Neurosurg. Psychiatr. 29, 446-450, (1966)
8. FEIGIN, J., G. BUDZILOVICH and J. OGATA: Edema of the grey matter of the human brain. J. Neuropath. exp. Neurol. 30., 206-215, (1971)
9. FREI, H. J., Th. WALLENFANG, W. PÖLL, H. J. FREI, R. SCHUBERT and M. BROCK: Regional cerebral blood flow and regional metabolism in cold induced brain edema. Acta Neurochirurg. (in press).
10. FRENCH, L. A. and J. H. GALICICH: The use of steroids for control of cerebral edema. Clinical Neurosurgery, 212-223 (1964)
11. GALICICH, J. H., A. A. FRENCH and J. C. MELBY: Use of dexamethasone in treatment of cerebral edema associated with brain tumors. J. Lancet, 31, 46-53 (1961)
12. GALICICH, J. H. and L. A. FRENCH: Use of dexamethasone in the treatment of cerebral edema resulting from brain tumors and brain surgery. Amer. Practit, 12, 169-174 (1961)
13. HADJIDIMOS, A., M. BROCK, M. HADJIDIMOS, J. P. DERUAZ and K. SCHÜRMANN: Die fokale und perifokale örtliche Hirndurchblutung bei cerebralen Tumoren. Prognostische Möglichkeiten durch Vergleich prä- und postoperativer Befunde im extratumoralen Hirngewebe. In: Ergebnisse der klinischen Nuklearmedizin, pp, 1020-1029, Stuttgart-New York, Schattauer 1971

14. HADJIDIMOS, A., U. STEINGASS, F. FISCHER, H. J. REULEN and K. SCHÜRMANN: The effects of dexamethasone on rCBF and cerebral vasomotor response in brain tumors. Preliminary Communication, Europ. Neurol., 10, 25-30, (1973)

15. HERRMANN, H. D., D. NEUENFELDT, J. DITTMANN and H. PALLESKE: The influence of dexamethasone on water content, electrolytes, BBB and glucose metabolism in cold injury edema. In: Steroids and Brain Edema, pp, 77-85, Berlin-Heidelberg-New York, Springer 1972

16. KULLBERG, G.: Clinical studies on the effect of corticosteroids on the ventricular fluid pressure. In: Steroids and Brain Edema, pp 253-258, Berlin-Heidelberg-New York, Springer 1972

17. KLATZO, I.: Pathological Aspects. Vortrag Kongress Deutsche Gesellschaft für Neurochirurgie im Mainz, April/Mai 1973

18. LASSEN, N. A.: The luxury perfusion syndrome and its possible relation to acute metabolic acidosis localized within the brain. Lancet 2, 1113-1115 (1966)

19. LONG, D. M., J. F. HARTMANN and L. A. FRENCH: The response of human cerebral edema to glucosteroid administration. Neurology, 16, 521-528 (1966).

20. MAXWELL, R. E., D. M. LONG and L. A. FRENCH: The clinical effects of a synthetic gluco-corticoid used for brain edema in the practice of neurosurgery In: Steroids and Brain Edema, pp 219-232, Berlin-Heidelberg-New York: Springer 1972

21. MAXWELL, R. E., D. M. LONG and L. A. FRENCH: The effects of glucosteroids upon cold-induced brain edema. In: Gross morphological and vascular permeability changes. J. Neurosurg. 34, 477-487 (1971)

22. MEINIG, G., H. J. REULEN and Ch. MAGAWLY: Regional cerebral blood flow and cerebral perfusion pressure in global cerebral edema induced by water intoxication. Acta neurochirurg. (in press)

23. MÜCKE, R.: Discussion in: Steroids and Brain Edema, pp 282-283, Berlin-Heidelberg-New York, Springer 1972

24. PALVÖGYI, R.: Regional cerebral blood flow in patients with cerebral tumors J. Neurosurg. 31, 149-163 (1969)

25. RANSOHOFF, J.: The effects of steroids on brain edema in man. In: Steroids and Brain Edema, pp 211- 217, Berlin-Heidelberg-New York, Springer 1972

26. REULEN, H. J., A. HADJIDIMOS, and K. SCHÜRMANN: The effect of dexamethasone on water and electrolyte content and on rCBF in perifocal brain edema in man. In: Steroids and Brain Edema, pp 239-252, Berlin-Heidelberg-New York, Springer 1972

27. REULEN, H. J. and H. G. KREYSCH: Measurement of brain tissue pressure in cold induced brain edema. Acta Neurochir. (in press)

28. REULEN, H. J., F. MEDZIHRADSKY, R. ENZENBACH, F. MARGUTH and W. BRENDEL: Electrolytes, fluids and energy metabolism in cerebral edema in man. Arch, Neurol. 21, 517-525 (1969)

29. SCHMIEDEK, P., A. BAETHMANN, E. SCHNEIDER, W. ÖTTINGER, R. ENZENBACH, F. MARGUTH and W. BRENDEL: The effect of aldosterone and an aldosterone antagonist on the metabolism of perifocal brain edema in man. In: Steroids and Brain Edema, pp. 203-210, Berlin-Heidelberg-New York, Springer, 1972

30. SPARACHIO, R., T. H. LINN and A. W. COOK: Methylprednisolone sodium succinate in acute craniocerebral trauma. Surg. Gynecol. Ostetr. 121, 1-516, (1965)

31. STEWARD-WALLACE, A. M.: A biochemical study of cerebral tissue and of the changes in cerebral edema. Brain, 62, 426-438, (1939)

32. WITHROW, C. D. and D. M. WOODBURY: Some aspects of the pharmacology of adrenal steroids and the central nervous system. In: Steroids and Brain Edema, pp 41-55, Berlin-Heidelberg-New York, Springer 1972

33. ZÜLCH, K. J.: Hirnschwellung und Hirnödem. Dtsch. Zschr. Nervenheilk. 170, 179-208 (1953)

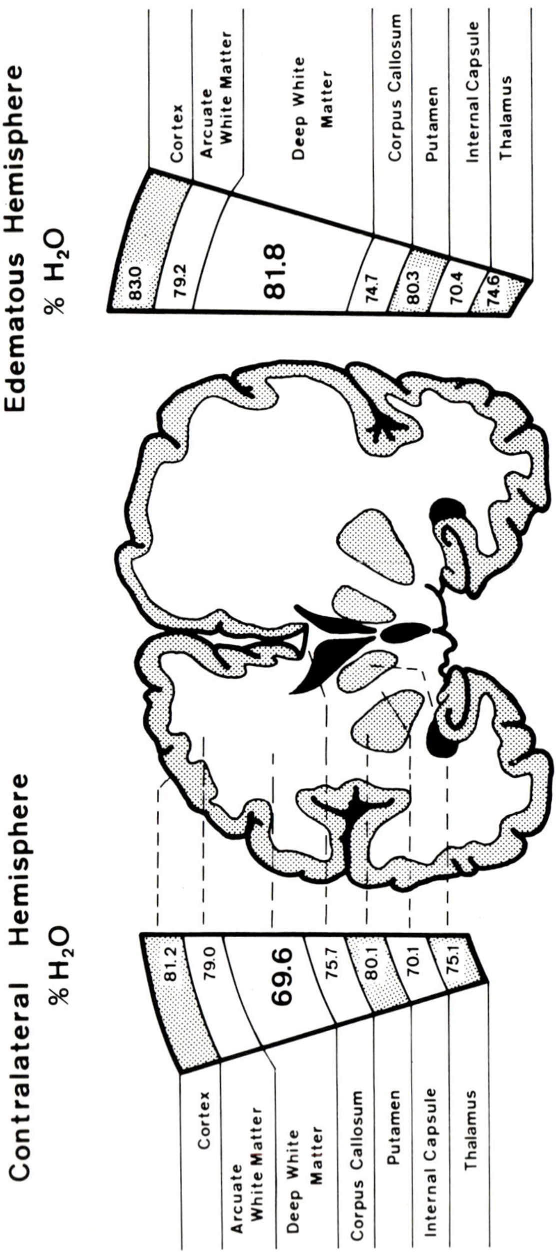

Fig. 1. Schematic representation of the changes in fluid content of various topographic brain regions in brain edema associated with brain tumors. Edematous hemisphere - tumor-bearing hemisphere

Fig. 3. Effect of dexamethasone on the water and electrolyte content of perifocal edematous cortex and white matter in patients with brain tumors. wt. wt. = wet weight; dry wt. = dry weight (26)

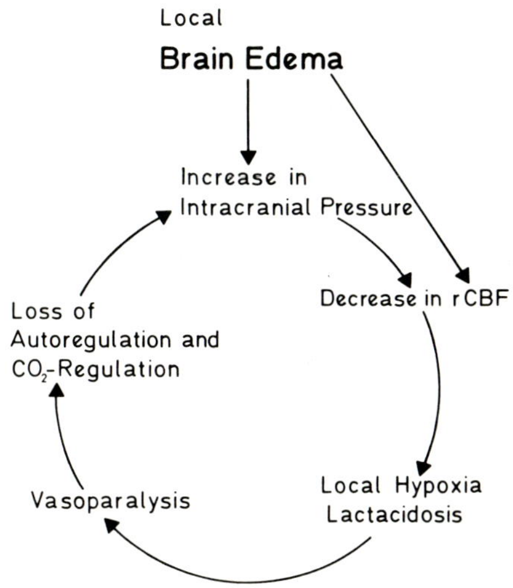

Fig. 2. Schematic representation of pathophysiological sequence of events in brain edema (see text)

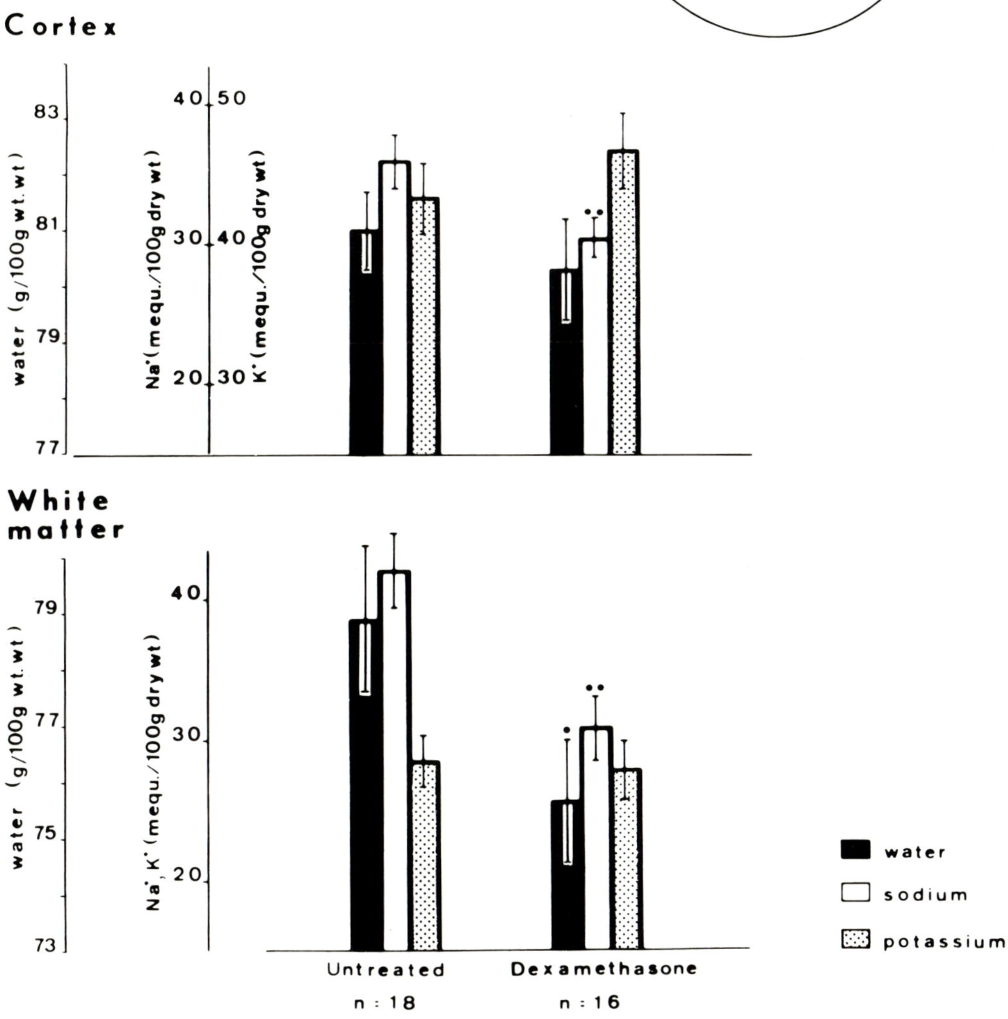

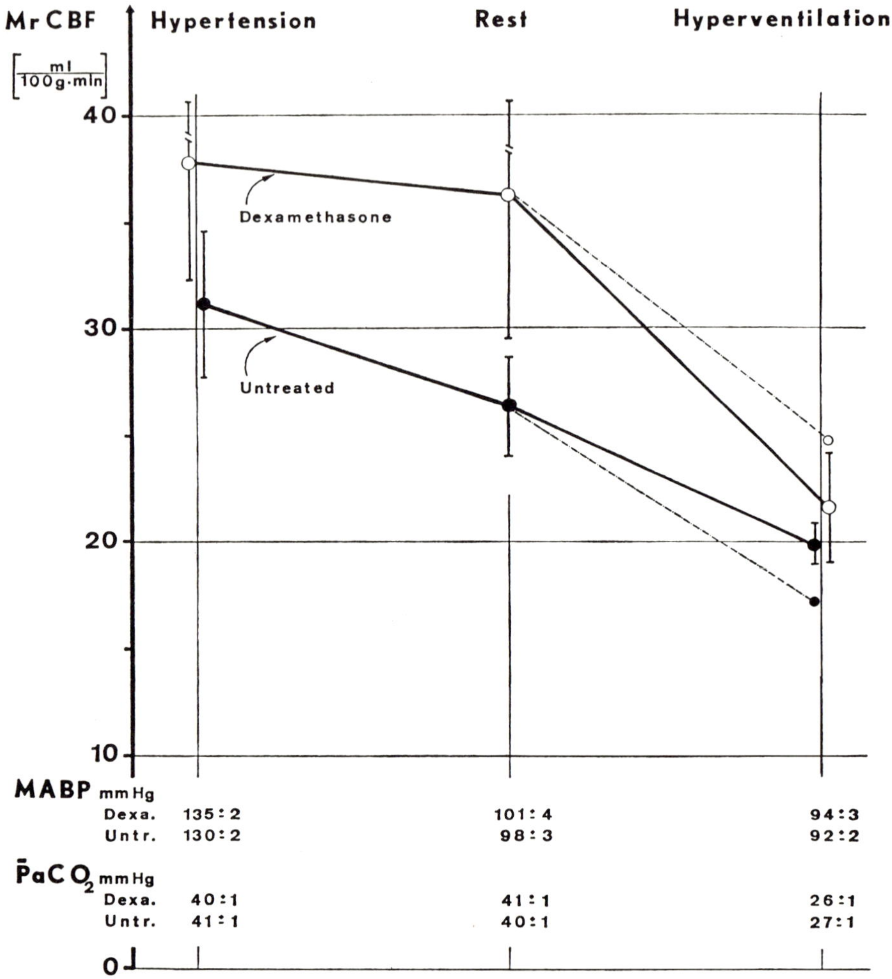

Fig. 4. Mean rCBF and vasomotor response in 6 patients with brain tumor before and after 5 - 7 days of dexamethasone administration (24 mg/day). Values at rest and during hypertension are corrected to a standard $PaCO_2$ of 40 mm Hg. The broken line shows the expected change of MrCBF following hyperventilation (26)

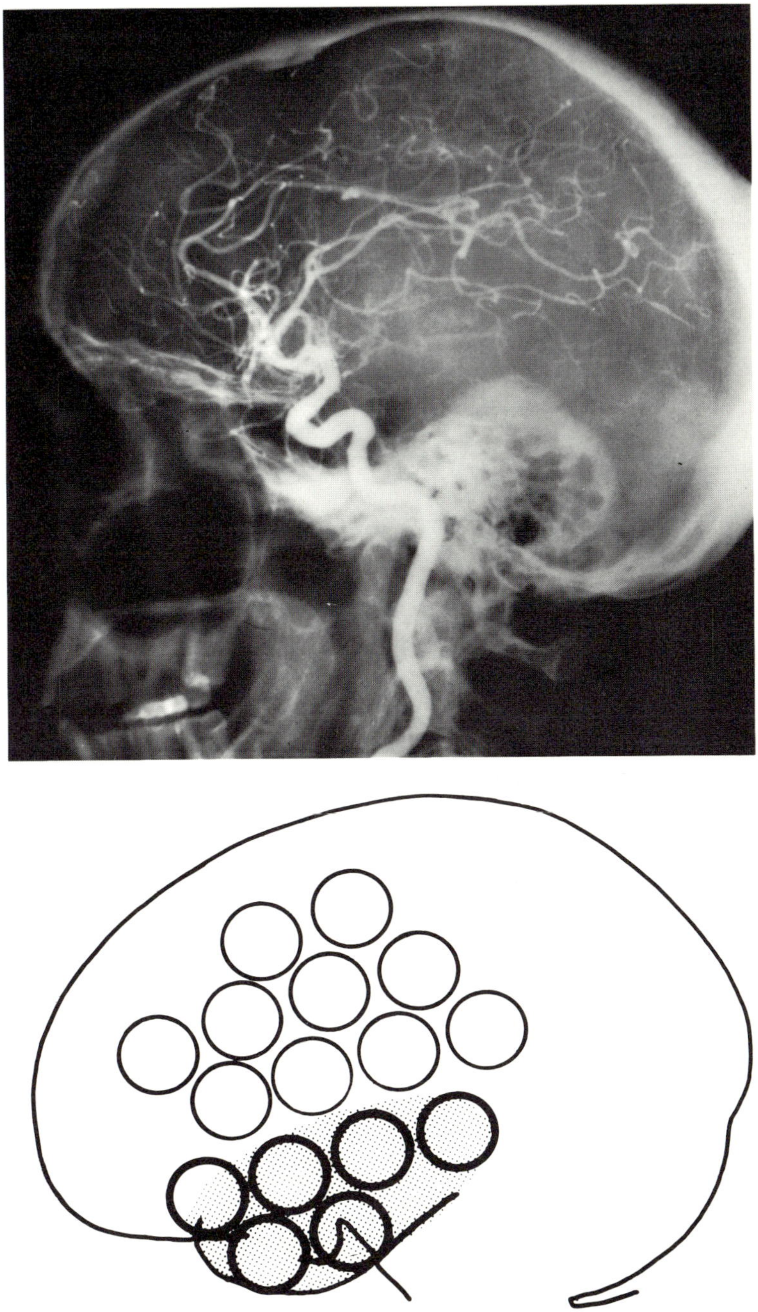

Fig. 5. Case report: Left sided temporal astrocytoma in a 60 year old male. Carotid angiogram and location of the scintillation probes for the measurement of rCBF

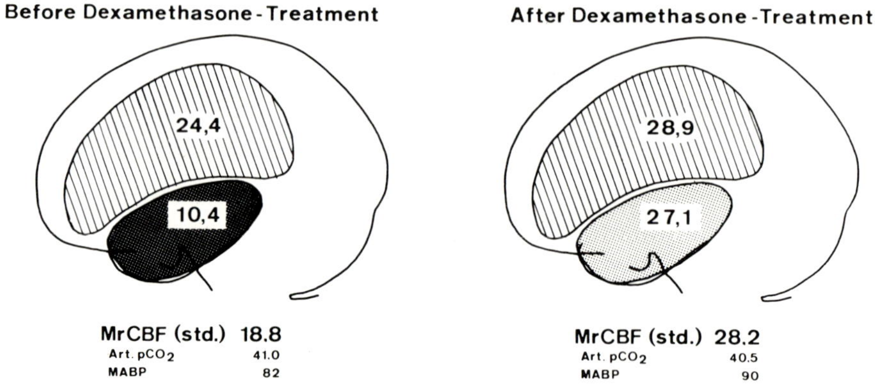

Fig. 6a. Case report: rCBF of the focus (tumor and perifocal edematous brain tissue) and of the residual hemisphere before and after dexamethasone therapy

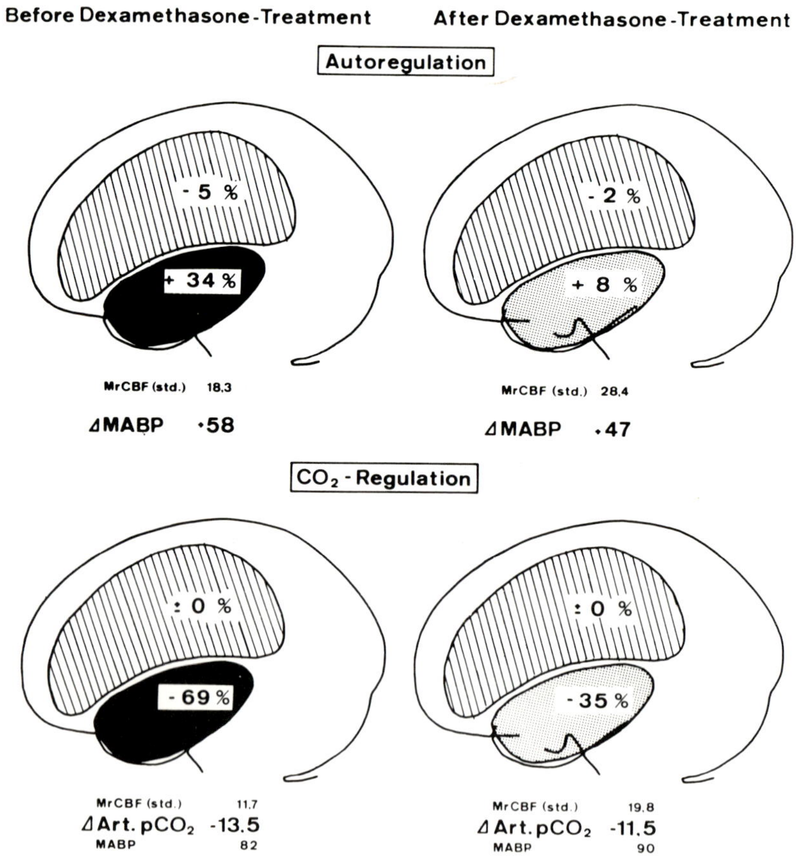

Fig. 6b. Case report: Vasomotor response of the focus (tumor and perifocal edematous brain tissue) and of the residual hemisphere before and after dexamethsone therapy

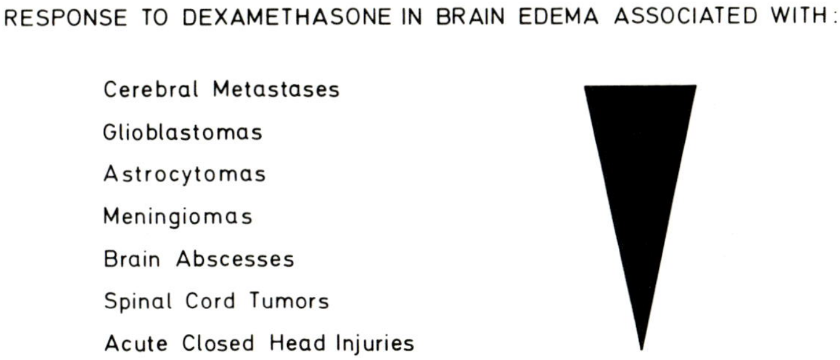

Fig. 7. Response to dexamethasone in brain edema associated with various cerebral diseases

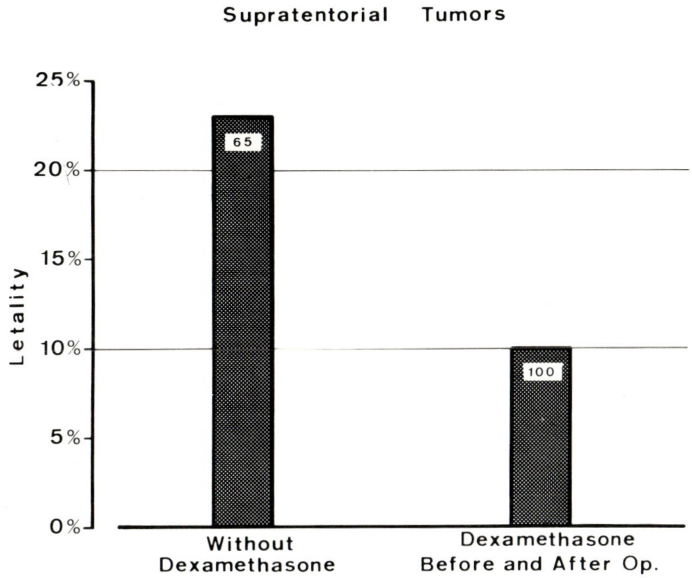

Fig. 8. Lethality of patients with supratentorial brain tumors treated with dexamethasone before and following operation (100 patients) as compared to patients (65) which were not treated with dexamethasone. Retrospective study

Electroencephalographical Findings During Therapy of Brain Edema with Dexamethasone

R. WÖRZ and H. RIEGER

Introduction

After the publications of GALICICH and FRENCH (2) several experimental and clinical investigations have confirmed the efficacy of dexamethasone treatment for cerebral edema (5, 6, 7, 10). At the same time they discussed several interesting problems. In order to gather more clinical information in man, we performed an electroencephalographic observation on the course before and during treatment with dexamethasone.

Materials and Methods

This study included 10 patients with supratentorial primary tumors, 8 with cerebral metastases and 2 others with pseudotumor cerebri. Primary neoplasms were 2 glioblastomas, 3 astrocytomas, 1 astroblastoma, 2 oligodendrogliomas, and 2 meningiomas. For the patients submitted to operation, the observation of the EEG course reached up to the date of the operation. For those, who had been palliatively treated, the study extended over several weeks and in some cases months. 15 patients received a daily dose of 24 mg of dexamethasone, 5 others were treated with 16 mg daily. In all cases, an EEG was recorded before treatment and compared in blind trial with another one which had been taken 4-5 days after the beginning of therapy. The interpreter of the EEG did not know the patient, the diagnosis nor the date of the recording. We used a 12-channel-instrument, mono-and bipolar techniques with several arrangements of the electrodes and performed a 4 minutes hyperventilation test.

Results

In the case of patients palliatively treated for a prolonged time with dexamethasone, a decrease of diffuse abnormalities was observed. At the beginning, focal EEG patterns became more prominent which in further development diminished in degree and spreaded. Monomorph delta groups as distant signs came less frequent or disappeared completely. In the cases, in which initially local findings had been observed, somewhat in the form of polymorphic delta activity, a diminution of degree amplitude, and spread in the neighbouring regions was noted.

The same observation was made in the case of sharp waves and spikes regarded as cerebral irritation signs.

In the blind trial, out of 20 EEGs, 16 which had been recorded during steroid therapy, were judged "improved" and 4 other "worse" compared to the initial curves. The observations on the course before treatment show, that the development of the tumor is accompanied with a tendency to worsening of EEG. We assumed the probability that within the period of investigation a worsening rather than an improvement of the EEG appears with p = 0.6 to p = 0.4. The 99 % score with 4 worsenings out of 20 pairs ranges from 0.04 to 0.51 and 95 % score from 0.06 to 0.44. Our assumed rate of worsening is beyond the 99 % score. With the clinically inadequate assumption of p = 0.5 to p = 0.5 there is a significance at the 5 % level of probability. In some cases, an 8-channel-EEG was stored on magnetic tape before and during dexamethasone treatment. In order to evaluate the inter-regional synchrony and certain spatio-temporal characteristics, the computation of cross correlation functions and their topographical mapping was applied, according to the technique described by RIEGER (11).

Fig. 3 shows the electrode positions; the activity observed by 7 bipolar EEG derivations are cross-correlated with the EEG of the "reference" - channel 1 on the midline. The seven cross-correlation functions are juxtaposed and intermediate values are interpolated.

Spatio-temporal maps of correlation functions can now be presented (Fig. 4 and 5).

Analysis conditions: Time resolution of (digital) EEG-measures: 1.6 ms (=step of lag). Maximal lag 409.6 ms. Number of sweeps for each correlation function: about 1 200, corresponding to an EEG duration of 8 to 10 min. One map is the result of computation of about 2 millions of individual measurements.

The patient presented in fig. 4 shows a modification of the spatio-temporal correlation structure during dexamethasone treatment which may be interpreted as an amelioration - although we still know little about spatio-temporal EEG features in brain tumors: In the upper map, the initial phase reversal (T=O) between positive and negative correlation areas is displaced to the left (affected) hemisphere. Similar observations are reported by CALISKA et al. (1), who applied the alpha average technique (REMOND et al.: 9) on brain tumors. During the treatment, the initial phase reversal returns to the normal site on the midline and the values of correlation coefficients are becoming higher (more level lines, especially in the initial part of the lower map).

Nevertheless, the systematic trend to EEG improvement during dexamethasone application observed in conventional records in our blind trial is not necessarily accompanied by a normalization tendency of correlation maps. The patient in fig. 5 shows - in spite of an amelioration in his EEG no modification in the very irregular, badly correlated spatio-temporal structure.

The two patients presented here show an unusual, irregular spatio-temporal pattern of correlation functions distinguishing them from the regular, symmetrical pattern of normal records. It is not surprising that a certain discrepancy can appear between conventional EEG and correlation maps: this method describes EEG qualities which are not detectable by visual analysis, especially the functional connection between the electrical activities of different regions.

Conclusions

Our conventional EEG findings during dexamethasone therapy may be interpreted as an expression of the diminution of the peritumoral edema. probably as consequence of this, of the decrease of raised intracranial pressure and of metabolic disturbances. Our results, however, do not allow us to state whether inhibitive or stimulative drug effects play a part in the growth of the tumor (3, 4, 8, 12, 13, 14).

They also show, that dexamethasone is at least effective in a part of the cases with pseudotumor cerebri.

The histological type of the tumor together with the extent of perifocal edema plays an important role whether striking or minor effects appear during treatment with dexamethasone.

Six of the eight cases with cerebral metastases, experienced a remarkable improvement; in 2 of them, in whom considerable pathological EEG patterns had been observed before treatment, there was an almost complete normalization. It may be assumed that this was due to small tumors accompanied by increased edema and considerable metabolic disturbances. One meningioma, 1 oligodendroglioma and 2 patients with metastases showed a worsening of the EEG.

Considering the neurological, psychopathological and other findings, the response of the growing intracranial process to dexamethasone provides useful clinical information on the extent of a perifocal edema.

Clinical or pharmacological investigations on the effects of drug have not yet been carried out using topographical methods. Our paper illustrates the fact that in the evaluation of the EEG in space-occupying processes and their treatment not only frequency and amplitude, but also topographical qualities are important parameters.

Further application of these methods of analysis seems desirable.

Summary

In 20 patients with evidence of cerebral edema, an electroencephalographic observation of the course before and during dexamethasone treatment was performed. In each case an EEG, recorded before the treatment, was compared in a blind trial with another one, which had been taken 4-5 days after the beginning of steroid therapy. 16 EEG records traced during the treatment period showed signs of improvement and 4 cases showed signs of worsening.

In patients with cerebral metastases who had been palliatively treated, an improvement of diffuse EEG abnormalities was seen at first. At this stage, focal signs tended to become more prominent. They diminished later on. When there were initially focal signs in the form of polymorphic delta activity, sharp waves or spikes, their degree, amplitude and spread improved substantially.

The histological type of the tumor together with the extent of perifocal or generalized edema plays an important role whether an impressive or a minor response appears to dexamethasone treatment.

Our findings also show that at least in part of the cases with pseudotumor cerebri dexamethasone has beneficial effects.

In several cases a chronotopographical analysis was performed. The cross correlation functions of 2 patients are topographically represented. The spatio-temporal maps illustrate that in brain tumor and edema topographical qualities are of interest.

REFERENCES

1. CALISKAN, A., J. GACHES, N. LESÈVRE and A. REMOND: Organisation spatio temperelle du alpha moyen chez des malades présentant des lésions expansives. Rev. Neurol., 123, 25 60 (1969)

2. GALICICH, J. H. and L. A. FRENCH: Use of dexamethasone in the treatment of cerebral edema resulting from brain tumors and brain surgery.

3. KODAMA, M., and T. KODAMA: Effect of steroid hormones on the in vivo incorperation of glycine -2-^{14}C into solid. Ehrlich tumor, kidney and liver. Cancer Res. 30, 228 (1970)

4. KOTSILIMBAS, D. G., L. MEYER, M. BERSON, J. M. TAYLOR and L. C. SCHEINBERG: Corticosteroid effect on intracerebral melanomata and associated edema. Some unexpected findings. Neurology 17, 223 (1967)

5. KULLBERG, G., and K. A. WEST: Influence of corticosteroids on the ventricular fluid pressure. Acta Neurol. Scand. Suppl. 13, 41:445 (1965(

6. LONG, D. M., F. J. HARTMANN and L. A. FRENCH: The response of human cerebral edema to glucosteroid administration. An electronmicroscopic study. Neurology 16, 521, (1966)

7. MAXWELL, R. E., D. M. LONG and L. A. FRENCH: The clinical effects of a synthetic gluco-corticoid used for brain edema in the practice of neurosurgery. In: H. J. REULEN and K. SCHÜRMANN (eds): Steroids and Brain Edema. pp 219, Berlin-Heidelberg-New York: Springer 1972

8. MEALEY, J., T. T. CHEN and G. P. SCHANZ: Effects of dexamethasone and methylprednisolone on cell cultures of human glioblastomas. J. Neurosurg. 34, 3:324 (1971)

9. REMOND, A., N. LESEVRE, J. P. JOSEPH, H. RIEGER and G. C. LAIRY: The alpha average. I. Methodology and description. EEG clin. Neurophysiol. 26, 245 (1969)

10. REULEN, H. J., A. HADJIDIMOS and K. SCHÜRMANN: The effect of dexamethasone on water and electrolyte content and on CBF in perifocal brain edema in man. In: H. J. REULEN and K. SCHÜRMANN (eds.):Steroids and Brain Edema pp 239, Berlin-Heidelberg-New York, 1972

11. RIEGER, H.: L'utilisation de la fonction de corrélation en recherche EEG topographique. French EEG Society Dec. 1972, in press in: Rev. EEG Neurophysiol. (Paris) 3, (1973)

12. TOOLAN, H. W.: Growth of human tumors in cortisone-treated laboratory animals: The possibility of obtaining permanently transplantable human tumors. Cancer. Res. 13, 389 (1953)

13. WILSON, C. B., M. BARKER, T. HOSHINO, A. OLIVER and R. DOWNIE: Steroid-induced inhibition of growth in glial tumors: a kinetic analysis. In: H. J. REULEN and K. SCHÜRMANN (eds.): Steroids and Brain Edema: pp 95, Berlin-Heidelberg-New York, Springer 1972

14. WRIGHT, R. L., B. SHAUMBA and J. KELLER: The effect of glucocorticosteroids in growth and metabolism of experimental glial tumors. J. Neurosurg. 30, 140 (1969).

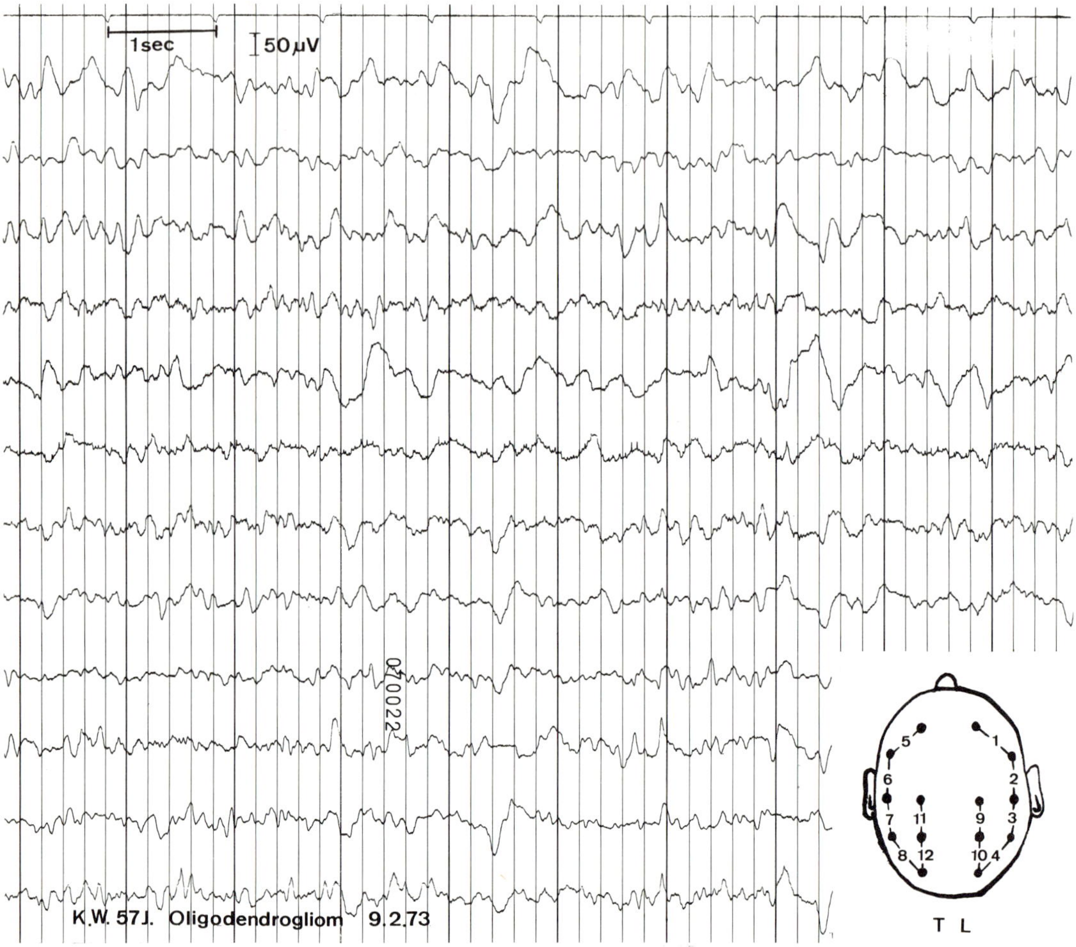

Fig. 1. K. W., 57 years old. Deep oligodendroglioma involving the left frontal lobe. Before treatment. EEG: There is a diffuse, continuous, and very irregular delta activity with predominance in the frontal regions. Alpha activity is present, but superimposed by irregular slow waves. The arrangement of electrodes is shown on the right, the numbers correspond to the EEG channels. The technique is the same as in fig. 1 - 2

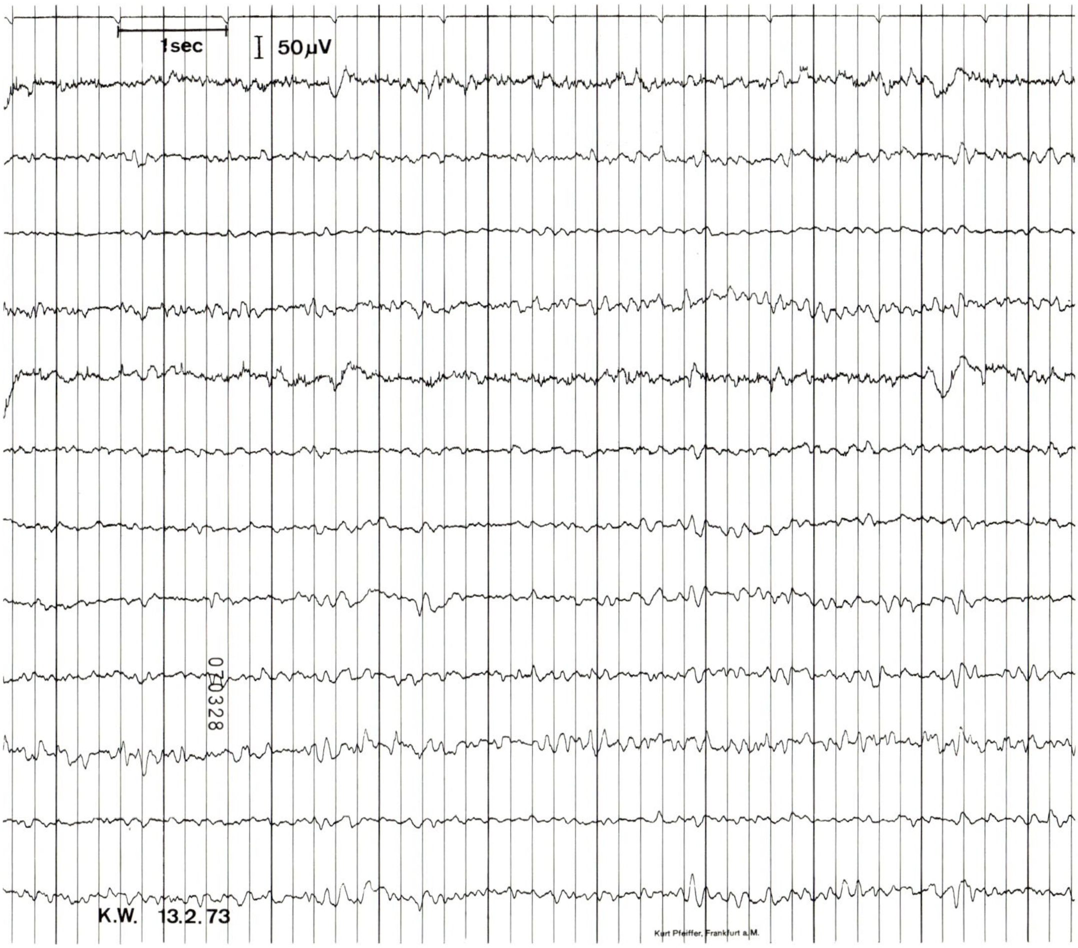

Fig. 2. Same patient as in fig. 1. During dexamethasone treatment. The frontal delta activity became sporadic, the general slowing is clearly less pronounced. Lability of frequencies in the alpha/theta range

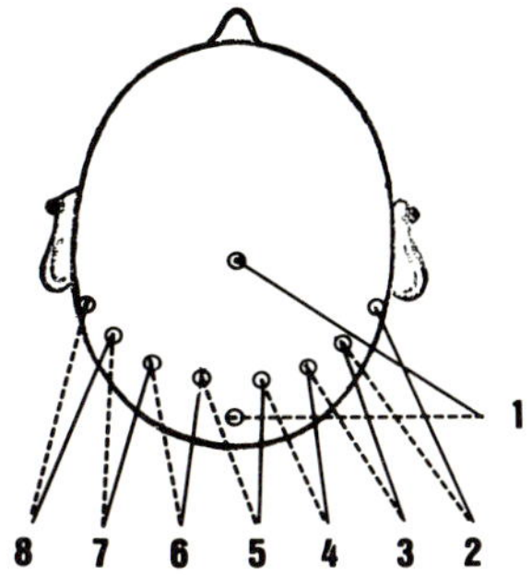

Fig. 3. Electrode arrangements for correlation analysis. Single electrode from right to left, crossing the midline 5 cm above the inion. The numbers indicate the 8 EEG channels. Channel 1 activity on the midline is correlated with all other channels

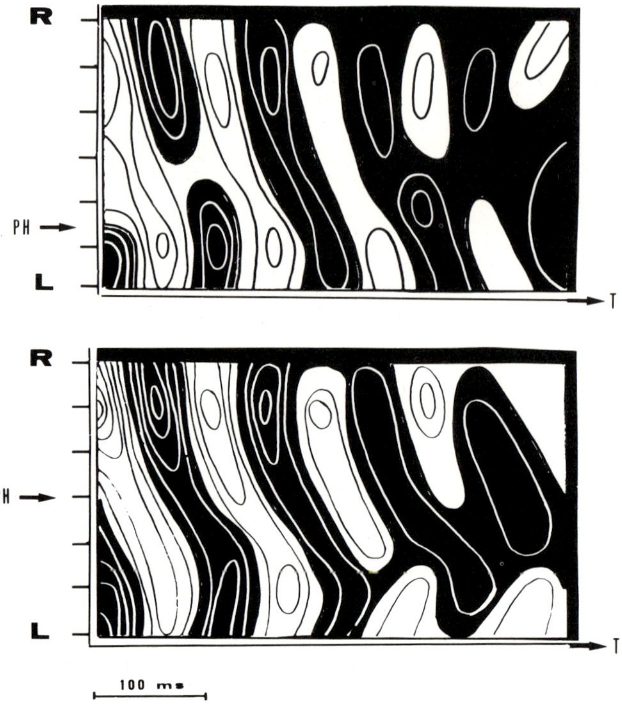

Fig. 4. Spatio-temporal representation of a series of cross-correlation functions in a patient with metastases in the left parietal region. Positive correlations correspond to dark, negative correlations to white areas. Neighbouring level lines differ by a correlation coefficient of 0.1; zero correlation exists on the limit between dark and white surfaces. The place of initial phase reversal (=zero correlation) is indicated by an arrow (pH). The ordinate represents the analysis time of 409.6 ms. On the abscissa the correlation functions obtained on the right hemisphere are represented on the upper part of each map, the corresponding functions of the left hemisphere in the lower part. The marks on the abscissa indicate the spacing of the original correlation functions: intermediate values are interpolated

Upper map: Oblique, slightly asymmetrical structure. The phase reversal is displaced to the left (affected) hemisphere

Lower map: Under dexamethasone treatment slightly higher correlations, same oblique structure. The initial phase reversal has returned to the midline

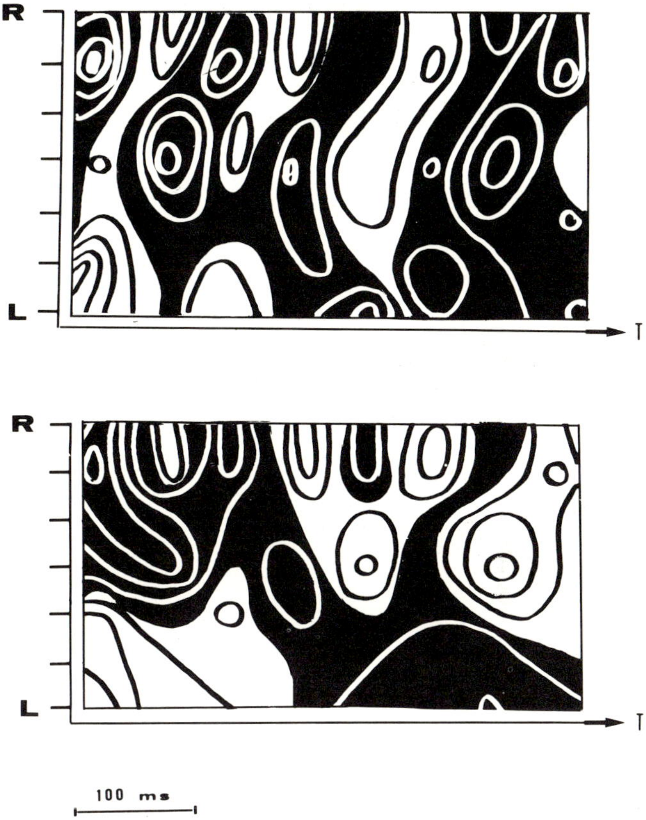

Fig. 5. Very irregular, almost random correlation maps of a patient with an astrocytoma (KII) of the left hemisphere (parieto-temporo-occipital expansion). Some regular "activity" is observed in the alpha range on the right hemisphere (R) only. On the left (L), very slow or irregular phenomena are present. Under dexamethasone treatment (lower map) no substantial change

Influence of Ventilation and Hyperventilation on Brain Edema and Intracranial Pressure

R. A. FROWEIN, A. KARIMI-NEJAD, and K. B. RICHARD

The task of reporting about hyperventilation in the sense of increased alveolar ventilation and its influence especially on the brain oedema seemed difficult from the neurosurgical point of view. There seem to be only few exact studies that are apt for clinical interpretation. For this reason, it seems necessary to accept the cerebrospinal fluid pressure (CSF pressure) as a further factor of intracranial pressure. In the course of a lumbar tapping, BARANY observed in 1912, that hyperventilation leads to a reduction in CSF pressure. After that it was especially LUNDBERG and co-workers (1959) who observed the ratio of ventricle fluid pressure (VFP) and the changes in the minute volume, for example, in the case of a 60-year old patient having a temporal glioblastoma. The average VFP of 30 mmHg, corresponding to approx. 400 mm H_2O, was measured under spontaneous breathing of 5-6 l/min. Artificial increase of the minute volume for 1 - 2 hours to 15 and more l/min. reduced the VFP to less than 275 mm H_2O.

For the neurosurgical judgement of a therapeutic application of hyperventilation in the presence of brain oedema and increased intracranial pressure - besides the effect volume - it is also the effect duration that is of importance: most studies are short-term observations: These will be discussed first. Thereafter, we shall discuss long-term hyperventilation and long-term discontinuous assisted ventilation (KARIMI-NEJAD, MASCHKE 1973).

Short-term observations

Since, 1960 the neurosurgery has known the short-term application of controlled hyperventilation with extreme negative endexpiratory pressure in the trachea, applied as positive-negative pressure ventilation in anaesthesia (HAYES et al. 1962, SCHETTINI et al. 1967, McCOMISH and BODLEY 1971). The resulting strong decrease of CSFP pressure and brain volume is exactly the reaction that is desired by the surgeon (Fig. 1).

COBB and co-workers 1931 already assumed - as many other investigations did later on - that this effect is caused, according to the kind of hyperventilation applied - by two mechanisms:

One is the decrease of pressure in the thorax and thus a better intracranial venous drain (HUBAY et al. 1954) and the other one is the reduced blood flow in the brain (see GOTOH and co-workers 1965, BROCK et al. 1969, FRAZER 1970, GOTTSTEIN 1970, CERVOS-NAVARRO et al. 1971, GAENSHIRT 1972), which is due to hypocapnia. According to the measurements taken by REULEN et al. 1970, this amounted to approx. 1/4 of the rest value at an arterial PCO_2 of 26 mmHg. At the same time, the regional brain flow in the region of a local brain lesion - infarct, oedema - can rise remarkably. LASSEN 1966, WUELLENWEBER 1967, LASSEN, PAL-

VOEGLY 1968, PALVOEGLY 1969, BROCK et al. 1970, REULEN 1971, SCHMIDT 1971 confirmed this so-called "inverse steal-effect". In an experiment on monkeys SOLOWEY (1968, 1970) caused a definite brain damage by media lock. As long as an hour before, a hyperventilation with arterial CO_2 pressure on 25 mmHg was begun and continued for another two hours after the lock. In the non-treated control group the media-infarct was definitely higher than under hyperventilation, If hyperventilation was not begun earlier than 1 hour after the media lock, no protective effect was obtained.

BROCK and co-workers 1970 were able to show that these short-term experimental observations are similar to the circumstances that occur during the operation of brain tumors in general anaesthesia with hyperventilation.

Long-term observations

The effects of therapeutic long-term hyperventilation in the acute stage of brain damage are less clear.

Above all,we may remind of the fact that, according to KARIMI-NEJAD, 1972, patients in an acute stage of brain damage caused by vascular lock, trauma, operation, etc., develop a spontaneous uneconomical hyperventilation under clinically recognizable respiratory disturbances in 92 % of all the cases.

In the arterial blood we find a wide-spread reduction of PCO_2 to an average of 30 mmHg (measurements taken from 161 patients, KARIMI-NEJAD 1970, KARIMI-NEJAD, FROWEIN 1971).

PLUM and SWANSON 1959, FROWEIN 1963, STEINBEREITHNER and co-workers 1967, showed - as we did - during the Meeting of our Society in Cambridge 1970 that this hyperventilation is one of the typical courses that respiratory disturbances take after acute brain damage. This peculiar feature distinguishes it partly from respiratory disturbances to be found in other patients in the stage of intense therapy and from the internal neurovegetative hyperventilation syndrome as well as from the hyperventilation connected with acute brain damage in the region of the rear cranial cavity and the central brain (SEEGER 1968). If, for this reason, an additional therapeutic hyperventilation is to be carried out in the stage of acute brain damage with spontaneous hypocapnia of 30 mmHg, a stronger reduction of the arterial carbonic acid pressure can only be expected if enforced measures are taken.

A selection of the latest papers (Tab. 1) shows that we, in fact, do have detailed experimental short-term studies, but that we do not have more than a very limited number of detailed clinical results of long-term hyperventilation or any other ventilation therapy.

In 40 patients having acute brain flow disturbances, CHRISTENSEN 1970 carried out hyperventilation in general aneasthesia and curarization up to a PCO_2 of 25 mm HG which was continued for the period of 3 days.

After 8 weeks the results obtained were as follows: 5 out of 20 patients were better, 9 were worse or dead. CHRISTENSEN obtained nearly the same result of a 50 % lethality when the 3-day-hyperventilation was not carried out with hypocapnia but with normocapnia and 3% CO_2 added to the breathing air. CHRISTENSEN comes to the conclusion that the result of this difficult hyperventilation treatment is not very encouraging, even if perhaps the hypocapnia-hyperventilation exerts a favour-

Table I. Ventilation under acute brain damage

Author		No. of patients	animal experiment	Ventilation type, duration	PCO_2 mm Hg	Type of Investigation and/or Result
HAYES, TINDALL	1969	13		HV, Narcosis	18 - 47	optimum range for arterial PCO_2 lies between 30 and 35 mm Hg
SOLOWAY et al	1968		dogs	HV 1^h ante, 2^h post	25	Media infarct less
	1970			HV 3^h post		no protective effect
CHRISTENSEN	1970	20		HV 3 days	40 25	acute strokes Lethality: normocapnia 11/20 hypocapnia 9/20
GORDON et al	1970	47		HV several days	25	brain traumata; Lethality: 3 %
VAPALAHTI	1970	13		HV several days	25	brain traumata; Lethality: 85 %
BROCK et al	1970	24		HV hours	26	brain operations
CERVOS-NAVARRO et al	1970				11 - 24	Dissociation of CBF in grey and white matter
GOSCH et al	1971		monkeys		23 - 25	blood flow in cortical area improved
BATTISTINIE et al	1971		cat		24	HV increase CBF in ischaemic lesions
MILLER and LEDINGHAM	1971		dogs	HV hours	19	increase in CSF lactate level
RAICHLE, POSNER PLUM	1971	4	dogs	HV, 5 hours	15 - 20	restoration of the CSF -pH
FREI et al	1971		cats	HV hours	16 - 27	increase of CBF in the region of lesion increase oflactate level in all brain sections

PAULSON	1971	5		HV until stabiliz.	25	CBF and CSF-pH return after several hours or days to values during normocapnia
CROCKARD et al.	1971	11		HV 3 - 5 days	26 - 30	brain traumata; lethality: 44 %
SCHETTINI et al	1972		dogs	HV 1 hour	15 - 7	no correlation between CSF and brain surface pressure
PAUL et al	1972	16		HV 5 - 120 min.	altering	3 types of responsiveness
KARIMI-NEJAD, FROWEIN	1973	595		discontinual assist. ventilation	30	brain traumata; lethality: 53 %

HV = Hyperventilation controls
CBF = cerebral blood flow
CSF = cerebro spinal fluid

able influence especially on secondary lesions, a fact which is difficult to judge because of the reduced number of investigations.

Similar criticism has to be shown when studying the results of hyperventilation treatment in the presence of traumatic brain damages.

GORDON 1970 is known to be the first to present a report about 51 patients with a hyperventilation of several days after severe brain traumata (group A). Hyperventilation was carried out without any regard to existing or non-existing respiratory disturbances. The lethality of only 10 % - and only 3 % in the years 1967 to 69 - can only be explained by the composition of the patients treated. In any case, the letality of group A is much lower than the approx. 30 % letality in 200 patients (group B), who had been trated in a diagnostically and therapeutically similar way in the previous years but without hyperventilation. The number of patients who recovered completely amounts to about 30 % in both groups. The number of more or less serious defects that were cured is, however, considerably higher with hyperventilation.

The emphasis GORDON puts on the difference between former treatment without any ventilation (B) and the modern treatment (A) is perhaps to be found not so much in the hyperventilation than in the mere fact of the existence of any ventilation at all in group A. In 1970, GORDON himself considered a group of 51 patients to be too small for a final judgement.

Following severe brain damages a great variety of factors becomes apparent which define the course: among these are unconsciousness, age and especially the severeness of respiratory disturbances, which are the most important ones. This becomes clearly visible with our own number of 680 patients having long-term consciousness disturbances: children and young patients on the average undergo a longer period of unconsciousness than middle-aged or elder patients do: the letality is lower than in the old age group (KARIMI-NEJAD 1972). These differences weigh especially heavily in smaller statistics and thus complicate to a great extent any comparison between different clinics.

If long-term ventilation is to be carried out in a larger number of patients - we generally do this for an average of 9 days - it must be feasible in a technically simple way. It must be investigated where the emphasis of the whole indication has to be laid. Is it only to be found in the aim of an arterial hypocapnia with the intention of intracranial pressure reduction? Or is it possible to reach an intracranial pressure reduction by applying other additional means and - at the same time - achieve by ventilation a normalization of the arterial oxygen pressure rather than a change in the carbon dioxide pressure, and as a consequence, improve the brain metabolism and thus the brain oedema? Here we will have to take into consideration the extraordinarily complicated pulmonary difficulties arising from a long-term ventilation that determine the course.

In order not to favour a bronchial-obstruction and an alveolar collapse (LYNCH 1959), pulmonologists demand, for long-term ventilation, a constant inflation of the lungs by intermittent positive ventilation applying - as has been demanded in recent times - a positive endexpiratory pressure "PEEP". In the acute stage of brain damage, however, the circulatory effects of this kind of ventilation are undesired, especially since they prevent venous drainage, as has been proved by many authors, e.g. COURNAND et al. 1948, MALONEY et al. 1953, SCHORER 1965, SILL and SIEMSSEN 1972.

In the acute and subacute stage of brain damage a type of ventilation will have to be applied that meets as many requirements as possible such as technical simplicity, normalization of arterial PO_2, intracranial pressure, reduction, consideration of pulmonary complications (WIEMERS and SCHOLLER 1973). The discontinuous ventilation with relatively low negative endexpiratory pressure - NEEP - has proved to be very satisfactory in this respect (KARIMI-NEJAD 1970, KARIMI-NEJAD and FROWEIN 1973). With our patients we were able to make 110 measurements of average improvements of the arterial oxygen pressure for the surviving - from 79 to 156 mm Hg - as well as for the lethal course - from 54 to 108 mm Hg (Tab.II). In all groups the average arterial carbon dioxide pressure was at about 30 mmHg. This arterial PCO_2 step proved to be optimal for the intracranial pressure reduction, also according to HAYES and TINDALL 1969, PAUL et al. 1972, KINDT and GOSCH 1972.

The therapeutic efficiency seems to be measurable on the CSF values,which parallel the situation in the brain tissue (FENCL et al. 1966, ZWETNOW 1970, METZEL and ZIMMERMANN 1971). In surviving patients an average increase in CSF-oxygen-pressure from 78 to 98 mm Hg was reached together with a steady PCO_2 of 39 : 36 mmHg. The average CSF acidosis with a pH of 7. 30 before the ventilation is of importance; in lethal cases this remained more or less unaffected; in survivors there was an amelioration of the CSF pH to 7. 32.

We do not know whether there exist any special investigations about the effects of long-term assisted ventilation on brain oedema.

The influence of intracranial pressure can be estimated best by measuring the ventricle-CSF pressure, even though it is not alway parallel to the brain-surface-pressure (SCHETTINI et al. 1972, SUNDBÄRG and NORSEN 1972, CORONEOS et al. 1972). May we - only for comparison - repeat the it is well known that the intraventricular CSF pressure decreases rapidly by lumbar or ventricle tapping, but that it reaches its starting point again within 5-60 minutes if the ventricle size is normal (HEMMER 1960, LORENZ 1972). After hyperosmolar infusion of Sorbitol 40 % the CSF pressure decreases less quickly but rises to - or even sometimes over - its starting point within 1 - 3 hours . Both measures cannot be repeated as often as desired (BRENNER 1973). A more frequent and longer high-resting of the patient's upper body and head can be carried out as long as his breathing and circulation allow this.

The decrease in CSF pressure levels up again within 1 - 2 hours (Fig. 2).

Different pressure is applied for long-term ventilation; with our patients this was in most cases an endexpiratory pressure of about 20 cm H_2O and a negative endexporatory pressure -NEEP- of 3 - 5 cm H_2O.

Measurements in the lateral ventricle at the Foramen Monroi showed in 80 % of the different phases of ventilation a reduction of CSF pressure ot 100 - 200 mm H_2O within 10 - 90 minutes (Fig. 3).

Emphasis must, however, be put on the fact that in some cases of heamorrhage - this pressure did not decrease, as has been shown in the studies by PAUL et al. 1972.

When patients showed positive reactions we interrupted the ventilation after 30-60 minutes. After that the CSF pressure increased again to its starting point within the course of 1-3 hours.

But the ventilation may be repeated regularly each hour and can be continued for several days - up to 3 - 4 weeks.

Table II. Influence of assisted ventilation (40 % O_2) on blood and CSF-gases

		Before Ventilation 4 l O_2/min		During Ventilation	
		Survivors 21	Fatalities 46	Survivors 27	Fatalities 83
arterial	PO_2 mm Hg	79 $\pm$ 50	54 $\pm$ 17	156 $\pm$ 104	108 $\pm$ 68
	PCO_2	33 $\pm$ 5	31 $\pm$ 6	33 $\pm$ 5	31 $\pm$ 7
	pH	7,46 $\pm$ 0,04	7,47 $\pm$ 0,o5	7,47 $\pm$ 0,05	7,47 $\pm$ 0,048
Jugular	PO_2	35 $\pm$ 9	31 $\pm$ 7	32 $\pm$ 10	34 $\pm$ 8
	PCO_2	38 $\pm$ 5	36 $\pm$ 7	37 $\pm$ 6	36 $\pm$ 6
	pH	7,41 $\pm$ 0,04	7,40 $\pm$ 0,05	7,43 $\pm$ 0,05	7,41 $\pm$ 0,04
CSF	PO_2	78 $\pm$ 31	70 $\pm$ 60	98 $\pm$ 36	76 $\pm$ 39
	PCO_2	39 $\pm$ 7	48 $\pm$ 12	37 $\pm$ 3,5	41 $\pm$ 9
	pH	7,30 $\pm$ 0,09	7,28 $\pm$ 0,09	7,32 $\pm$ 0,11	7,29 $\pm$ 0,08

In the case of a 56-year-old patient the discontinuous assisted ventilation with negative endexpiratory pressure was continued for 8 days (Fig. 4).

The continued registration shows that during the whole course the reduction of ventricle-fluid-pressure was achieved symptomatically during each ventilation phase. The slow increase of the minimum value is due to the worsening of the basic process which could not be influenced in this case.

Definite indications on the average effects of this ventilation can only be obtained from extensive statistics for longer periods: if lethality is taken as a criterion, we find that there was a decrease of lethality from 75 % to 35 % in 595 patients who were treated with discontinuous long-term ventilation during the years 1966 - 1971 (KARIMI-NEJAD, FROWEIN 1973). This will certainly be due to several factors, but one may be quite sure that it is the discontinuous long-term ventilation that is one of the most important factors contributing to this amelioration (KARIMI-NEJAD and MASCHKE 1973).

Table III.
Results of discontinuous long-term ventilation in 592 patients with acute brain damage

Year	1966	1967	1968	1969	1970	1971
No. of patients	78	84	86	108	113	123
Lethality	75%	67%	66%	63%	54%	53%

Summary

Hyperventilation with strong arterial hypocapnia was originally applied in order to achieve a reduction of intracranial pressure. It is one of the steady and approved means of anesthesia in neurological surgery.

The value of the ventilation therapy in its widest sense - in the presence of acute brain damage - is fully accepted.

The therapeutic value of a continued controlled long-term hyperventilation during the whole stage of brain edema seems, however, to be questionable.

In contrast to this, the discontinuous long-term ventilation with negative end expiratiory pressure is technically much simpler and pulmonary less complicated and can be repeated as often as desired. Its foremost aim is the amelioration of the blood gases.

An irregular, but progressive reduction in intracranial pressure, which could be repeated for days, was demonstrated. Because of this and other short-term experimental results a positive influence on the brain edema seems to be possible.

REFERENCES

1. BARANY, R.: Messung des Minimums des Liquordrucks teta oto-lyryng. 5, 390-391 (1923)

2. BATTISTINI, N., M. CASACCHIA, C. FIESCHI, M. NARDINI and S. PASSERO: Treatment of experimental cerebral infarction with passive hyperventilation In: Ross Russell, Brain and Blood Flow, 102-106, 1971

3. BRENNER, H.: Hypertonic and diuretic therapy of brain edema. 24 Jahrestagung Deutsche Gesellsch. Neurochirurgie, Mai 1973

4. BROCK, M., A. HADJIDIMOS, J. P. DERUAZ and K. SCHÜRMANN: Regional cerebral blood flow and vascular reactivity in cases of brain tumor (London 1970). In: Ross Russell, Brain and Blood Flow, 1971

5. CERVOS-NAVARRO, J., E. VALENCAK and M. LEIPERT: Circulatory disturbances and ultrastructural correlates in hyper- und hypoventilation. In: Head Injuries. Proceedings of an Intern. Symp. 1970, Edinburgh and London, Churchill Livingstone, 1971

6. CHRISTENSEN, M. S.: Stroke treated with prolonged hyperventilation. In: Ross Russell, Brain and Blood Flow, 358-364, 1971

7. COBB, S. and F. FREMONTSMITH: The cerebral circulation. Arch. Neurol. Psychiat. 26, 731-736, (1931)

8. CORONEOS, N, J., D. G. MCDOWALL, V. W. PICKERODT, N. P. KEANY, and R. M. GIBSON: A comparison on intracranial extradural pressure with subarachnoid pressure. Br. J. Anasth., 43, 1198 (1971)

9. COURNAND, D. A., H. L. MOLTEY, L. WERKO and D. W. RICHARDS: Physiological studies of the effects of intermittent positive pressure breathing on cardiac output in man. Amer. J. Physiol. 152, 162, (1948)

10. CROCKARD, H. A. et al.: The inportance of blood-CO_2, levels in head injury management: Improvement with hyperventilation. Br. J. Surg. 58, 857, (1971)

11. FEND, V., T. B. MILLER, and J. R. PAPPENHEIMER: Studies on the respiratory response to disturbances of acid-base balance with deductions concerning the ionic composition of cerebral interstitial fluid. Amer. J. Physiol. 210, 459-479, (1966)

12. FRAZER, R. A. R., B. M. STEIN, S. K. HICAL, R. E. BARRETT and J. L. POOL: Cerebrovascular reactivity: Blockade of acute and chronic vascular spasm and hypocapnic constriction. In: Ross Russell, Brain and Blood Flow, 236-243, 1971

13. FREI, H. J., W. PÖLL, H. J. REULEN, M. BROCK and K. SCHÜRMANN: Regional energy metabolism, tissue lactate content and rCBF in old injury oedema In: Ross Russel, Brain and Blood Flow, 125-129, 1971

14. FROWEIN. R. A.: Zentrale Atemstörungen bei Schädel-Hirn-Verletzungen und bei Hirntumoren. Monogr. Ges. Geb. Neurol. und Psychiat. H. 101, Berlin-Göttingen-Heidelberg, 1963

15. FROWEIN, R. A. und A. KARIMI-NEJAD: Sauerstoffversorgung des Hirngewebes nach schweren Hirnschädigungen. Acta Neurochir. 19, 1-31, (1968)

16. GÄNSHIRT, H.: Der Hirnkreislauf. Stuttgart, Thieme, 1972

17. GORDON, E.: The effects of controlled ventilation on the clinical course of patients with severe traumatic brain injury. Ross Russell, Brain and Blood Flow, 1971

18. GOSCH, H. H., J. MCGANLEY and G. W. KINDT: Arterial pCO_2-reduction in the treatment of acute increased intracranial pressure. Surg. Forum 22, 427-429, (1971)

19. GOTOH, F., J. S. MEYER and Y. TAKAGI: Cerebral effects of hyperventilation in man. Arch. Neurol. 12, 410-423, (1965).

20. GOTTSTEIN, V., W. BERGHOFF, K. HELD, H. GABRIEL, Th. TEXTOR and V. ZAHN: Cerebral metabolism during hyperventilation and inhalation of CO_2. In: Ross Russell, Brain and Blood Flow, 170-173 (1970)

21. HAYES, Th. M. and G. T. TINDALL: Effects of altering arterial carbon dioxide pressure on internal carotid blood flow and cerebrospinal fluid pressure in man. Surg. Forum 20, 421-424 (1969)

22. HAYES, G. J., C. HARVEY and MC. SLOCUM: The achievement of optimal brain relaxation by hyperventilation technics of anesthesia. J. Neurosurg. 19, 65-70, (1962)

23. HEMMER, R.: Der Liquordruck, Thieme, Stuttgart, 1960

24. HUBAY, C. A., R. C. WALTZ, G. A. BRECHER, J. PRAGLIN and R. A. HINGSON: Circulatory dynamics of venous return during positive-negative pressure respiration. Anesthesiology 15, 445, (1954)

25. KARIMI-NEJAD, A.: Atemgasdruck- und Säure-Basen Veränderungen im arteriellen und hirnvenösen jugularen Blut sowie im Liquor cerebrospinalis im akuten und subakuten Stadium einer Hirnschädigung und ihre therapeutischen Konsequenzen. Thesis, Köln, 1970

26. KARIMI-NEJAD, A.: Advantages and limitation of longtern ventilation. Acta Neurochir. 26, 364-365, (1972)

27. KARIMI-NEJAD, A.: Disorders of respiratory regulation in acute stage of diffuse brain damage. Abstracts of Symposion: Central rhythmic and regulations, circulation, respiration, extrapyramidal motorsystem, Berlin, July 13th-15th, 1972

28. KARIMI-NEJAD, A. and R. A. FROWEIN: The effects of central respiratory disorders on blood and CSF gases. In: Modern aspects of Neurosurgery, Vol. I, 74-85, 1971, Excerpta Medica, Amsterdam

29. KARIMI-NEJAD, A. and R. A. FROWEIN: Langzeitbeatmung nach akuter Hirnschädigung. Zbl. Neurochir. 34 (1973)

30. KARIMI-NEJAD, A. and H. MASCHKE: Einfluß diskontinuierlicher Langzeitbeatmung auf die Lungenfunktion bei akuter Hirnschädigung. In: Wiemers und Scholler, 208-215, 1973

31. KINDT, G. W. and H. H. GOSCH: Arterial pCO_2 effect at various levels of intracranial pressure. In: Brock und Dietz, Intracranial Pressure, Berlin-Heidelberg, Springer, 210-213, 1972

32. LASSEN, N. A.: The luxury-perfusion syndrome and its possible relation to acute metabolic acidosis localized within the brain. Lancet, 2, 1113 (1966)

33. LASSEN, N. A. and R. PALVÖLGYI: Cerebral steal during hypercapnia and the inverse reaction during hypocapnia observed by the 133Xenon technique in man. Scand. J. clin. Lab. Invest. Suppl. 102, XIII:D (1968)

34. LORENZ, R. and E. GROTE: Relations between cerebrospinal fluid pressure elasticity of the dura and volume of the CSF. In: Intracranial Pressure, ed. BROCK und DIETZ, Springer, Berlin, 265-270, 1972

35. LUNDBERG, N. A. KJÄLLQUIST and Ch. BIEN: Reduction of increased intracranial pressure by hyperventilation. Acta Psych. Neurol. Scand. Suppl. 34, 139, (1959)

36. LYNCH, S., A. LEVY and K. ELLIS: Effects of alternating positive and negative endotracheal pressure on the caliber of bronchi. Anesthesiology 20, 325, (1959)

37. MALONEY, J. V., J. O. ELAM, S. W. HANDFORD, G. A. BALLS, D. W. EASTWOOD, E. S. BROWN and R. H. TEPNAS: Importance of negative pressure phase in mechanical respirators. J. Amer. med. Ass. 152, 212, (1953)

38. MC COMISH, P, B. and P. O. BODLEY: Anaesthesia for Neurological Surgery London, Lloyd-Luke, 1971

39. MC DOWALL, D. G., W. FITCH, V. W. A. PICKERODT, N. J. CORONEOS, and N. P. KEANEY: Hemodynamic effects of experimental intracranial space-occupying lesions in passively-ventilated dogs and baboons. Eur. Neurol. 8, 92-96, (1972)

40. METZEL, E. and W. E. ZIMMERMANN: Changes of oxygen pressure, acid-base balance, metabolites and electrolytes in cerebrospinal fluid and after cerebral injury. Acta neurochir. (wien) 25, 177-188, (1971)

41. MILLER, J. D. and I. McA. LEDINGHAM: Reduction of raised intracranial pressure: hyperbaric oxygen versus hyperventilation. Brit. J. Surg. 56, 630, (1969)

42. MILLER, J. D. and I. McA. LEDINGHAM: Reduction of increased intracranial pressure: comparison between hyperbaric oxygen and hyperventilation. Arch. Neurol. 24, 210-216, (1971).

43. PALBÖGLY, R: Regional cerebral blood flow in patients with intracranial tumors. J. Neurosurg. 31, 149-163, (1966)

44. PAUL, R. L., O. POLANCO, S. Z. TURNEY, T. CRAWFORD and R. A. COWLEY: Intracranial pressure response to alterations in arterial CO_2 pressure in patients with head injuries. J. Neurosurg. 36, 714-720, (1972)

45. PAULSON, O. B: Restoration of autoregulation by hypocapnia. In: Ross Russell, Brain and Blood Flow, 313-321, 1971

46. PLUM, F. and A. G. SWANSON: Central neurogenic hyperventilation in man. Arch. neurol. psychiat. (Chicago) 81, 535-549, (1959)

47. PLUM, F. and H. W. BROWN: The effect on respiration of central nervous system disease. Ann. N. J. Acad. Sci. 109, 915, (1963)

48. RAICHLE, M. E., J. B. POSNER and F. PLUM: Cerebral blood flow during and after hyperventilation. In: Ross Russell, Brain and Blood Flow, 223-228, 1971

49. REULEN, H. J.: Veränderungen der regionalen Hirndurchblutung beim zerebralen Ödem und ihre therapeutische Beeinflussung durch Hyperventilation. Z. Prakt. Anaesth. Wiederbelebung, 6, 426-430, (1971)

50. REULEN, H.J. and K. SCHÜRMANN: Steroids and Brain Edema. Berlin-Heidelberg-New York, Springer, 1972

51. ROSS RUSSELL: Brain and Blood Flow. Proceedings of the 4th intern. symposium on the regulation of cerebral blood flow, London 1970, London, Pitman, 1971

52. SCHETTINI, A., A. W. COOK and E. S. OWERE: Hyperventilation in craniotomy for brain tumor. Anesthesiology 28, 363, (1967)

53. SCHETTINI, A., L. MC KAY, J. MAHIG and J. H. MODELL: The response of brain surface pressure to hypercapnia hypoxia and hyperventilation. Anaesthesiology, 36, 4-12, (1972)

54. SEEGER, W.: Atemstörungen bei intrakraniellen Massenverschiebungen. Acta Neurochir. Suppl. XVII, Wien, Springer, 1968

55. SCHORER, R.: Untersuchungen zum Netto-Effekt der "respiratorischen Kreislaufpumpe". Fortsch. Med. 83, 745-748, (1965)

56. SILL, V. and S. SIEMSSEN: Hämodynamische Nebenwirkungen bei der Beatmung mit positiven endexpiratorischen Drucken. Der Anaesthesist, 21m 305-310, (1972)

57. SOLOWAY, M., W. NADEL, M. S. ALBIN and R. J. WHITE: The effect of hyperventilation on subsequent cerebral infarction. Anaesthesiology 29, 975-980, (1968)

58. SOLOWAY, M., G. MORIATRY, J. G. FRASER and P. J. WHITE: The effect of delayed hyperventilation on experimental middle cerebral artery occlusion. In: Ross Russell, 98-101, 1971

59. STEINBEREITHNER, K. and O. WAGNER: Untersuchungen über das Verhalten des Säurebasenhaushaltes und der Atemgase in Liquor und arteriellem Blut bei schweren Schädeltraumen mit besonderer Berücksichtigung des Hyperventilationssyndroms. Klin. Wchschr. 1, 126-133, (1967)

60. SUNDBÄRG, G. and H. NORNES: Simultaneous recording of the epidural and ventricular fluid pressure. In: M. BROCK and H. DIETZ (eds.) Intracranial Pressure, Berlin, Springer, 1972

61. VAPALAHTI, M.: Intracranial pressure, acid base status of blood and cerebrospinal fluid, and pulmonary function in the prognosis of severe brain injury. Helsinki, Kopiopalveln oy, 1970

62. WIEMERS, K. and K. L. SCHOLLER: Lungenveränderungen bei Langzeitbeatmung. Intern. Symposion in Freiburg 1971, Thieme, Stuttgart, 1973

63. WÜLLENWEBER, R., U. GÖBB and J. SCANTO: Beobachtungen zur Regulation der Hirndurchblutung. Acta neurochir. 16, 137-153, (1967)

64. ZWETNOW, N. N.: Effects of increased CSF pressure on the blood flow and on the energy metabolism of the brain. Acta Physiol. Scand. Suppl. 339 (1970)

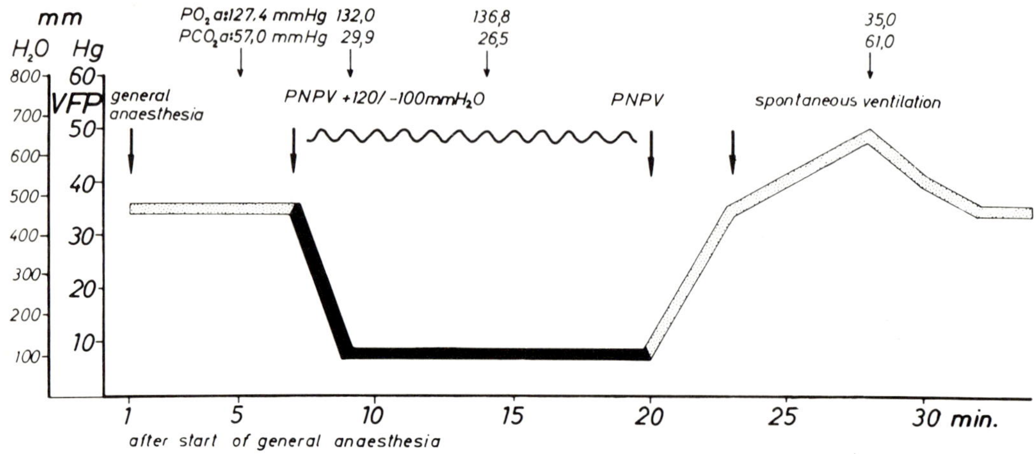

Fig. 1. Mean ventricular fluid pressure (VFP) and blood gases before, during and after positive-negative-pressure ventilation (PNPV) in halothane-nitrous oxide-O_2-anesthesia. 5, 5 year-old boy, having papillary congestion of unknown origin

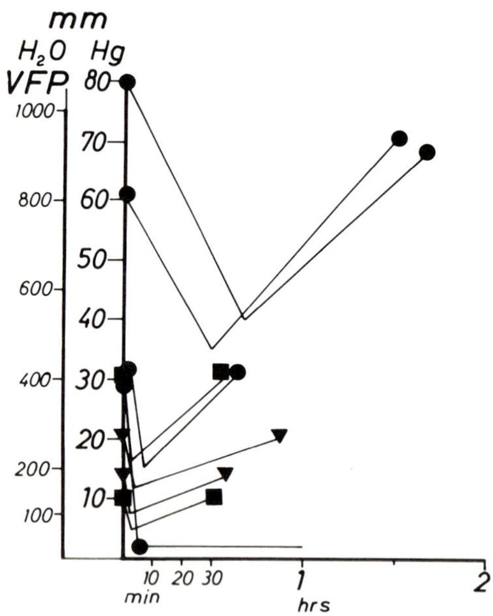

Fig. 2. Effects of high head-resting on ventricular fluid pressure (VFP) ▼10° higher, ■ 20° higher● 30° higher

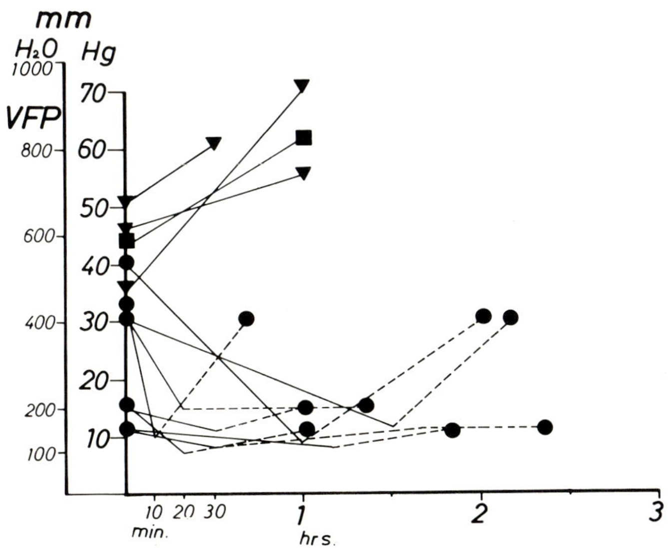

Fig. 3. Effects of assisted ventilation with "NEEP" on ventricular fluid pressure (VFP) ● cerebellar tumor, ▼ frontal glioblastoma, ■ early and acute subdural hematoma

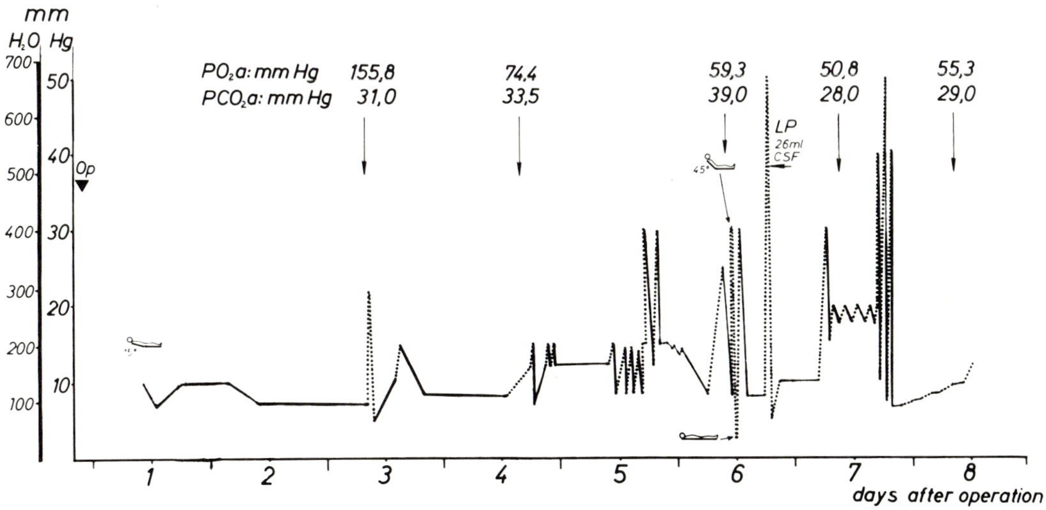

Fig. 4. Discontinuous assisted ventilation with "NEEP" in a 47-year-old female patient after operation for a cerebellar tumor. • • • • Portex tube + humidifier, ———— respirator "NEEP"

Artificial Ventilation in Cerebral Edema – A Critical Analysis of Manometric and Gazometric Conditions

A. KÜHNER, B. ROQUEFEUIL, E. VIGUIE, PH. FREREBEAU, M. BAZIN, J. M. PRIVAT, and C. GROS

Artificial ventilation is one of the dominant therapeutic factors in the treatment of cerebral edema since it ensures the control of arterial PCO_2 which, in its turn, plays an important role in intracranial hypertension.

However, many studies have shown that artificial ventilation may impose a mechanical block on CSF drainage. The aim of this work is to critically analyse the manometric and gazometric effects of artificial ventilation during cerebral edema.

Pathophysiological review

The role of CO_2 as a causative factor of vasogenic edema has been known for a long time (4, 6). All hypercapnias cause an immediate rise of intracranial pressure by direct, in situ, cerebral vasoparalysis and by an increase in cardiac output and systemic blood pressure. The main merit of a permanently controlled ventilation is precisely to prevent all hypercapnic crises.

Independently of its effects on $PaCO_2$, artificial ventilation may act on intrapulmonary and systemic hemodynamics (2, 3, 7). Many important studies have defined the techniques for artificial ventilation in cerebral edema; they have attributed much importance to the regulation of ventilation.

In physiological states and in apnea the graph of CSF is modulated by arterial systolic and diastolic waves (physiologic pulsogram).

In spontaneous respiration, there is a low amplitude modulation of PCSF synchronised with the respiratory phase. The CSF is lower during inspiration (venous return is favored by the negative pressure) and it increases slightly during expiration due to the increase in intrathoracic pressure which reduces venous return.

In artificial ventilation we find an inversion of this phenomenon. A slight increase in intrathoracic pressure during insufflation gives a higher PCSF than is measured during exsufflation. Thus, in a patient under controlled ventilation even with intermittent positive pressure, there is the risk of ICP variations related to the insufflation peak, the length of insufflation time and an eventual negative expiratory pressure.

Experimental studies have shown that in the case of cerebral edema the most favorable adjustment of the regulation is that which, for a satisfactory alveolar ventilation, requires the lowest insufflation pressures, the shortest ratio, and a moderate negative pressure to bring the mean intrathoracic pressure close to zero.

It seems that the problem with artificial ventilation in cerebral edema resides in the conciliation of two opposed imperatives : to control hypercapnia by a satisfactory alveolar ventilation, knowing that this causes or may cause unfavorable mechanical conditions.

The aim of this work is to elucidate, as much as possible, the true importance of these gazometric and manometric conditions.

Study conditions

a) The choice of patients

The recordings were made on ten patients in the acute phase of head trauma. Each one presented a "brain stem" type of symptomatology with cerebral edema manifested by increased intracranial pressure

b) Methods and material

The study of the effects of artificial ventilation on ICP required, in addition to measures of CSFP, the measurement of tracheal pressure, and arterial and venous pressures as well as the determination of blood gases.

Ventricualr CSF pressure was recorded with an intraventricular probe.

Intratracheal pressure was measured by means of a needle probe in the intubation catheter or in the tracheotomy opening connected to a pressure cell by a catheter.

Central venous pressure was measured in the superior vena cava by a catheter introduced by either the subclavian or humeral route. The CVP measurement required a perfect catheter patency with distinct respirator oscillations.

Arterial pressure: We used a "Grandjean type" arterial microcatheter which has the following advantages:

minimal trauma to the artery
good tolerance of the artery even over several days
easy maintenance due to permanent rinsing
no risk of hemorrhage even in the event of an accidental disconnection

A bidirectional stopcock at the extravascular catheter rip permitted the easy withdrawal of the arterial blood for the measurement of blood gases.

The catheter and the probe are connected to "Statham type" pressure transducers, Each transducer has a biconic head closed by two, three-way stopcocks. One cone was connected to the pressure-measuring catheter; the other, a lateral cone, was for tissue and zeroing before each measurement.

To establish a reference (zero) point, the four transducers were fixed at the level of the right atrium with the patient on his back.

The pressures transmitted by the transducers were recorded on a four-track "Roche-Dassault" monitor;each pressure was recorded on its appropriate base-level in mmHg.

25 or 50 for tracheal pressure
200 for arterial pressure
12, 5 or 25 for CVP
12, 5 or 25 or 50 for CSF pressure

For this study of the influence of artificial ventilation on ICP we used the most perfected volumetric respirators (SF4 Robert et Carrière-Engstrom 3000).

The parameters successively envisioned were:

the influence of $PaCO_2$

the influence of insufflation pressure during constant alveolar ventilation
a study of the ratio $\frac{\text{insufflation}}{\text{exsufflation}}$

the effects of negative pressure and positive expiratory pressure (REEP).

Results and discussion

A. Gasometric ventilatory factors with an effect on ICP

Artificial ventilation has a primordial role in controlling vasogenic edema by lowering $PaCO_2$ (Fig. 1). By itself, in cerebral edema, it lowers the initial PCSF by 62 %. This easily equals the results obtained with the most efficient osmotic treatments.

An analysis of the tracing of intracranial hypertension which we have (10 cases) shows that a lowering of the $PaCO_2$ by 1 mmHg induces a lowering of the initial ICP by 5 %.

We had the opportunity to verify on the wards, in a reproducible manner, the immediate effect of hypercapnia on ICP. The ICP rises as soon as the patient unhooks himself from the respirator or if the respirator is not well regulated (Fig. 2).

B. Mechanical ventilatory factors with an effect on ICP

We re-undertook the study of the different mechanical adjustments of a volumetric respirator and their effects on ICP.

1. A study of the insufflation pressure (Fig. 3)

During constant alveolar ventilation isolated variations of the pressure factor affect the level of CSF pressure. This effect is, however, moderate. A lowering of the insufflation pressure by 10 mm Hg only lowers the PCSF by 3 mmHg. By taking an average of the tracings, we calculated that a lowering of insufflation pressure by 1 mmHg only lowers the initial CSFP by 1 to 2 %.

The variations in CVP are negligeable. The mean blood pressure remains the same in constant alveolar ventilation.

2. The effect of negative pressure (Fig. 4)

The use of a negative expiratory pressure increases venous return and decreases the $PaCO_2$. Fig. 4 shows the effect of adding progressive negative pressures with a decrease in arterial pressure by a lowering of left cardiac output caused by hypercapnia. The CSFP shows a greater fall due to the summation of the two preceding factors. Thus, by the summation of its hemodynamic and gazometric effects, the use of a negative expiratory pressure is an effective means of controlling cerebral edema. However, the effectiveness of a negative pressure is limited and there is nothing to be gained by lowering the $PaCO_2$ below 20 mmHg. Quite to the contrary, in certain patients an excessively negative expiratory pressure may cause bronchiolar collapse and, thus, an increase in intraalveolar pressure and hypercapnia (Fig. 5).

The importance of a negative pressure in artificial ventilation in cerebral edema is certain, but, in the lowering of CSFP obtained, we must take into account the mechanical factor and the inevitable hypocapnia. In taking an average of the recorded tracings, a negative pressure of 1 mmHg lowered theCSFP by 7 %, but after taking into account the gazometric factor the actual lowering caused by the negative pressure was 1.5 % to 3 %.

3. Study of the exsufflation ratio

The study of this parameter is difficult to realise if we want to maintain a constant alveolar ventilation and a constant insufflation pressure.

The CSFP is a direct function of the duration of insufflation. The variations in CVP are synchronous to those of CSFP. In figure 6, the obstacle to venous return and, consequently, to CSF drainage due to the increase in duration of insufflation is undeniable and confirms the classical findings of intra-pulmonary hemodynamics, but is of relatively limited importance.

We noted in all our tracings a mean increase in CSFP of 8 - 10 % above its initial value when the I ratio was increased from 1/3 to 1/1.

The danger of a blind manipulation of the I ratio is clearly shown in figure 7. When the insufflation time becomes equal to the exsufflation time the hemodynamic situation can deteriorate and cardiac tamponade occur with venous hypertension due to an increase in intrathoracic pressure, low left cardiac output and a collapse of systemic arterial pressure. The CSFP then collapses due to a decrease in cerebral perfusion pressure and a slight hypocapnia in spite of maximal mean tracheal pressure and CVP. The dissociation between the retrograde mechanical effects, theoretical factors of CSF hypertension, and the gazometric effect is striking.

4. The influence of positive end expiratory pressure (PEEP)

The risks and limitations of negative pressures have been stressed by many authors (7, 8,). The alveolar mixture (the quality of the ratio ventilation to perfusion) is one of the primary concerns of artificial ventilation specialists.

The bronchi and bronchioles kept in slight positive pressure during expiration maintain a sufficient diameter and a good gaseous exchange with an increase in $PaCO_2$.

PEEP is used in situations where bronchiolar collapse is to be avoided: such situations are met with in neurosurgery. The possibility of using a PEEP is found in certain respirators. We used it once with the follwing results (Fig. 8):

an increase in the mean intra-alveolar pressure
an increase in mean CSF pressure
a slight increase in mean CVP.

However, in this case, the $PaCO_2$ also increased and thus there was also an increase in mean arterial pressure; the increase in CSFP is due to the conjugated variations in the mean tracheal pressure and the ratio of cerebral perfusion. Because of this effect on CSFP the use of PEEP is indicated only in exceptional and well studied circumstances.

Thus, in all of our tracings the predominant role of CO_2 over the mechanical conditions is certain as soon as there is a variation in alveolar ventilation. We have seen that hypercapnia CSF hypertension is produced immediately in a patient who is disconnected from the respirator or whose respiration is not well regulated; the mechanical conditions become more favourable:

increase in venous return during hypercapnia (high cardiac output)
decrease in the mean intrathoracic pressures.

Inversely, the reventilation of the patient instantly corrects CSF hypertension and this correction appears even though the mechanical factors are less favorable.

The most typical and most indiscutable example of the predominance of the gazometric factors over the mechanical factors is found in the tracing of cardia tamponade (fig. 7).

Conclusion

It seems that the technology of artificial ventilation, the circulatory effects of which are well known (1) should take into consideration, concerning its effects on cerebral edema, mechanical factors whose influence is moderate, but undeniable and the CO_2 factor which has a great and direct effect on the levels of intracranial pressure.

The ideal artificial ventilation in dealing with cerebral edema consists in working with a mean intratracheal pressure as near as possible to zero. This is accomplished by a rapid insufflation under low positive pressure followed by a prolonged exsufflation under a slight negative pressure. These should be sufficient to assure a good alveolar ventilation with hypocapnia.

Thus, because it allows the patient to rest, restore normoxic conditions and stabilize the level of CO_2, artificial respiration has a role equal to that of hypertonic solutions in the treatment of cerebral edema.

Summary

We studied the influence of artificial ventilation on intracranial pressure in an attempt to establish the best ventilatory conditions for cerebral edema.

Artificial ventilation acts on intracranial pressure both by variations in gazometric and manometric conditions. The role of $PaCO_2$ on the perfusion pressure and on cerebral vasodilatation is well known. The decrease in intracerebral pressure during artificial hyperventilation is immediate and very important: a mean lowering of 61 % of the initial value.

Artificial ventilation also influences intracranial pressure by its effect on intrathoracic hemodynamics. Ideal conditions for artificial ventilation in cerebral edema have been defined as follows:

mean pressure as close to zero with low insufflation pressure and moderately negative exsufflation pressure;
the ratio I/E (insufflation time/exsufflation time) should be equal to or less than 1/2.
We have found that the role of these manometric factors has been greatly exaggerated.

Under constant alveolar ventilation we have found:

a lowering of the maximal insufflation pressure by 10 mm Hg only diminishes the mean CSF pressure by 3 mmHg;
a negative exsufflation pressure of -1 mmHg only lowers the mean CSF pressure by 3 %. At lower pressure we get bronchiolar collapse with air trapping;
a variation of the I/E ratio from 1/1 to 1/3 (with a constant insufflation pressure) only lowers the mean CSF pressure by 1.5 mmHg, or increasing I/E ratio from 1/3 to 1/1 increases CSFP by 10 %;
an opportune observation of cardiac tamponade with extremely high venous pressure confirms the negligeable role of manometric conditions.
Nevertheless a prolonged respiratory alkalosis induced by long-term hyperventilation could cause non-desirable metabolic side-effects.

REFERENCES

1. DU CAILAR, J., Ch. TRIADOU, B. ROQUEFEUIL and P. MALZAC: Effects de la ventilation artificielle sur la circulation: Agressologie 10-55 (1969)
2. COURNAND, A.: Physiological studies of the effect of intermittent positive pressure on cardiac output in man: Amer. J. Physiol. 152-162 (1948)
3. GILBERT, RGB., GF. BRINDLE and A. GALINDO: Anesthesia for neurosurgery: IAC n°4: Little Brown and Company Boston (1966)
4. KETY, S. S. and CF. SCHMIDT: The effects of passive and active hyperventilation on cerebral blood flow, cerebral oxygen consumption cardiac output and blood pressure of normal young men: J. Clin. Invest., 25-107 (1946)
5. LAZORTHES, G. and L. CAMPAN: L'oedème cérébral: 1 vol. MASSON Paris (1963)
6. LUNDBERG, N.: Reduction of increased intracranial pressure by hyperventilation. A therapeutic aid in neurosurgery: Acta Psych. Scand. Suppl. 34, 139, (1965)
7. SABATHIE, M.: Le problème de l'aide expiratoire: Agressologie 12 B, 153-160 (1961)
8. TORRI, G.: Notions de transfert des gaz et de perfusion alvéolaire: Agressologie 12 B, 83, (1971)

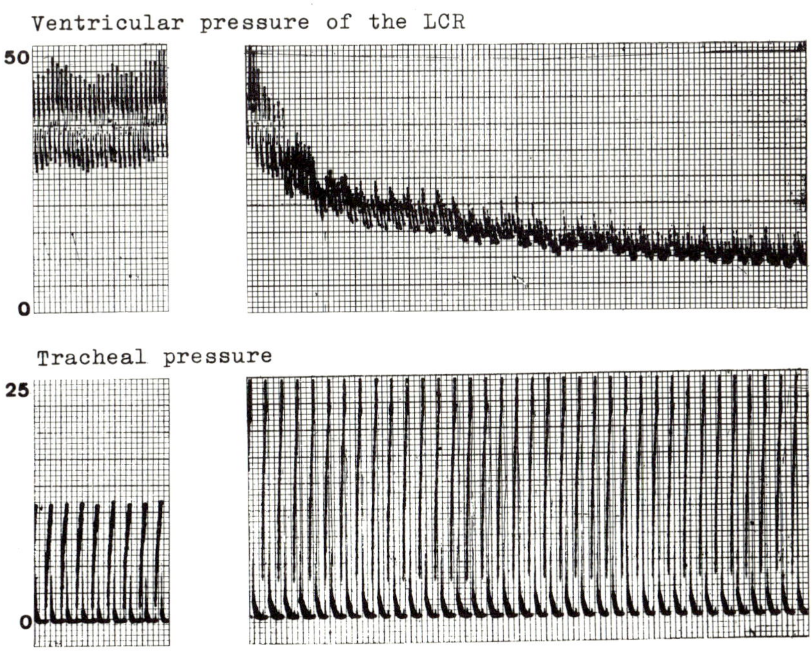

Fig. 1. Effect of hyperventilation

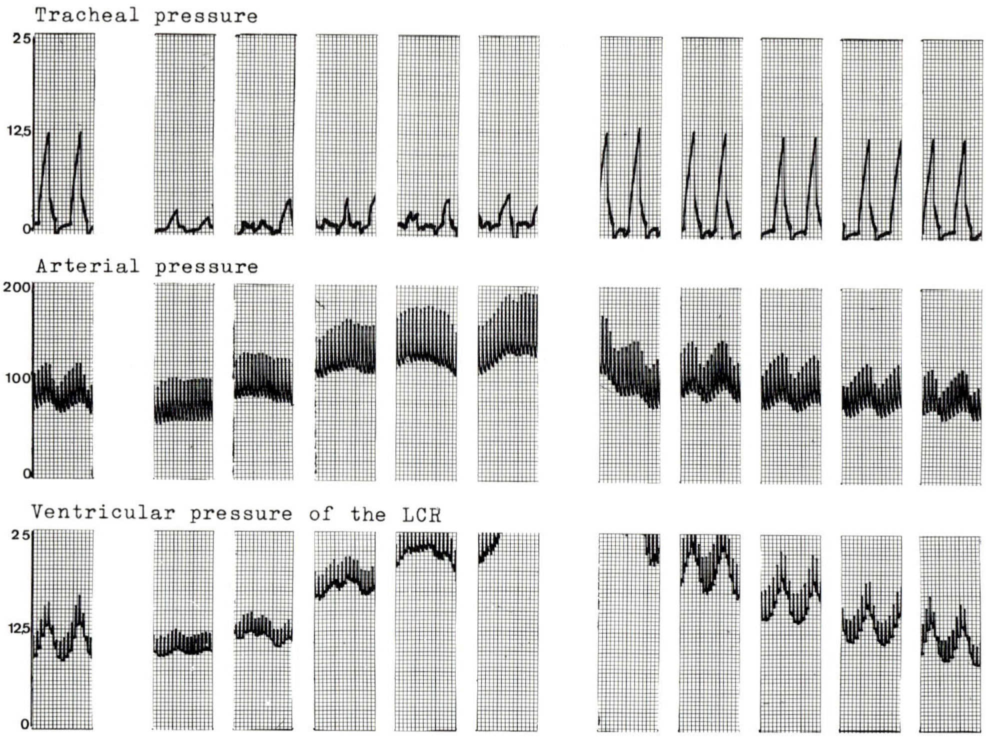

Vol/min	14 l	6 liters	14 liters
pH	7.45	7.38	7.45
P_{CO_2}	33	43	33
P_{O_2}	63	48	60

Fig. 2. Effect of accidental hypercapnia (respirator dysregulated)

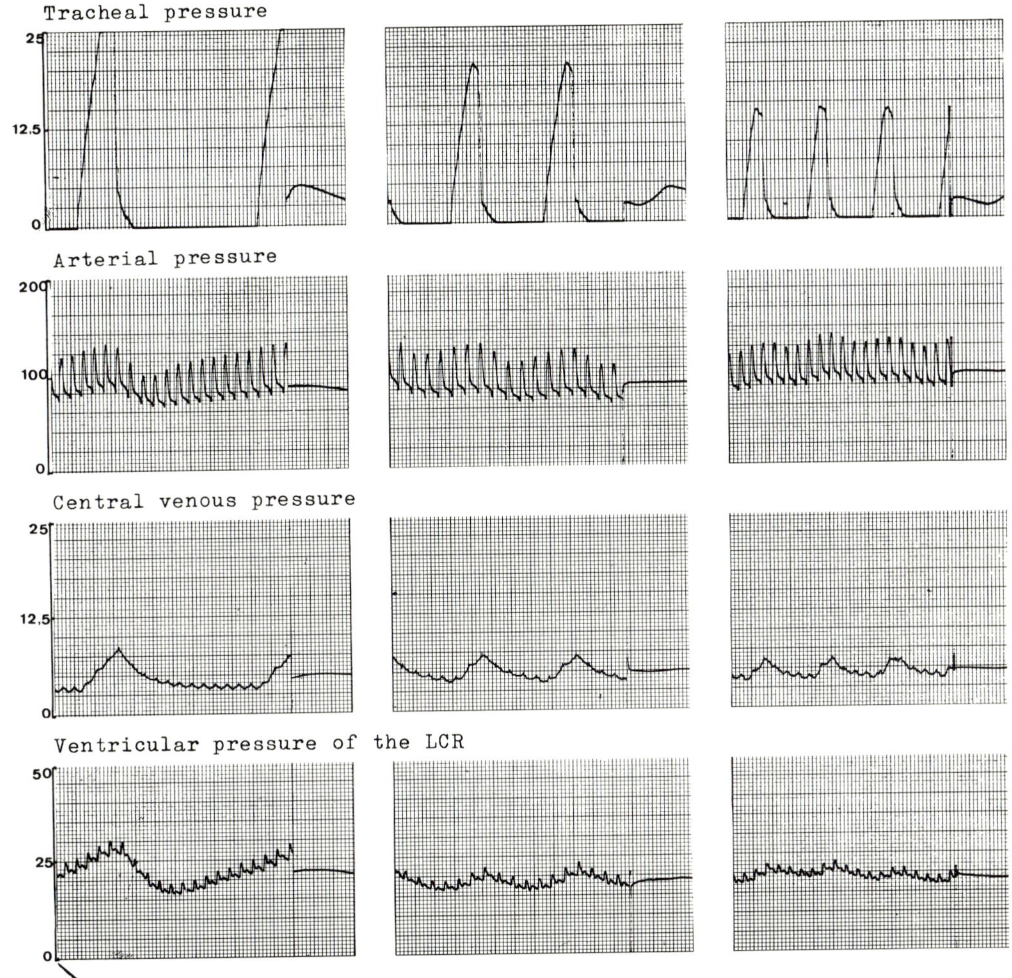

Pressure	0 + 25	0 + 20	0 + 15
pH	7.50	7.53	7.53
P_{CO_2}	27	26	26
P_{O_2}	84	93	96
F	10	20	30
I/E	1/3	1/2	1/2

Fig. 3. Effect of progressive lowering of the insufflation pressure with constant alveolar ventilation

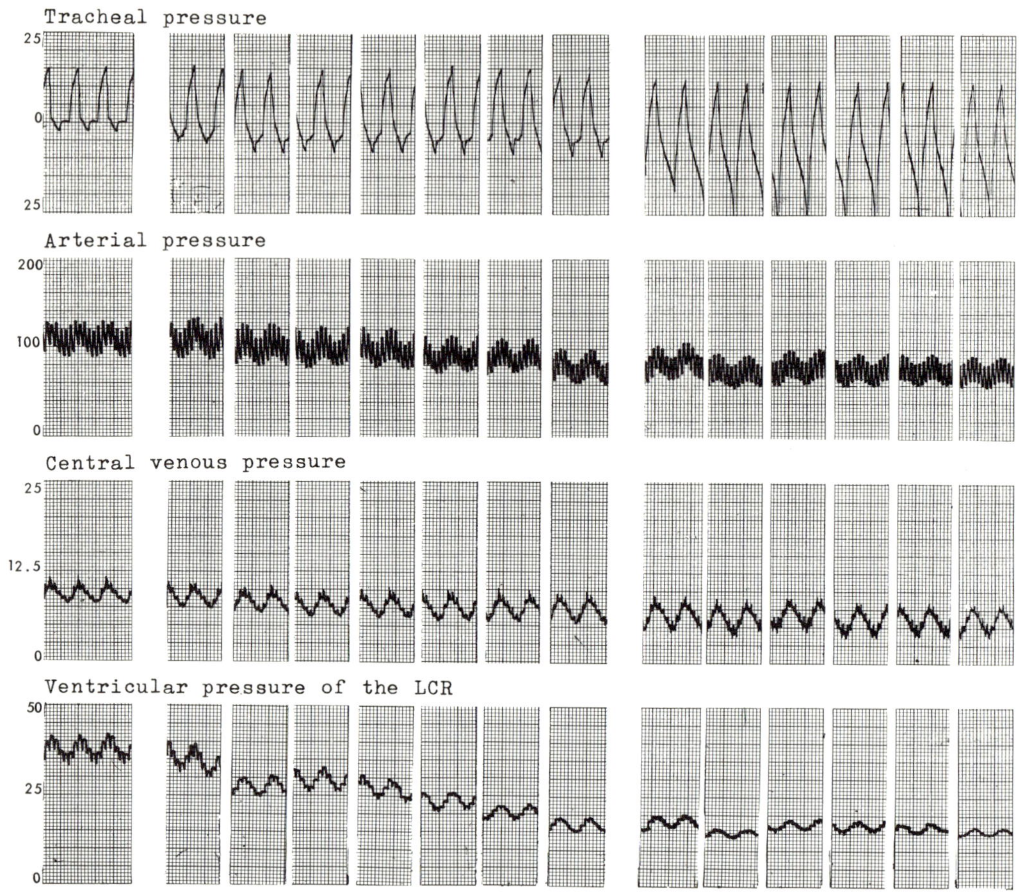

		0 10″ 20″ 1′ 2′ 3′ 4′	0 10″ 20″ 1′ 2′ 3′
Level of negative pressure		Slight negative pressure	Significant negative pressure
pH	7.45	7.56	7.61
P_{CO_2}	31	23	19
P_{O_2}	127	76	78

Fig. 4. Effects of different negative expiratory pressures

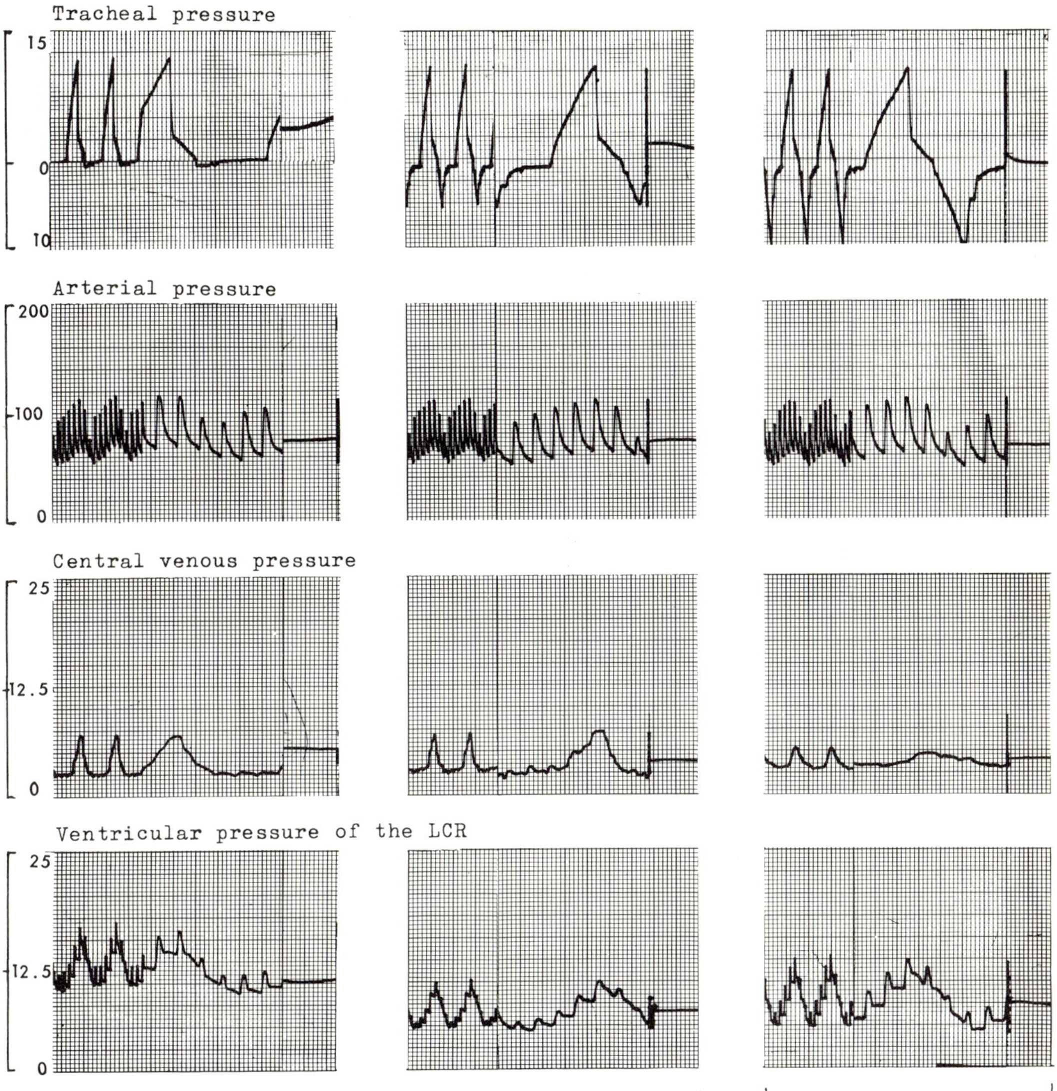

Pressure	0 +12	− 5 +11	− 10 +10
pH	7.45	7.52	7.49
P_{CO_2}	33	29	31
P_{O_2}	63	70	65

Fig. 5. Bronchiolar collapse and increase of CSFP by excessive negative pressure

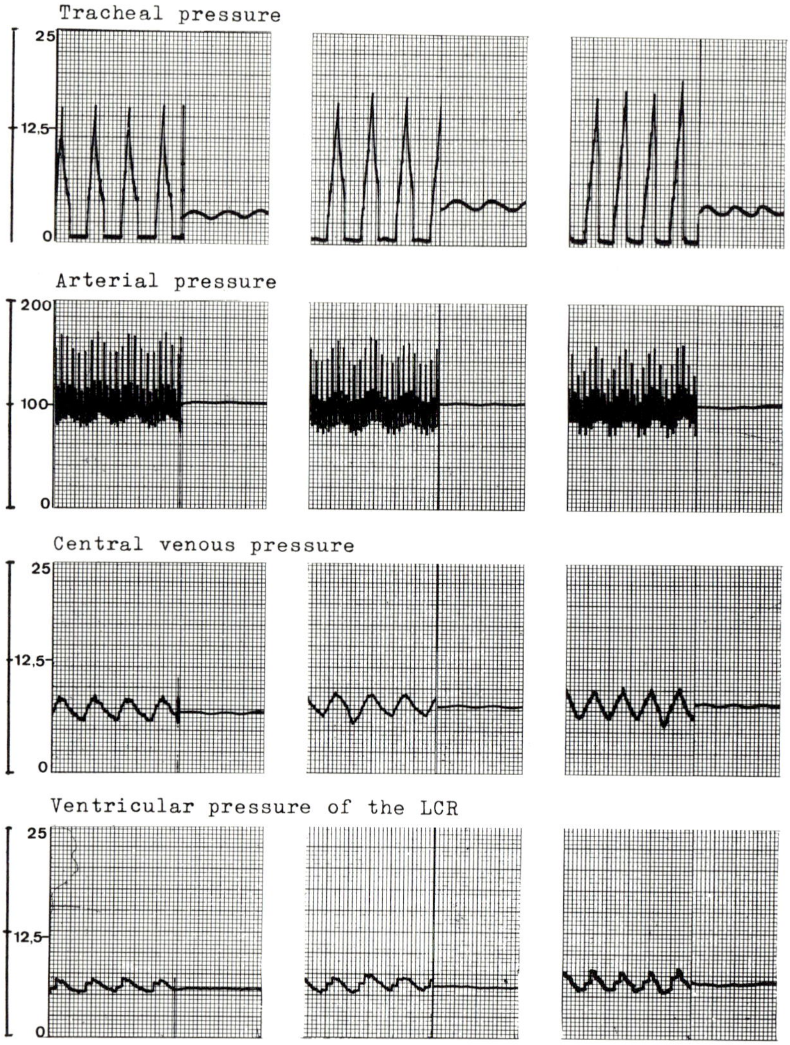

I/E	1/3	1/2	1/1
pH	7. 53	7. 55	7.53
P_{CO_2}	36	37	39
P_{O_2}	60	62	70
F	22	20	24
Vol/min	14 liters	13. 5 lit.	13 liters

Fig. 6. Influence of the variation of the I/E-ratio

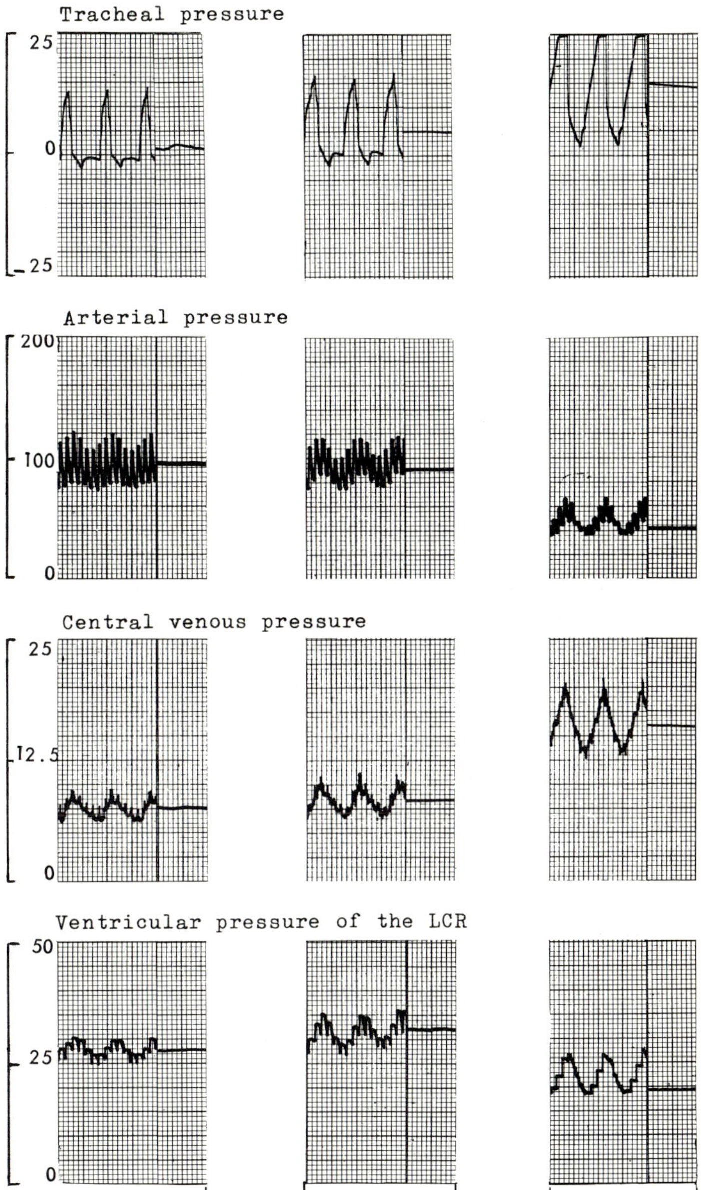

I/E	1/3	1/2	1/1
pH	7.44	7.45	7.51
P_{CO_2}	32	31	25
P_{O_2}	144	127	160

Fig. 7. Cardiac tamponade at an I/E-ratio of 1/1: "paradoxal" lowering of CSFP by hypocapnia and hypotension

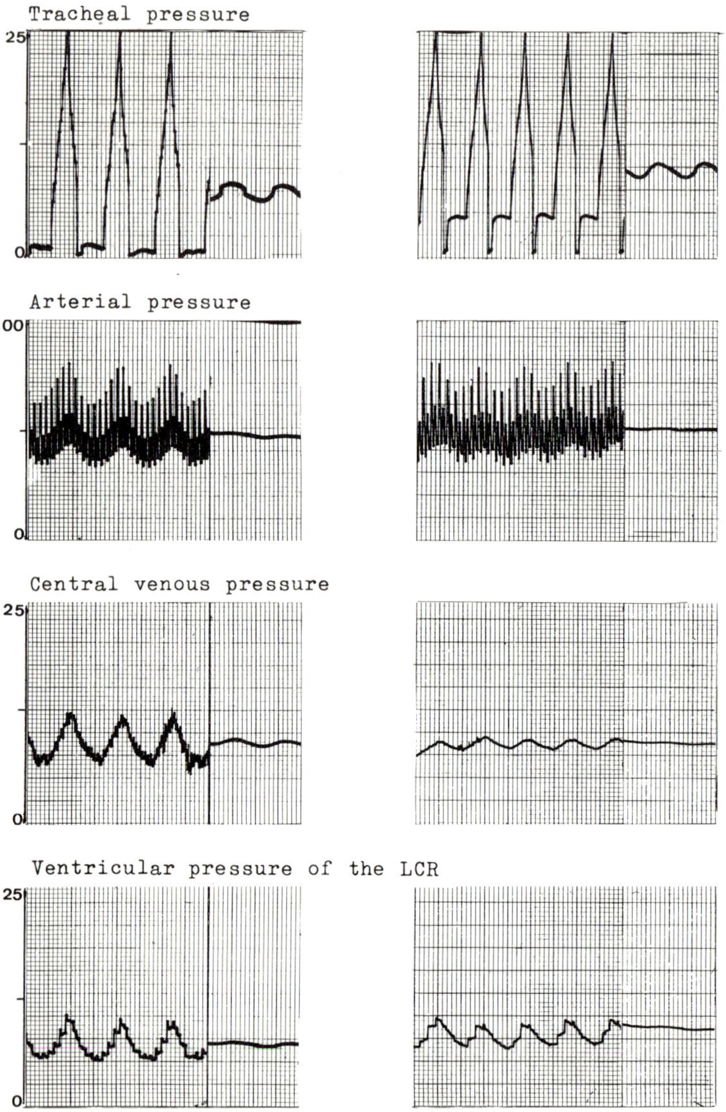

P	0+25	5 + 25
pH	7.52	7.51
P_{CO_2}	39	44
P_{O_2}	62	95

Fig. 8. The effect of PEEP: slight increase of CSFP by increase of CVP and PCO_2

The Influence of Ventilatory Changes on CSF Lactate and CSF L/P-Ratio in Brain Injury

R. SCHUBERT, T. WALLENFANG, H. J. REULEN, and K. SCHÜRMANN

Diagnostic and prognostic evaluation of patients with severe head injury by means of measurable values in an urgent and not yet satisfactorily fulfilled clinical need. In recent years changes in CSF lactate and pyruvate concentrations in patients with head injury have been pointed out by various authors with the suggestion to apply them to clinical diagnosis and prognosis. Lactacidosis and increased lactate/pyruvate ratio in CSF have been demonstrated in the pressure of serious damage of brain tissue, e. g. in patients with severe head injuries. CROCKARD and TAILOR (1) observed a correlation between the amount of CSF lactacidosis and prognosis, indicating that patients whose CSF-pH decreased below a certain level did not recover.

This study may elucidate if the CSF lactate concentration, respectively the lactate/pyruvate ratio, is a constant parameter for a certain pathological situation or if it may be additionally influenced by respiratory changes such as hyperventilation.

Method

In 40 cats a cold injury was inflicted to the right frontal cortex. 24 h later, at the culmination of the edema, the animals were kept under controlled ventilation. Groups of 10 cats were either normoventilated, hypoventilated or moderately or severely hyperventilated. Acid base status and mean arterial blood pressure were continously controlled. After a control period under normocapnia conditions pCO_2, pO_2, lactate and pyruvate in blood and CSF were determined. Following this the animals were ventilated appropriately for 2 hours. At the end of the examination the aforementioned samples were withdrawn and brain was momentaneously frozen with liquid nitrogen. Then lactate and pyruvate were measured in CSF and arterial blood as well as in the following brain areas such as 1. lesion; 2. adjacent region, 3. remote area; 4. in the uninjured contralateral hemisphere.

Results

Fig. 1 demonstrates the influence of ventilatory changes of the arterial pCO_2 on pCO_2 and CSF pH. Under normoxic normocapnic conditions the arterial pCO_2 is 28.9 mmHg, the pCO_2 of CSF is 31.6 mmHg and CSF pH is 7.441. Under hypocapnia the pCO_2 rises and the pH decreases, however, in case of moderate, as well as pronounced hypocapnia, a decrease of pCO_2 and an increase pH occurs.

Changes in lactate and pyruvate as well as in lactate/pyruvate ratio of CSF are represented in fig. 2. Under normoxic normocapnia ventilation a lactate concentration of 1.43 m Mol/lH_2O, a pyruvate of 0.14 m Mol/l H_2O and a lactate/pyruvate ratio of 11.2 was obtained. It is seen that the lactate concentration rises progrediently under moderate and pronounced hypocapnia. A rise of the arterial and CSF pCO_2 to approximately 70 mmHg causes a slight decrease of the pyruvate concentration whereas lactate remains unchanged. Because of these unproportional changes of both metabolites the lactate/pyruvate ratio increases significantly during hypocapnia, whereas during hypercapnia a moderate increase is observed.

In fig. 3 the lactate concentrations of the different brain areas are represented. The lowermost curve is to show the CSF lactate for purpose of comparison. The figure provides the relevant information that under normal, therefore normoxic, normocapnic conditions the highest lactate value occurs in the lesion area proper and in the directly adjacent tissue of the damaged hemisphere. Remote to the lesion, the lactate concentration is slightly increased in comparison to the contralateral undamaged hemisphere. In case of moderate and pronounced hypocapnia the lactate increases in all brain areas as well as in CSF. In reverse, CSF lactate remains unchanged under hypocapnia compared to normal conditions, whereas tissue lactate decreases in all regions. These results allow the conclusion that most likely the cause of the CSF lactacidosis is the local edema, which lead to a local decrease in blood supply and a local hypoxia. This edematous focus sustains the lactacidosis constantly.

These experimental results in animals were confirmed on various patients with severe head injuries whose intracranial pressure was continously controlled following operation by means of LUNDBERG's method as shown in the last figure. A moderate hypocapnic, a pronounced hypocapnic as well as a normoxic normocapnic and finally, a hypercapnic ventilation was performed under controlled conditions. Specimens of CSF were measured at intervals of 1 to 3 hours. Here also a clear tendency towards an increase under hypocapnia as well as a decrease under hypercapnia of the CSF lactate concentration becomes apparent. The lactate/pyruvate-ratio is lowest in moderate hypocapnia and rises in case of any other ventilatory change such as pronounced hypocapnia, normoxic normocapnia or hypercapnia.

Summary

The CSF lactate level is influenced not only by the extent of the head injury but also by the type of ventilation, i.e. the arterial pCO_2. In cases of low CO_2-values and increased pH a higher lactate is observed and, in reverse, a CSF lactate decrease is seen in the pressure of raised CO_2 values and decreased CSF pH. A diagnostic and prognostic statement by means of CSF metabolite concentrations should only be made if the type of ventilation is considered simultaneously, which means that a raised or decreased lactate concentration cannot be prognostically evaluated unless the arterial pCO_2 remains unchanged.

REFERENCES

1. CROCKARD, H.A. and A.R. TAYLOR: Arterial CSF lactate/pyruvate values as a guide to prognosis in head injury coma. In: Cerebral Blood Flow and Intracranial Pressure. S. Karger, Basel (1972)

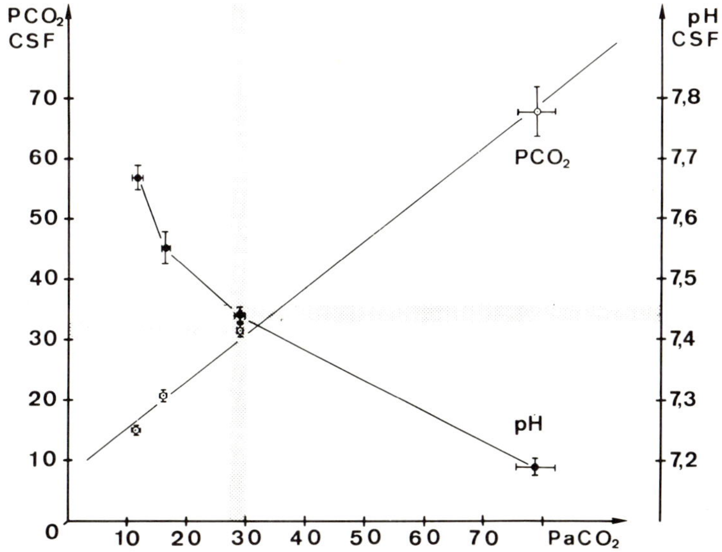

Fig. 1. CSF pH and CSF pCO_2 at an arterial pCO_2 of 11.5 mmHg, 16 mmHg, 29 mmHg, 76.6 mmHg

Fig. 2 and 3: see page 144/145

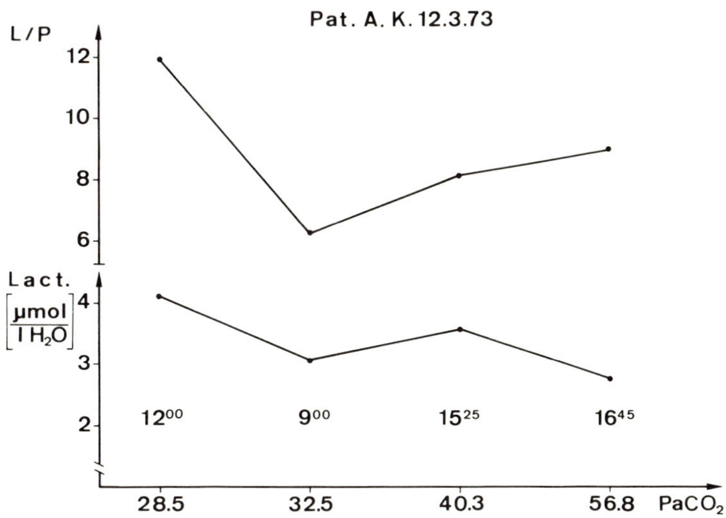

Fig. 4. CSF lactate concentration and CSF L/P-ratio of a patient, determined continuously under different ventilation types

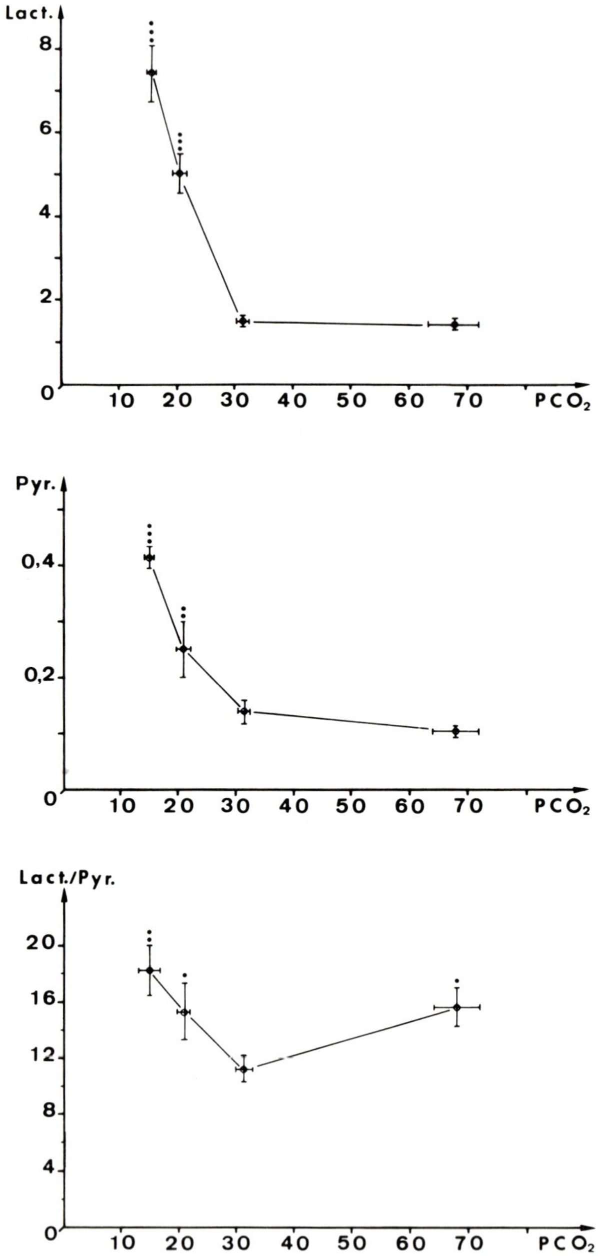

Fig. 2. Lactate and pyruvate concentrations mMol/l H_2O under changed ventilatory conditions. Lowest curve: L/P ratio. Significance: (Student t- test) + = P 0.05

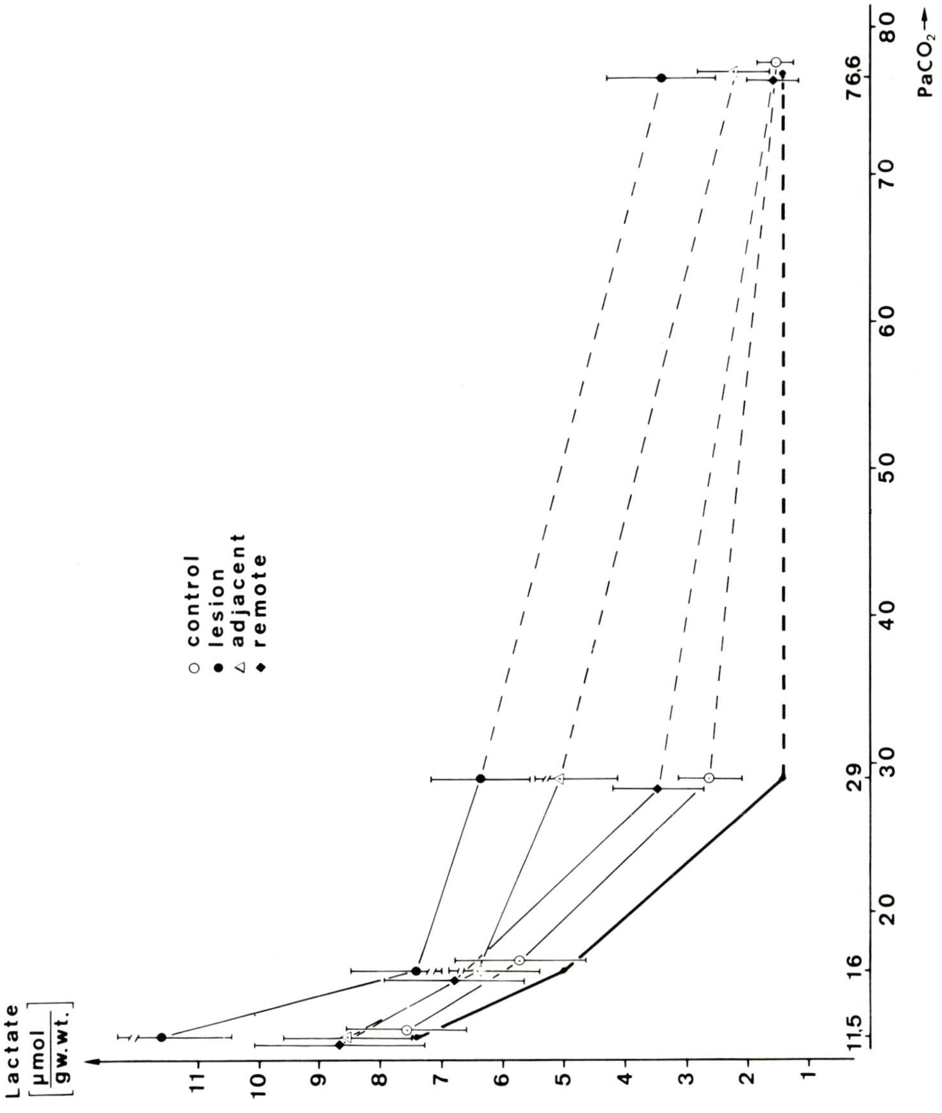

Fig. 3. Lactate concentration uMol/g w. wt. of the different brain areas. Lowest curve CSF lactate concentrations uMol/ml H_2O

Treatment of Cerebral Acidosis in Posttraumatic and Postoperative Cerebral Edema
Influence on CBF, EEG, and Clinical Status

E. METZEL, H. SCHRADER, H. D. SEITZ, M. HIRSCHAUER, H. ZIMMERMANN, W. E. ZIMMERMANN, and F. MUNDINGER

Severe cerebral acidosis, which is often accompanied by normal or only slight alterations in arterial blood-gas or acid-base levels, is shown by animal experiments to have three main causes:

1. respiratory, through hypoxia
2. cerebral, owing to a decrease in the cerebral blood flow (anoxidative metabolism)
3. direct lesion of brain tissue

Anyone of these three can by itself cause cerebral acidosis, which is always followed by a more or less pronounced cerebral edema. In the case of craniocerebral injuries acidosis is often caused by all three noxae.

For reasons of expediency we have divided our patients into three clinical stages. Fifty patients were examined altogether, and 10 patients in whom a suboccipital puncture had been performed for other reasons, were used for comparison.

Clinical stages of craniocerebral injuries

Stage I	No neurological symptoms brief unconsciousness no or only slight negetative symptoms normal EEG
Stage II	unconsciousness within 48 hours slight neurological symptoms moderate vegetative symptoms pathological EEG
Stage III	Coma severe neurological and vegetative symptoms severe pathological EEG

Fig. 1 shows the correlations between arterial and cerebrospinal fluid CSF values, the shaded areas indicating the respective normal range. With regard to pO_2 it is noteworthy that the seriously injured in particular show a reduction in oxygen tension. pH drops mainly in the CSF, wereas the arterial pH level may well stay within normal limits or even be raised. In severe cases the lactate is usually increased, more so in the CSF than in the arterial blood. In our experience the determination of the CSF lactate permits a prognosis to be made. The patients with a CSF lactate over 40 mg% either did not survive or developed extremely severe sequellae in the form of an apallic or dyspallic syndrome.

In some cases pCO_2 is decreased paralleling a syndrome of hyperventilation, or raised in the case of already impaired diffusion of ventilation.

+)Supported by Deutsche Forschungsgemeinschaft SFB 70 (IIIe)

Since, in our experience, it is not yet possible to ascertain the chief cause of acidosis in severe craniocerebral trauma on the basis of these parameters, therapy should aim at interrupting the vicious circle:

peripheral ventilation disturbances and/or cerebral edema cerebral hypoxia cerebral acidosis

from two sides.

1. The conventional methods of preserving and supporting the circulatory and respiratory functions usually permit normalization of gas tension levels in the CSF, but have hardly any effect on cerebral acidosis. There still remains a striking discrepancy between blood pH and CSF pH and also in the lactate levels.

2. While these parameters can be satisfactorily normalized in the arterial blood as a result of treatment, cerebral acidosis persists as an expression of the disturbed cerebral metabolism or of major lesions of cerebral tissue.

In case of severe persistent CSF acidosis we therefore attempted, after preliminary experiments with animals, to influence the CSF acidosis directly by giving sodium bicarbonate intrathecally. 35 patients have so far been treated in this way, in 10 of whom we measured rCBF by the clearance method. 6 patients have partially or completely recovered, one of whom is at present still under treatment. Only 4 of these patients are apallic.

All these cases were desolate patients, in which the severe clinical symptoms and the persistent metabolic CSF acidosis led us to expect an unfavourable outcome.

After being given sodium bicarbonate intrathecally these patients were controlled

1. clinically
2. by the Xe^{133}-rCBF clearance method according to LASSEN and INGVAR, 120 regions of one hemisphere being studied with a multicrystal camera
3. by EEG and EISA controls

In accordance with the findings of BALDY-MOULINIER and FREREBEAU et al. we observed a marked reduction of 45 % on average in the supply of blood to the brain in the acute stage of craniocerebral trauma. This was clearly related to the severity of the coma and to the CSF lactacidosis.

Following conversion of the flow-weighted intercepts of the biexponential X^{133}-clearance curves, it was seen that a reduction of the relative weight of the grey matter to half the norm was essentially responsible for the decrease in the mean total blood flow; evidently parts of the cortex assume the circulatory properties of the white matter.

Following intrathecal administration of sodium bicarbonate a marked blood flow increase to nearly every part of the brain can be seen. A decrease in cerebral blood flow was found in only 1 of 10 patients; in all other cases there was a more or less marked increase (Fig. 4). In the case of the one patient showing a decrease, however, the total blood flow had risen above the initial value 24 hours later.

The increase in blood circulation was demonstrated equally in both the grey and white matter. A tendency for the displaced relative weights to be normalized towards the fast compartment, however, was not observed.

Following the administration of bicarbonate the EISA showed a desynchronization lasting up to 2 hours with a decrease in the proportion of slow frequencies. Both are registered by the changes in the frequency spectrum and by the narrowing of the EEG tape.

EEG controls show that this effect disappears again after 2-3 hours and the slow frequencies then once more predominate.

This phenomenon has yet to be interpreted, just as the observed increase in blood circulation cannot be explained. The latter is difficult to reconcile with the common hypothesis that cerebral perfusion is solely dependent on pH. Animal experiments have shown that while intrathecal doses of sodium bicarbonate can increase blood circulation, giving THAM has but little effect and physiological saline solution none at all. To what extent CSF-regulating centres in the brainstem - as postulated by SHALIT et al. - may play a part here through neurogenic activation of the cerebral cortex need further elucidation.

Summary

1. In case of severe craniocerebral trauma a disturbance of the cerebral metabolism usually takes place in the form of lactate acidosis, caused on the one hand by the direct destruction of tissue with secondary hypoxia, and/or a ventilation disturbance as a result of unconsciousness, which again can lead to cerebral hypoxia. Cerebral hypoxia is,in its turn, closely related to cerebral edema.

2. Metabolic cerebral acidosis is closely correlated to the clinical state, cerebral blood flow and changes in EEG.

3. CSF and brain lactacidosis cannot be corrected by treatment in the periphery i. e. there may be alkalosis in the peripheral blood but marked acidosis in the CSF.

4. Intrathecal administration of sodium bicarbonate is a possible direct method of normalizing cerebral or CSF acid-base balance.

5. Intrathecal administration of sodium bicarbonate increases CBF significantly.

6. The patients examined to date indicate that the prognosis of unfavourable or even without any chance cases can be improved by means of this treatment.

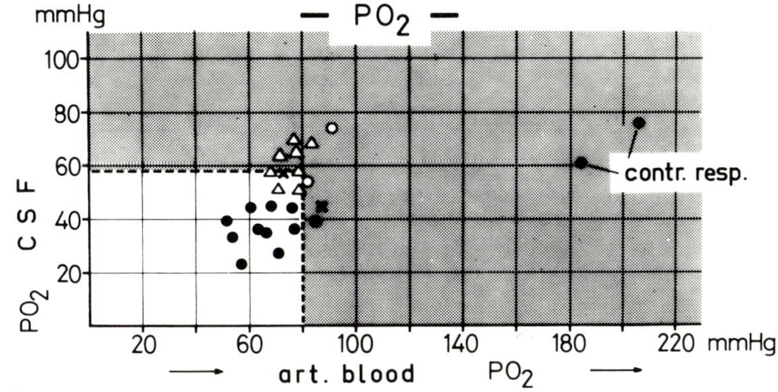

Fig. 1.a

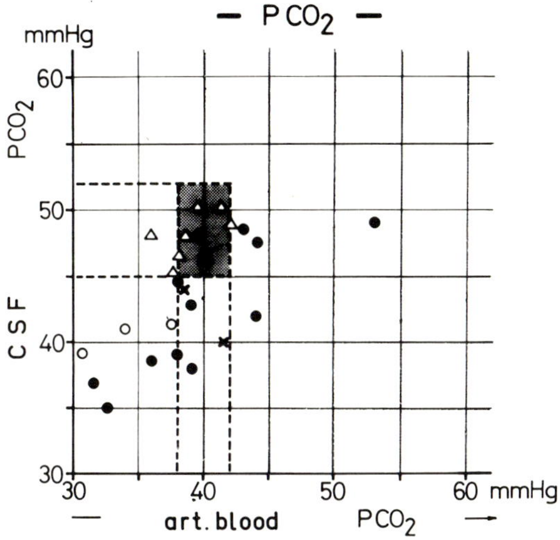

Fig. 1.b

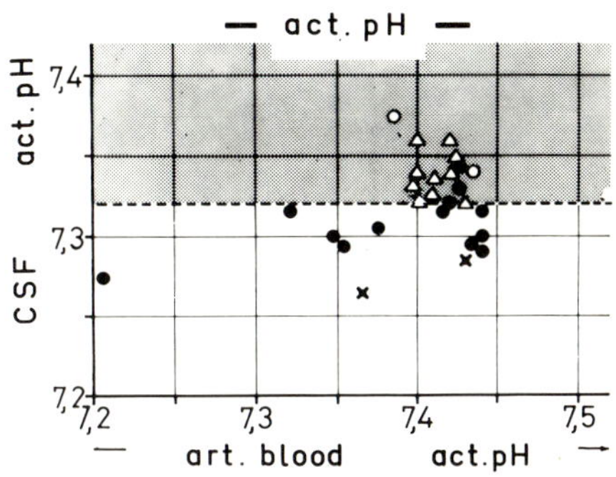

Fig. 1.c

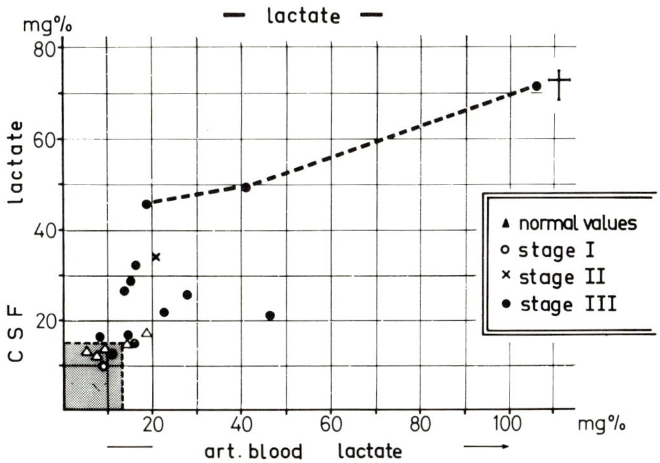

Fig. 1.d

Fig. 1. Correlations between CSF (ordinates) and arterial (abscissa) parameters in craniocerebral trauma of varying severity (2-3 days after injury)

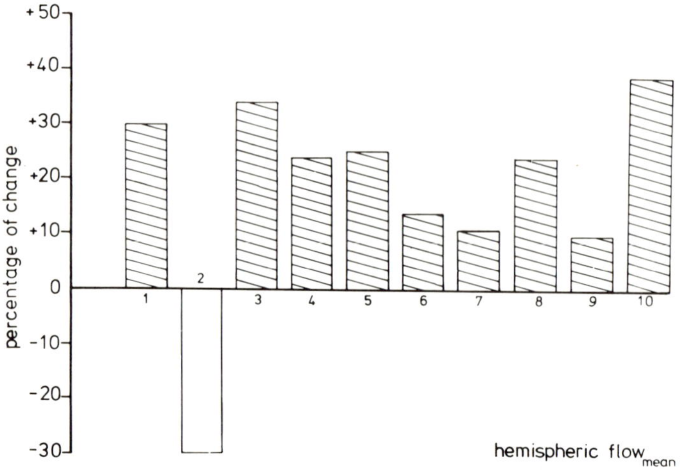

Fig. 2. Mean change in cerebral blood flow in 10 patients following treatment with sodium bicarbonate

Effect of Hyperbaric Oxygen on Intracranial Pressure in Brain Edema

D. MILLER

Introduction

Although hyperbaric oxygen (OHP) was considered early on in the treatment of generalised and focal cerebral ischemia it was only in 1966 that OHP was suggested as a therapeutic agent in the management of patients with increased intracranial pressure (ICP) and cerebral edema (1, 2, 18). The first claims for the efficacy of OHP in the treatment of brain edema and raised ICP were based on a reduction of mortality in experimental animals (rats and dogs) in which edema-causing brain lesions had been made. Clinical studies (4, 10, 19) reported temporary improvement in patients with various types of brain lesion, including trauma, associated with raised ICP.

In considering possible effects of OHP on the brain in states of raised ICP associated with brain edema, 3 possible mechanisms, operating simultaneously, may determine the final result. The first effect is of increased oxygen tension and content of the blood in reversing tissue hypoxia (for this to occur, tissue blood flow is necessary). The second possible effect of OHP is on the cerebral blood vessels themselves, rather than the parenchyma. OHP is known to have a mild vasoconstricting effect in several regions studied (9); although the mechanism of action of OHP on cerebral blood flow (CBF) has been disputed, vasoconstriction occurs (7, 8). The reduction of cerebral blood volume lowers ICP. Finally, high concentrations of oxygen in the tissues may have a toxic effect on metabolism at the cellular level, suggested by in vitro studies (5).

Five series of experiments have been undertaken by the author and his colleagues to investigate the second of these possible mechanisms, namely the physiological effects of OHP in experimental animals in which ICP had been artificially increased. Measurements were made of arterial blood pressure (BP), ICP, arterial and cerebral venous blood gases and CBF. All of the investigations were carried out in anesthetised, artificially ventilated mongrel dogs and took place in a large pressure chamber in the Hyperbaric Unit of the Western Infirmary, Glasgow, in which the investigators could remain with the experimental animal throughout the study. The dogs breathed a mixture of oxygen and nitrogen equivalent to a 20% oxygen mixture at normal atmospheric pressure (air equivalent), which could be changed to 100% oxygen under normo or hyperbaric conditions while maintaining normocapnia. In addition, at intervals throughout each experiment, 5% CO_2 was added to the inspired gas mixture to test reactivity of the cerebral vessels to carbon dioxide by observing the response of ICP, cerebral venous blood gases and, on occasions, CBF. The results of these investigations (11-14) may conveniently be summarised here.

Results

First series: ICP was increased by the inflation of an extradural balloon in 10 dogs. Administration of 100% oxygen at 2 atmospheres absolute (ATA) for periods of 15 minutes increased arterial PO_2 from 100 to over 1000 mmHg., raising arterial oxygen content by 3 ml/100 ml blood, and significantly reduced the high ICP by 37%. This reduction of ICP was accomplished without any significant alteration in BP or arterial PCO_2, but it did appear to depend upon retention of responsiveness of the cerebral blood vessels to changes in PCO_2. At a late stage in the experiments, when ICP was more than 70 mmHg. and inspired CO_2 failed to produce any further increase of ICP, then OHP failed to reduce ICP. At an earlier stage in the experiment, when inspired CO_2 did cause an increase in ICP, OHP invariably reduced ICP.

Second series (Table I): In this group of 7 dogs ICP was increased by application of a container filled with liquid nitrogen to the dura mater (1). OHP at 2 ATA was administered for 15 or 30 minute periods in the 6 hours following the production of the cryogenic brain lesion. The tenfold increase in the arterial PO_2 was associated with a 35% reduction in ICP, without any significant change in arterial PCO_2 of BP, but again this decrease in ICP occurred only in dogs who were able to respond to inhaled CO_2 by an increase in ICP. When OHP was successful in reducing ICP there was a significant increase in cerebral arterio-venous oxygen content difference, which, assuming a constant cerebral metabolic rate, was equivalent to a 19,5% decrease in total CBF.

Table I. Effect of OHP at 2 ATA for 30 minute periods. Results of 25 runs in 7 dogs with cerebral cold injury

	Air =	P value	OHP
ICP mmHg (M ± SE)	43.1 ± 2.9	<0.001	27.6 ± 2.2
MAP mmHg	114.2 ± 2.2	N.S.	114.1 ± 2.6
Arterial PCO_2	40.6 ± 0.6	N.S.	39.8 ± 0.5
Arterial PO_2	110.0 ± 2.7	<0.001	1208.0 ± 20.0
Cerebral arterio-venous oxygen content difference ml/100 ml	3.89 ± 0.59	<0.005	4.83 ± 0.62
Cerebral arterio-venous PCO_2 difference	9.42 ± 0.99	<0.001	12.04 ± 1.02

Third series (Table II): In a further 7 dogs cryogenic brain lesions were produced as described, but in addition, regional cerebral cortical blood flow was measured by [85]Krypton clearance in the hemisphere opposite to the cryogenic lesion during breathing of air equivalent and OHP and 2 ATA. In these experiments OHP was administered for 1 hour periods and was found to reduce ICP by 33% in the 5 CO_2-responsive dogs; this decrease in ICP was associated with a 19% decrease in cortical blood flow. When OHP was successful in reducing ICP, however, there was a significant increase in cerebral perfusion pressure (CPP = BP - ICP), since BP did not significantly change. It was thereby calculated that the fall in ICP and CBF due to OHP at 2 ATA was caused by a 42% increase in cerebrovascular resistance. Since this occurred without any change in arterial PCO_2 this was evidence of a direct vasoconstrictor action of OHP on responsive cerebral blood vessels during raised ICP and brain edema.

Table II. Effects of OHP at 2 ATA for 1 hour periods. Results of 13 runs in 5 dogs with cerebral cold injury

	Air =	P value	OHP
ICP mmHg (M ± SE)	43.0 ± 4.0	<0.001	30.0 ± 4.0
MAP mmHg	119.0 ± 3.0	N.S.	116.0 ± 2.0
CPP mmHg	76.0 ± 4.0	<0.001	86.0 ± 5.0
Arterial PCO_2 mmHg	40.5 ± 1.1	N.S.	40.4 ± 0.8
Arterial PO_2	105.0 ± 4.0	<0.001	1196.0 ± 29.0
rCBF ml/G/min	0.9 ± 0.13	<0.001	0.76 ± 0.11
rCVR mmHg/ml/100G/min	0.91 ± 0.09	<0.02	1.29 ± 0.23

Fourth series: Having shown that OHP reduced increased ICP by cerebral vasoconstriction, the purpose of this series was to compare OHP with another method of obtaining cerebral vasoconstriction, namely hypocapnia. Three groups of dogs were compared, 5 normocapnic, normoxic controls, 6 normocapnic dogs which received OHP for 4 hours commencing 1 hour after a cryogenic brain lesion, and 6 normoxic dogs which were hyperventilated to a mean arterial PCO_2 of 20 mmHg for 4 hours commencing 1 hour after the production of the brain lesion.

ICP rose slowly in controls over 6 hours, but was reduced by 26% in the OHP group and 34% in the hyperventilated group. CBF, calculated from arterio-venous oxygen content differences, was reduced by 13% in the OHP group and by 39% in the hyperventilated dogs. CSF lactate increased to 3 times the starting value in the control animals, by the same amount in the OHP group, but in the hyperventilated dogs CSF lactate rose twice as much as noted in other experiments involving hypocapnia(16, 17).

It was concluded that OHP at 2 ATA was a weaker cerebral constrictor than severe hypocapnia; the effects of OHP could be increased by accompanying hypocapnia and, more important, completely reversed by even mild hypercapnia. Hyperventilation, though more effective in reducing ICP, caused a greater reduction of CBF.

Fifth series (Table III): To test whether further increase in arterial PO_2 would intensify the vasoconstricting effects of oxygen, comparison was made in 5 dogs with cryogenic brain lesions of the effects of OHP at 2 ATA and at 3 ATA. When administering 100% oxygen, an increase in the ambient pressure from 2 ATA to 3 ATA increases arterial PO_2 from 1000 to approximately 2000 mmHg. This increases the dissolved oxygen content of the blood from 3 to 6 ml O_2/100 ml blood. (This is equivalent to the normal cerebral arterio-venous oxygen content difference).

OHP at 2 ATA caused, as before, a 30% decrease in ICP with a significant increase in cerebral arterio-venous PCO_2 and pH differences, consistent with a reduction in CBF. OHP at 3 ATA, on the other hand, caused only a transient decrease in ICP, which returned to control levels within 15 minutes despite the continued administration of OHP. There was no change in cerebral arterio-venous blood gas differences, suggesting that cerebral vasoconstriction was not occurring with OHP at 3 ATA. This final study showed that further increasing the arterial PO_2, far from intensifying the vasoconstricting action of OHP, actually abolished it.

Conclusions

OHP at 2 ATA produces a significant reduction in ICP which has been artificially increased in experimental animals both by inflation of intracranial balloons and by cerebral cold injury. This reduction of ICP is caused by cerebral vasoconstriction which is produced directly in the absence of changes of arterial PCO_2 or blood pressure. The reduction of CBF causes a fall in cerebral volume. The relation between this fall in volume and the resultant fall in ICP is determined by the intracranial volume/pressure curve (15). In addition, the effect of OHP on ICP depends on the presence and degree of vascular reactivity in the brain (as demonstrated by the effect of carbon dioxide on ICP). Finally, when the vessels are reactive, small increases in arterial PCO_2 can override the vasoconstrictor effect of OHP.

OHP at 3 ATA does not reduce CBF in normal dogs (9) and did not reduce ICP in the present study; it is possible that toxic effects of very high PO_2 levels cause anerobic glycolysis in the brain (5, 6), and by producing tissue acidosis reverse the cerebral vasoconstriction.

These experimental findings can be applied to recommendations for the use of OHP therapy in patients. For OHP to be effective in reducing ICP, cerebrovascular reactivity must be present and this points to the need for functional testing during continuous ICP monitoring of the effects of hypocapnia on ICP and of the intracranial volume/pressure status (15). Secondly, during administration of OHP, arterial PCO_2 must not be allowed to increase, as this will reverse the effects of OHP.

Lastly, the experimental findings suggest that a combination of moderate hypocapnia and OHP may be better than either agent alone.

Table III. Effect of OHP at 2 ATA (7 runs) and 3 ATA (13 runs) in 5 dogs with cerebral cold injury

	2 ATA			3 ATA		
	Air =	P	OHP	Air =	P	OHP
ICP mmHg (M ± SE)	42.1 ± 4.3	<0.005	28.3 ± 3.6	39.4 ± 3.4	N.S.	35.2 ± 2.6
MAP mmHg	111.0 ±12.0	N.S.	110.0 ±12.0	119.0 ± 7.0	N.S.	111.0 ± 7.0
CPP mmHg	69.0 ±10.0	<0.005	82.0 ± 9.0	80.0 ± 7.0	N.S.	76.0 ± 7.0
Arterial PCO_2 mmHg	38.2 ± 1.2	N.S.	38.8 ± 1.2	39.2 ± 0.7	N.S.	39.2 ± 0.6
Arterial PO_2 mmHg	94.9 ± 2.9	<0.001	1227.0 ±10.0	96.4 ± 1.7	<0.001	1891.0 ± 5.0
Cerebral venous PO_2 mmHg	48.0 ± 1.4	<0.02	78.4 ± 6.1	51.3 ± 2.0	<0.001	430.0 ±41.0
Cerebral a-v PCO_2 difference	8.5 ± 1.1	<0.05	12.2 ± 1.6	10.6 ± 0.6	N.S.	11.2 ± 0.9
Cerebral a-v pH difference	0.062 ± 0.013	<0.01	0.075 ± 0.011	0.060 ± 0.005	N.S.	0.057 ± 0.009

REFERENCES

1. CLASEN, R.A., D.L.BROWN, S.LEAVITT et al: The production by liquid nitrogen of acute closed cerebral lesion. Surg.Gynec. 96, 605-616 (1953)

2. COE, J.E. and T.M.HAYES: Treatment of experimental brain injury by hyperbaric oxygenation. Amer.Surg. 32, 493-495 (1966)

3. DUNN, J.E. and J.M. CONNOLLY: Effects of hypobaric and hyperbaric oxygen on experimental brain injury. In Proceedings of the 3rd International Conference on Hyperbaric Medicine, 447-454. Edited by I. W. BROWN and B.G. Cox. National Academy of Science: Wahington 1966

4. FASANO, V.A., G.BROGGI, R.URCIUOLI et al: Clinical applications of hyperbaric oxygen in traumatic coma. In Proceedings of the 3rd International Congress of Neurological Surgery. Edited by A.C. de Wets. Excerpta med. (Amsterdam) 110, 502-505 (1966)

5. HAUGAARD, N.: Cellular mechanisms of oxygen toxicity. Physiol.Rev. 48, 311-373 (1968)

6. HOLBACH, K.H., F.K.SCHRÖDER and S.KÖSTER: Alterations of cerebral metabolism in cases with acute brain injuries during spontaneous respiration of air, oxygen and hyperbaric oxygen. Europ.Neurol. 8, 158-160 (1972)

7. JACOBSON, I., A.M.HARPER and D.G.McDOWALL: The effects of oxygen under pressure on cerebral blood flow cerebral venous oxygen tension. Lancet 2, 549 (1963)

8. LAMBERTSEN, C.J., R.H.KOUGH, D.Y.COOPER et al: Oxygen toxicity: effects in man of oxygen inhalation at 1 and 3, 5 atmospheres upon blood gas transport, cerebral circulation and metabolism. J.appl.Physiol. 5, 471-486 (1953)

9. LEDINGHAM, I.McA: Hyperbaric oxygen. In "Scientific Foundations of Neurology". Edited by M. Critchley, J.O' Leary and B. Jennett. Heinemann London. 260-266 (1972)

10. LEDINGHAM, I.McA., D.C.McDOWALL and A.M.HARPER: Cerebral cortical blood flow under hyperbaric conditions; in Brown and Cox Hyperbaric medicine. Proc. 3rd Int.Conf.Publ.No. 1404, pp.243-248 (Nat.Acad.Sci.Natl.Res. Council, Washington) 1966

11. MOGAMI, H., T.HAYAKAWA, N.KANAI et al: Clinical application of hyperbaric oxygenation in the treatment of acute cerebral damage. J.Neurosurg. 31, 636-643 (1969)

12. MILLER, J.D., W.FITCH, I.McA.LEDINGHAM et al: The effect of hyperbaric oxygen on experimentally increased intracranial pressure. J.Neurosurg. 33, 287-296 (1970a)

13. MILLER, J.D., I.McA.LEDINGHAM and W.B.JENNETT: Effects of hyperbaric oxygen on intracranial pressure and cerebral blood flow in experimental cerebral edema. J.Neurol.Neurosurg.Psychiat. 33, 745-755 (1970b)

14. MILLER, J.D. an I.McA.LEDINGHAM: Reduction of increased intracranial pressure. Arch.Neurol.Chicago 24, 210-215 (1971)

15. MILLER, J.D.: The effects of hyperbaric oxygen at 2 and 3 atmospheres absolute and intravenous mannitol on experimentally increased intracranial pressure. Europ.Neurol. In Press

16. MILLER, J. D., J. GARIBI and J. D. PICKARD: The effects of induced changes of cerebro-spinal fluid volume during continuous monitoring of ventricular fluid pressure. Arch. Neurol. 28, 265-269 (1973)

17. PLUM, F. and J. B. POSNER: Blood and CSF lactate during hyperventilation. Amer. J. Physiol. 212, 864-870 (1967)

18. PLUM, F., J. B. POSNER and W. W. SMITH: Effect of hyperbaric, hyperoxic hyperventilation on blood, brain and CSF lactate. Amer. J. Physiol. 215, 1240-1244 (1968)

19. SUKOFF, M. H., S. A. HOLLIN, O. E. ESPINOSA et al: The protective effect of hyperbaric oxygenation in experimental cerebral edema. J. Neurosurg. 29, 236-241 (1968)

20. WÜLLENWEBER, R., U. GÖTT and K. H. HOLBACH: rCBF during hyperbaric oxygenation. In "Cerebral Blood Flow". Edited by M. Brock, C. Fieschi, D. H. Ingvar, N. A. Lassen and K. Schürmann. Springer Berlin, 1969, 271-272

Effect of Hyperbaric Oxygenation (HO) in Severe Injuries and in Marked Blood Flow Disturbances of the Human Brain

K.-H. HOLBACH

The real indication for the hyperbaric oxygenation therapy (HOT) in our specialty is the deficiency of oxygen in the brain tissue, since brain hypoxia is an essential factor of the following circulus vitiosus: primary brain lesion - hypoxia - hypoxic sequela (especially brain edema) - increased secondary hypoxia - secondary hypoxic brain lesions.

In order to minimize or prevent brain damage due to hypoxia more than 600 sessions of HOT were administered to patients with life-threatening brain injuries, mainly acute cerebrovascular lesions and severe postoperative cerebral edema, since 1967.

At the same time, various investigations were conducted and among other things the following results were obtained:

I. Hyperbaric oxygenation causes a marked rise in arterial oxygen pressure (Fig. 1) reaching the 8 to 10-fold at an inspiratory oxygen pressure of 1, 5 ata and about the 12 fold at an inspiratory oxygen pressure of 2, 0 ata as compared to the arterial oxygen pressures measured during spontaneous air breathing. On the other hand the oxygen pressure in the jugular bulb venous blood rises only slightly, resulting in marked increase in cerebral arteriovenous oxygen difference. This is an important factor for the tissue oxygen supply.

II. In the same group of patients we also studied the effect of the hyperbaric oxygenation on cerebral glucose metabolism (Fig. 2) as the essential source of the energy production in the brain.

Normally the cerebral arteriovenous difference (AVD) for oxygen is ~ 7, 0 vol %, for glucose ~ 10, 0 mg % and the negative AVD for lactate is ~ 0, 8 mg %. Subtracting AVD-lactate from AVD-glucose gives the amount of glucose that is oxydized by the amount of taken up oxygen. 1, 34 mg % of glucose are oxydized by 1 ml of oxygen, and therefore the normal glucose oxydation quotient (GOQ), expressing the ratio of AVD-glucose minus AVD-lactate divided by AVD-oxygen is 1, 34. On the other hand, we found during the initial phase of this study that while the patients breathed air spontaneously there was a low AVD-O_2 as compared to the exceedingly high amount of oxydizable glucose that remains available after subtracting the markedly increased AVD-lactate from the AVD-glucose.

On account of this uncompensated balance of the cerebral glucose metabolism the GOQ is far above its normal value demonstrating a reduced oxydative glucose metabolism and a compensatory increase of the unoxydative glucose metabolism, i. e. of the glycolysis. This indicates a deficient oxygen supply of the brain tissue resulting in a hypoxic hypoxydosis, i. e. an insufficient oxydative energy production of the brain tissue.

Compared to the initial state, we found during the second period - 10 min after changing from air to oxygen breathing - a significantly increased AVD-O_2 and a very distinct and significant decrease of AVD-glucose and of AVD-lactate. Therefore the GOQ was reduced. This change of the cerebral glucose metabolism is best characterized as the "Pasteur effect", the inhibition of glycolyses by oxygen.

During the third period of this study - 10 min after reaching an inspiratory oxygen pressure of 1, 5 ata - a well compensated balance of the cerebral glucose metabolism was found as indicated by the normal GOQ of 1, 35 showing that the AVD-O_2 corresponds to the available amount of oxydizable glucose. The biochemical pattern of the second and also of the third phase of this study indicates a sufficient oxygen supply and oxydative energy production of the brain.

Against that, we again found in the 4th period - 10 min after reaching an inspiratory oxygen pressure of 2, 0 ata - a much too high AVD-glucose respectively a too great amount of oxydizable glucose in relation to the AVD-O_2, resulting in an uncompensated balance of the cerebral glucose metabolism and in a marked rise of the GOQ. This, as already seen in the initial period again shows a marked stimulation of the glycolysis and indicates a disturbance of the oxydative glucose metabolism and an insufficient energy production of the brain, i.e. an hypoxydosis.

In contrast to the hypoxic hypoxydosis of the initial phase the hypoxydosis of this 4th phase cannot be caused by too low oxygen pressure but must be caused by the high oxygen pressure leading to an oxygen toxicity of the brain, especially because higher oxygen pressures have an inhibitory effect on the oxydative metabolic pathways. Therefore this probably refers to a hyperoxic hypoxydosis, showing, that patients with severe brain lesions at least to some extent do not tolerate an inspiratory oxygen pressure of 2, 0 ata resulting in alterations of the cerebral glucose metabolism.

As a typical, immediately appearing sequela of this hyperoxic hypoxydosis we find during the 5th phase of the examination - 10 min after complete decompression continuously respiring oxygen - and especially during the last period - 10 min after changing from oxygen to air breathing - a much too low AVD-glucose in relation to the AVD-O_2.

This indicates a disturbance of the cerebral glucose uptake and thus shows a disturbed function of the blood brain barrier.

III. Furthermore we simultaneously studied the acid base balance in this group of patients and especially found that the lactate concentration (La) and the lactate-pyruvate-quotient (L/P) of the cerebrospinal fluid (CSF) (Fig. 3a) reflected the alterations of the cerebral glucose metabolism seen under the different inspiratory oxygen pressures (IOP). For we observed a considerable decrease of the La and of the L/P up to an IOP of 1, 5 ata. This indicates an increase of the oxydative glucose metabolism and a reduction of the unoxydative glycolysis, thus showing an improvement of the oxygen supply of the brain tissue.

Against that the La and L/P enormously rise at an IOP of 2, 0 ata and thus show like the corresponding alteration of the cerebral glucose metabolism the hyperoxic hypoxydosis. After complete decompression we observed in the 5th and in the last period of the examination a fading away of these metabolic changes in the CSF.

As the examinations of the cerebral metabolism in another group of patients with severe traumatical brain lesions showed (Fig. 3b) such an oxygen toxicity, i.e. a hyperoxic hypoxydosis does not occur if the IOP is not elevated above 1, 5 ata. But in doing so we found a continuous reduction of La and of L/P in the CSF.

This indicates an increasing and continuing improvement of the cerebral oxygen supply and thus also an improved oxydative, more energy producing, cerebral glucose metabolism.

IV. These laboratory findings also correspond to the following clinical results obtained by the application of HOT and already comprised in 1971. At this time we had given 267 courses of HOT to 102 patients. From these 102 patients 52 had been treated with an IOP of 2-3 ata and 50 with an IOP of 1, 5 ata. Comparing the results of these two groups we find only in 25 % a marked and in 52 % no improvement in the patients that were treated with IOP of 2-3 ata. Against that, we observed in the 50 cases that were treated with an IOP of 1, 5 ata a considerable improvement in 48 % and no improvement in 36 %. This comparison showed a statistically significant, much more favourable clinical result to the patients who had been treated with the lower IOP of 1, 5 ata.

V. We also investigated the effect of HO on the regional cerebral blood flow (rCBF) in another group of patients with traumatic brain lesions using a fluvograph. The rCBF measurements (Fig. 4) were made with a needle thermocouple deeply implanted in the affected brain hemisphere. The results showed a decrease of rCBF during the rise of the IOP and an increase of rCBF during the decrease of the elevated IOP. This demonstrates the cerebral vasoconstriction caused by the increasing IOP, especially since the arterial PCO_2 and the arterial pH and the arterial blood pressure practically remained unchanged.

On account of these laboratory findings and of the clinical results we can assume that patients with considerable brain lesions having a hypoxic hypoxydosis of the brain can well be treated with an IOP of 1, 5 ata improving the clinical course of their condition. However, exposing such patients to an IOP higher than 1, 5 ata will at least partly result in adverse effects, affecting the oxydative glucose metabolism and the cerebral glucose uptake. For the favourable effect of HO the following factors are of considerable importance:

1. HO improves the oxygenation of the brain tissue by the enormous rise of the arterial oxygen pressure.

2. HO reduces the brain pressure by cerebral vasoconstriction. This is very favourable for the perfusion and oxygenation of the affected, hypoxic edematous regions of the brain.

3. The improved oxygenation of the brain tissue causes an increase of the oxydative glucose metabolism and thus also a rise of the cerebral energy formation. At the same time the unoxydative cerebral metabolism, the glycolysis is reduced causing a decrease of the La and of the L/P and therefore also a reduction of the cerebral lactacidosis.

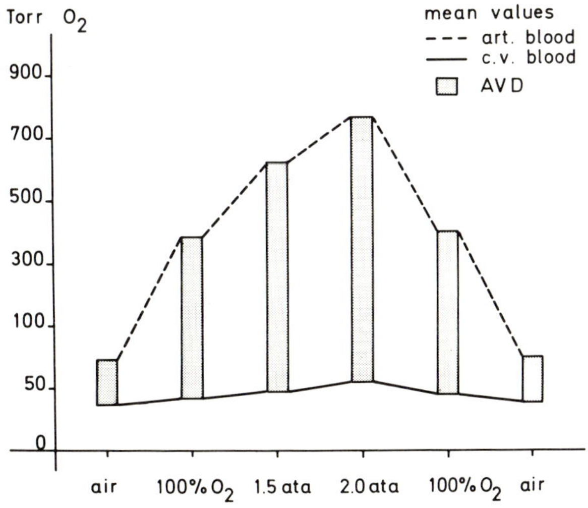

Fig. 1. Mean arterial and cerebral venous oxygen pressure (PO_2) at different inspiratory PO_2 in a group of 13 patients treated with HO

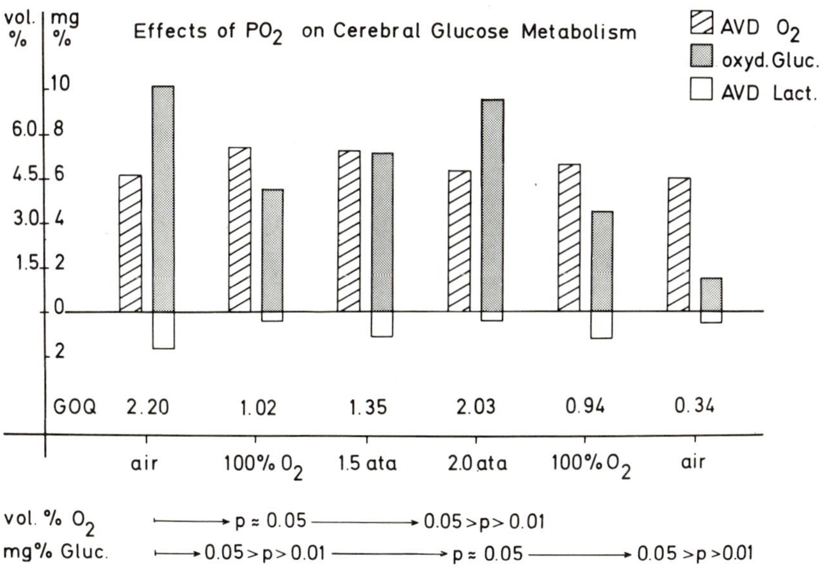

Fig. 2. Mean arterio-cerebral venous differences (AVD) of oxygen represented by the columns with diagonal lines and of glucose and of lactate. The AVD-glucose is represented by the total columns next to the ones of AVD-O_2. From the total AVD-glucose the AVD-lactate is substracted and indicated within the AVD-glucose columns beneath the baseline. After that the amount of oxydizable glucose remains and is indicated by small dots within the columns of AVD-glucose above the baseline

We chose the measure on the ordinate for AVD-O_2 (vol %) and for AVD-glucose (mg %) so that each volume of oxygen taken up by the brain simultaneously indicates the amount of glucose that can be oxydized by it. This makes it possible to visualize the balance of the cerebral glucose metabolism also being reflected by the corresponding GOQ

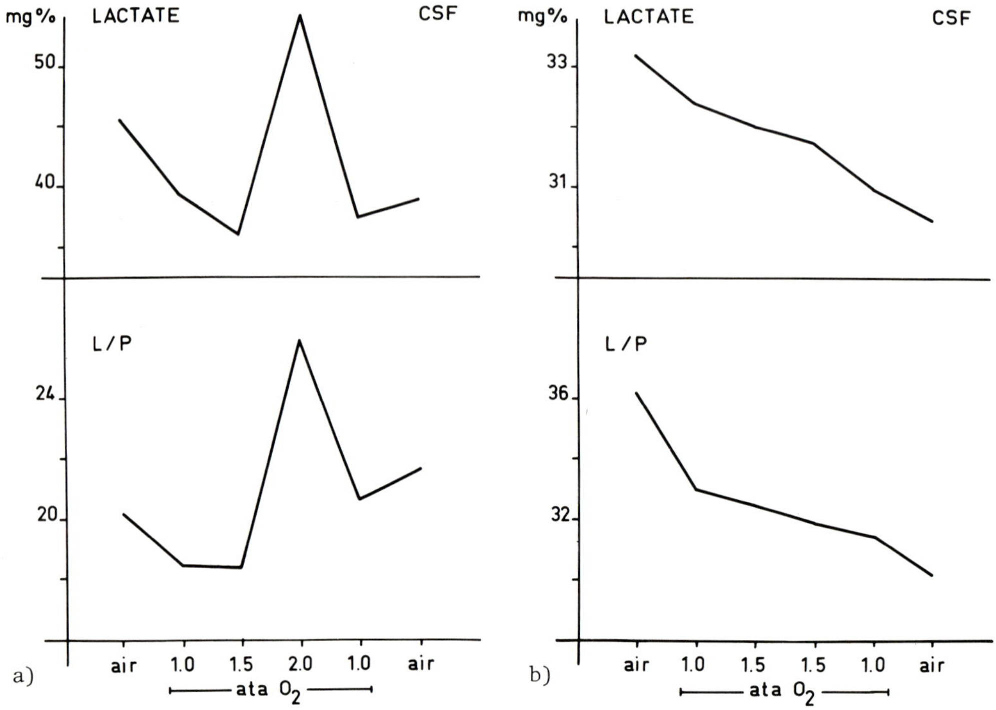

a) b)

Fig. 3. a) In the same group of patients we simultaneously measured the lactate and pyruvate concentration in the CSF and calculated the L/P

b) In another group of posttraumatic cases only exposed to an inspiratory oxygen pressure of 1, 5 ata the same parameters were studied

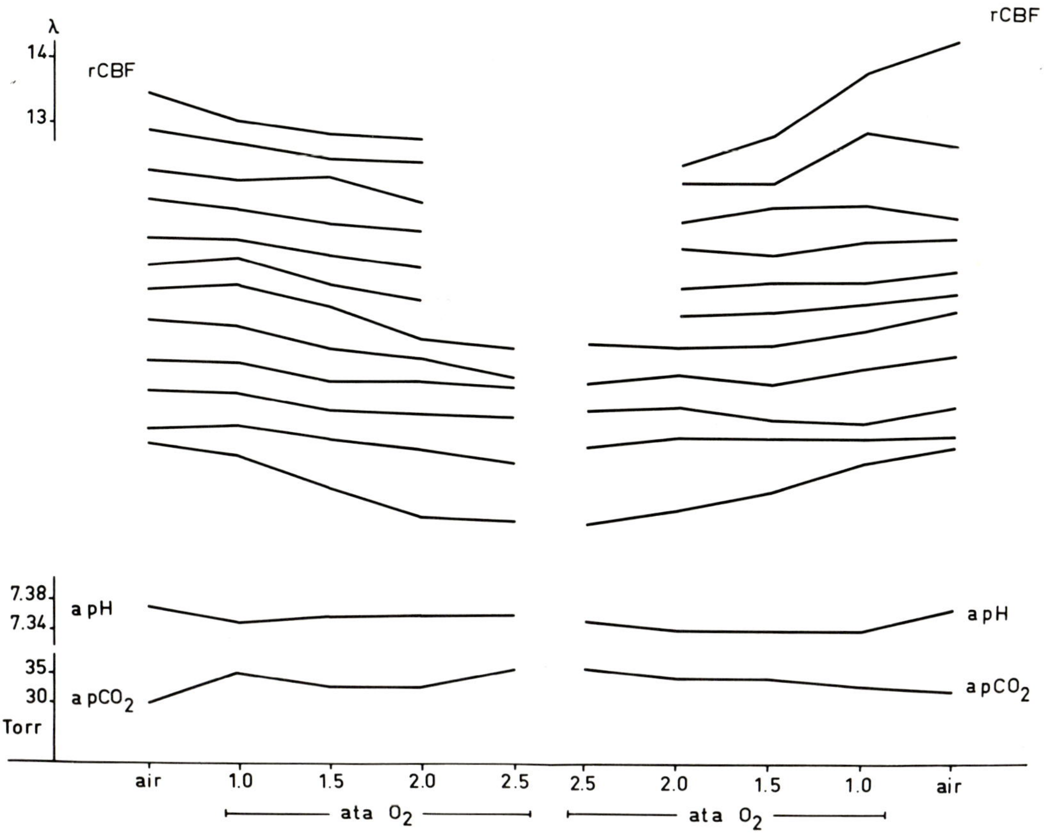

Fig. 4. In a further group of posttraumatic cases rCBF, $aPCO_2$, apH and also aBP (the latter is not shown in the figure) were simultaneously measured during courses of HOT

Chapter III.

Intracranial Pressure, Cerebral Blood Flow and Metabolism

The Effects of Hypercarbia on Cerebral Blood Flow and Carbohydrate Metabolism in Deep Normovolemic Arterial Hypotension

J. HAMER, S. HOYER, H. STOECKEL, E. ALBERTI, and P. PACKSCHIES

In the last decade both clinical studies and animal investigations have shown that lowering the systemic arterial blood pressure to values of about 50 mmHg will leave cerebral blood flow (CBF) unchanged due to a decrease of the cerebro-vascular resistance (LASSEN 1959, HIRSCH and KÖRNER 1964, RAPELA and GREEN 1964, HÄGGENDAL and JOHANSSON 1965, HARPER 1965, 1966). The ability of the brain to keep the blood flow constant over a certain range of falling cerebral perfusion pressure (CPP) has been termed autoregulation (AR) of the cerebral circulation. In addition, COHEN et al. 1964, WOLLMAN et al. 1964, ALEXANDER et al. 1965, RAICHLE et al. 1970 and GOTTSTEIN et al. 1971 could demonstrate that with a decrease of CBF in hypocapnia the cerebral arterio-venous differences of oxygen and glucose will increase in a compensatory fashion, thus keeping the corresponding cerebral metabolic rates ($CMRO_2$ and CMR glucose) constant.

The present investigations contribute to the question as to how these important parameters of the oxydative cerebral metabolism change below the autoregulatory range and, in particular, how hypercapnia influences CBF, the av-differences of O_2 and glucose and the cerebral output of lactate in this stage.

Material and methods

In 10 halothane (0, 5 vol. %) anesthetized, artificially ventilated normoxic-normocapnic mongrel dogs CPP (defined as the difference between mean systemic arterial blood pressure and mean intracranial CSF-pressure) was decreased in a stepwise fashion to values of about 70 mmHg (stage I) and to 40 mmHg (stage II) by controlled intravenous injections of Trimethaphan (Arfonad^{R}). After maintaining steady state conditions over 30 minutes, the following measurements were carried out in the resting state and in the two mentioned CPP-stages:

1. CBF, 2. av oxygen and glucose differences, 3. cerebral lactate output. Cerebral blood flow was determined by means of the KETY-SCHMIDT technique modified by BERNSMEIER and SIEMONS (1953). The volume of oxygen was measured by gas chromatography, the concentrations of glucose and lactate enzymatically. pH, PCO_2, base excess and standard bicarbonate were determined in the Astrup apparatus and controlled before and immediately after the single measurements. Blood samples were taken from the femoral artery and from the superior sagittal sinus. At stage II (mean CPP 43 mmHg), the abovementioned measurements were also performed under hypercapnic conditions, after inhalation of 5 % CO_2. During the investigations the body temperature of the experimental animal was kept at a normothermic level. Statistical calculations were based on the FRIEDMAN- and the STUDENT-test.

Results

Table I contains the mean values (n=10) of CBF and of the corresponding parameters of cerebral carbohydrate metabolism at different steps of decreased CPP and at a normocapnic level (mean $PaCO_2$:34, 3 Torr) and at a hypercapnic state (mean $PaCO_2$:82, 6 Torr). Statistical significances are marked by asterisks. While decreasing mean CPP from 98 mmHg to 71 mmHg, under normocapnic conditions, neither CBF nor $(A-V)O_2$ and $CMRO_2$ were altered. Glucose utilization and cerebral output of lactate, however, were increased. A further fall of CPP to a mean value of 41 mmHg was accompanied by a highly significant decrease of CBF for about 51 % of the corresponding resting values. Although the av oxygen and glucose differences increased, O_2 and glucose utilization was not sufficient, with regard to the sharp drop of CBF, to keep the corresponding cerebral metabolic rates constant.

Table I

	$PaCO_2$ 34, 3 Torr			$PaCO_2$ 82, 6 Torr
CPP , (mm Hg)	98, o	71, o	41, o	43, o
CBF , (ml/100g min)	65, 6	64, 1	32, 2^{+++}	64, 6^{+++}
$(A-V)O_2$, (vol. %)	6, 63	6, 94	9, 13^{+}	6, 69^{+}
$CMRO_2$, (ml/100g min)	4, 19	4, 38	2, 89^{+}	4, 17^{++}
(A-V)glucose , (mg%)	7, 3	9, 5	10, 5^{+}	3, 8^{+++}
CMRglucose , (mg/100g min)	4, 6	6, 2	3, 3^{+}	2, 6
(V-A)lactate , (mg%)	0, 45	2, 56^{++}	3, 75	o, 96^{+}
CMRlactate , (mg/100g min)	0, 33	1, 62^{+}	1, 14	o, 63^{+}

$^{+}P < 0,005$; $^{++}P < 0,01$; $^{+++}P < 0,001$

Furthermore, the cerebral formation of lactate was markedly augmented in this pressure stage (II): In contrast to 7 % of glucose metabolized to lactic acid in the resting state, the glycolytic formation rate amounted to 34 % at a CPP of about 40 mmHg.

With raising of the $PaCO_2$ to 82, 6 Torr on an average, CBF increased in 9 of 10 preparations, reaching almost the resting values or even exceeding them. Whereas $CMRO_2$ improved according to the rise of CBF, (A-V)glucose decreased significantly in all preparations under hypercapnic conditions, and CMR glucose was further lowered in spite of improved blood flow (see figures 1 and 2). Furthermore, hypercapnia induced a significant decrease of (V-A) lactate (see figure 3).

Discussion

The present investigations have shown that at a CPP of about 40 mmHg AR is abolished and the carbohydrate metabolism of the brain is severely disturbed. On the contrary, at a moderate reduction of CPP to values of about 70 mmHg, AR is still effective, probably due to a compensatory rise of cerebral lactate production. The autoregulatory mechanisms, however, do not bring about maximal vasodilatation, since, below the autoregulatory range, cerebral vessels may still be responsive to increased $PaCO_2$ and thus be further dilated (see figure 4). Although hypercarbia may have a beneficial effect on CBF, it will cause, on the other hand, a considerable inhibition of glucose metabolism. In this regard, our investigations are consistent with the experimental results of DOMONKOS and HUSZAK 1959, COHEN et al. 1964, WEYNE et al. 1970 and JAMES et al. 1971.

We have demonstrated, in another experimental study on normoxic normotensic dogs (ALBERTI et al., unpublished data), that the inhibitory effect of hypercapnia on cerebral carbohydrate metabolism seems to be dependent on the degree of raised $PaCO_2$. Below a $PaCO_2$ of about 60 mmHg, there is apparently no inhibition of cerebral metabolism. The underlying mechanisms of this inhibitory effect of hypercarbia are still poorly understood. Possibly, with falling arterial pH in respiratory acidosis, the intracellular pH-optimum for enzymatic reactions of carbohydrate metabolism may be deteriorated and thus glucose uptake inhibited (SIESJÖ et al. 1972). On the other hand, the possibility of CO_2-fixation in intermediary metabolism should be discussed (WAELSCH et al. 1964). It is well known by the so-called Ochoa-reaction that, due to a reducing carboxylation, pyruvate can be changed to malate which easily converts to oxalacetate which, together with acetyl-CoA, reacts at the beginning of the TCA-cycle. If in hypercarbia the Ochoa-reaction were accelerated, the reducing carboxylation of pyruvate would explain why in hypercapnia lactic acid, the product of reduced pyruvate in glycolysis, must be decreased and why, furthermore, a hypercapnic influence on the TCA-cycle may result in lowered cerebral metabolism of glucose.

The decrease in lactate formation under hypercapnia and, vice-versa, an increased output of lactate in hypocapnia have been found by many investigators (BAIN and KLEIN 1949, DOMONKOS and HUSZAK 1959, ALEXANDER et al. 1965, LEUSEN et al. 1966, WEYNE et al. 197o). In particular, the fundamental experimental studies of DOMONKOS and HUSZAK and of LEUSEN and coworkers have provided evidence of an intracellular pH-dependence of lactate formation in the brain. Thus, lactic acid seems to have a rather important biochemical regulatory function in the cerebral acid-base equilibrium.

With special regard to raised intracranial pressure, cerebral vasodilatation and further increase of intracranial blood volume under hypercapnic conditions, below the autoregulatory range, may be of great clinical importance. LANGFITT and associates (1965) have shown that the intracranial pressure-volume relationship is not linear, but corresponds to an exponential function. Thus, from a certain point on the pressure-volume curve, a relatively small increase of intracranial volume may provoke an unproportional rise in intracranial pressure. Therefore, hypercarbia may have deleterious effects in cases of raised intracranial pressure.

In accordance with the clinical observations of BRUCE, LANGFITT and MILLER (1973), our results suggest that an increase of CBF cannot always be regarded as an absolutely reliable criterion for improvement of the cerebral metabolic state. Further pertinent determinations of other metabolic parameters as $CMRO_2$ and

CMRglucose and output of lactate etc. will better help to understand the complex changes in cerebral functions.

REFERENCES

1. ALEXANDER, C.S., P.J. COHEN, H. WOLLMAN, T.C. SMITH, M. REIVICH and R.A. van der MOLEN: Cerebral carbohydrate metabolism during hypocarbia in man. Studies during nitrous oxide anesthesia. Anesthesiology 26, 624-632 (1965)

2. BAIN, J.A. and J.R. KLEIN: Effect of carbon dioxide on brain glucose, lactate, pyruvate and phosphates. Am. J. Physiol 158, 478-484 (1949)

3. BERNSMEIER, A. und K. SIEMONS: Die Messung der Hirndurchblutung mit der Stickoxydulmethode. Pflügers Arch. ges. Physiol. 258 249-162 (1953

4. BRUCE, D.A., T.W. LANGFITT, J.D. MILLER, H. SCHUTZ, M.P. VAPALAHTI, A. STANEK and H.I. GOLDBERG: Regional cerebral blood flow, intracranial pressure, and brain metabolism in comatose patients. J. Neurosurg. 38 131-144 (1973)

5. COHEN, P.J., H. WOLLMAN, S.C. ALEXANDER, P.E. CHASE and Ph.D. BEHAR: Cerebral carbohydrate metabolism in man during halothane anesthesia. Effects of $PaCO_2$ on some aspects of carbohydrate utilization. Anesthesiology 25, 185-191 (1964)

6. DOMONKONS, J. and I. HUSZAK: Effects of hydrogen-ion concentration on the carbohydrate metabolism of brain tissue. J. Neurochem. 4, 238-243 (1959)

7. GOTTSTEIN, U., W. BERGHOFF, K. HELD, H. GABRIEL, M. TEXTOR and U. ZAHN: Cerebral metabolism during hyperventilation and inhalation of CO_2. Brain and Blood Flow. Proceedings of the IV. International Symposium London, Sept. 197o. Pitman Medical and Scientific Publishing Co Ltd. London 1971, p 170-173

8. HÄGGENDAL, E. and B. JOHANSSON: Effects of arterial carbon dioxide tension and oxygen saturation on cerebral blood flow autoregulation in dogs. Acta physiol. scand. 66, 27-53 suppl. 258 (1965)

9. HARPER, A.M.: The inter-relationship between $aPCO_2$ and blood pressure in the regulation of blood flow through the cerebral cortex. Acta neurol. scand. suppl. 14, 94-103 (1965)

10. HARPER, A.M.: Autoregulation of cerebral blood flow: Influence of the arterial blood pressure on the blood flow through the cerebral cortex. J. Neurol. Neurosurg. Psychiat. 29, 398-403 (1966)

11. HIRSCH, H. und K. KÖRNER: Über die Druck-Durchblutungs-Relation der Hirngefäße. Pflügers Arch. ges. Physiol. 280, 316-325 (1964)

12. JAMES, I.M., C. YANALATOS and S. NASHAT: The effect of CO_2tension and blood pressure on cerebral metabolism and blood flow after isoprenaline infusion. Brain and Blood Flow. Proceedings of the IV. International Symposium London, Sept. 1970. Pitman Medical and Scientific Publishing Co Ltd. London 1971, p 229-232

13. KETY, S.S. and C.F. SCHMIDT: The determination of cerebral blood flow in man by the use of nitrous oxide in low concentrations. Am. J. Physiol. 143, 53-66 (1945)

14. LANGFITT, T.W., J.D.WEINSTEIN and N.F.KASSELL: Cerebral vasomotor paralysis produced by intracranial hypertension. Neurology 15, 622-641 (1965)

15. LASSEN, N.A.: Cerebral blood flow and oxygen consumption in man. Physiol. Rev. 39, 183-238 (1959)

16. LEUSEN, I., G.DEMEESTER and E.LACROIX: Lactate and pyruvate in the brain of rats during changes in acid-base balance. Archives Internationales de Physiologie et de Biochemie 74, 528-531 (1966)

17. RAICHLE, M.E., J.B.POSNER and F.PLUM: Cerebral blood flow during and after hyperventilation. Arch.Neurol. 23, 394-403 (197o)

18. RAPELA, C.E. , H.D.GREEN: Autoregulation of canine cerebral blood flow.

19. SIESJÖ, B.K., J.FOLBERGROVA and V.MACMILLAN: The effect of hypercapnia upon intracellular pH in the brain, evaluated by the bicarbonate-carbonic acid method and from the creatin phosphokinase equilibrium. J.Neurochem. 19, 2483-2495 (1972)

20. WAELSCH, H., S.BERL, C.A.ROSSI, D.D.CLARKE and D.D.PURPURA: Quantitative aspects of CO_2 fixation in mammalian brain in vivo. J.Neurochem. 11, 717-728 (1964)

21. WEYNE, J., G.DEMEESTER and I.LEUSEN: Effects of carbon dioxide, bicarbonate and pH on lactate and pyruvate in the brain of rats. Pflügers Arch.ges. Physiol. 314, 292-311 (197o)

22. WOLLMAN, H., S.C.ALEXANDER, P.J.COHEN, P.E.CHASE, E.THELMAN and Ph.D.BELAR: Cerebral circulation of man during halothane anesthesia. Effects of hypocarbia and of d-tubocurarine. Anesthesiology 25, 180-184 (1964)

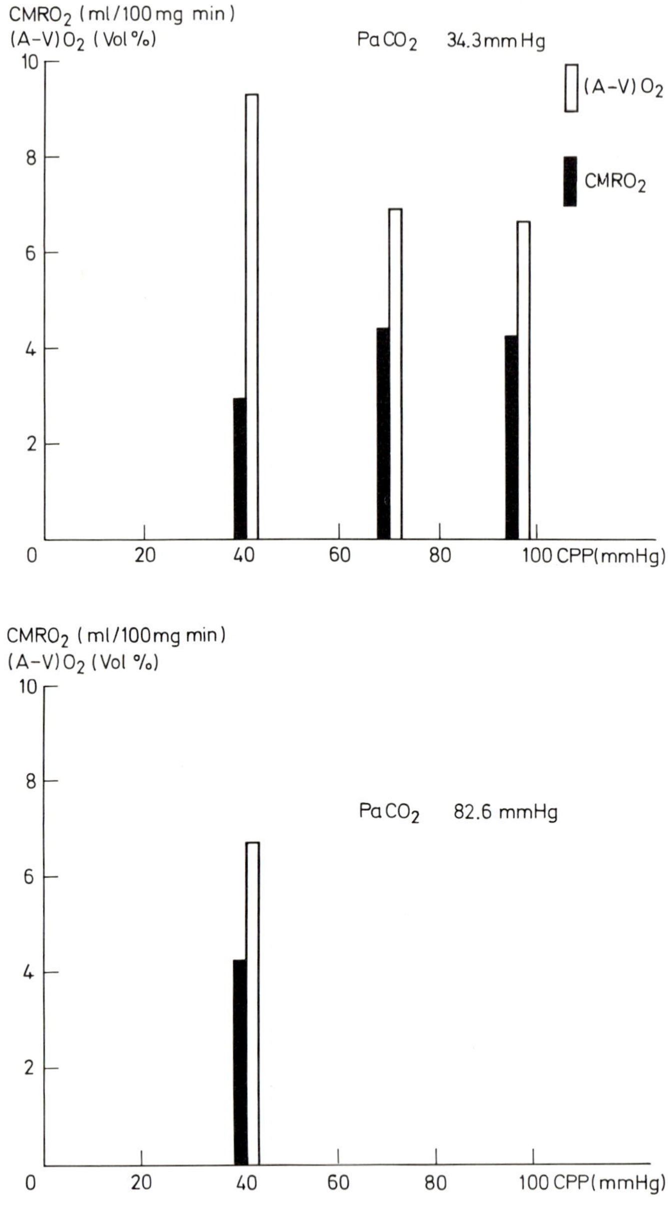

Fig. 1. (see text)

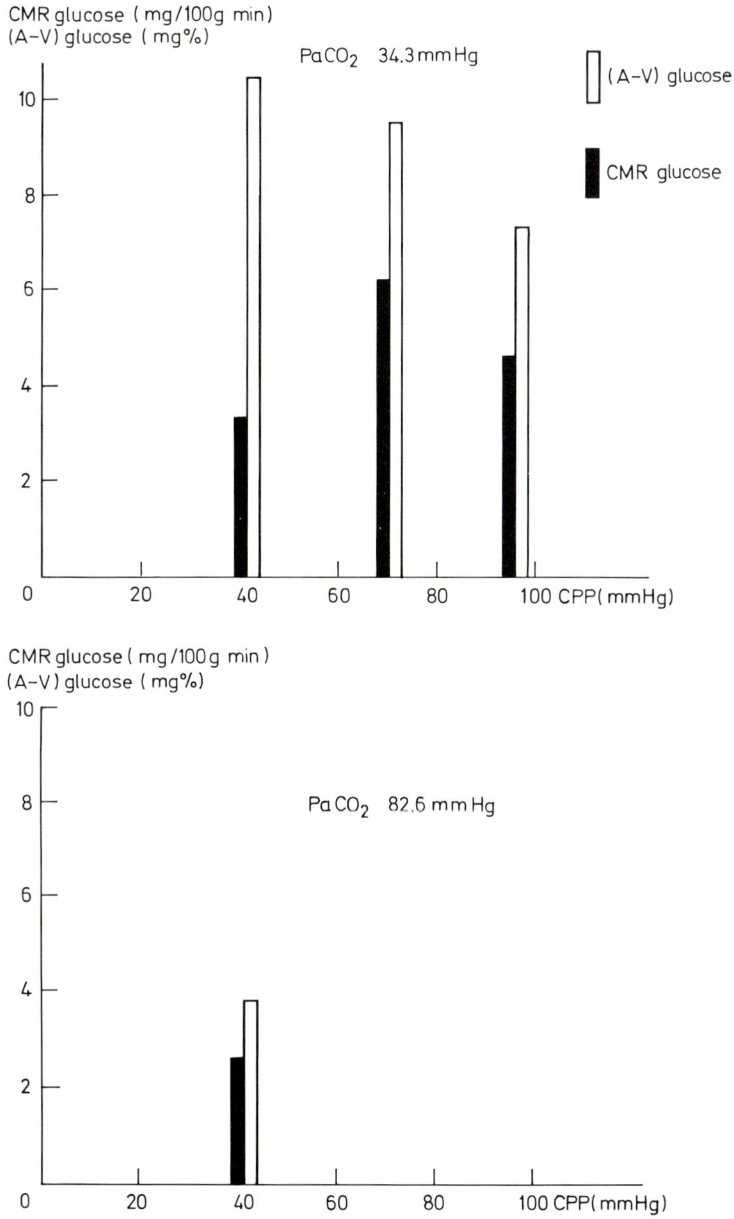

Fig. 2. (see text)

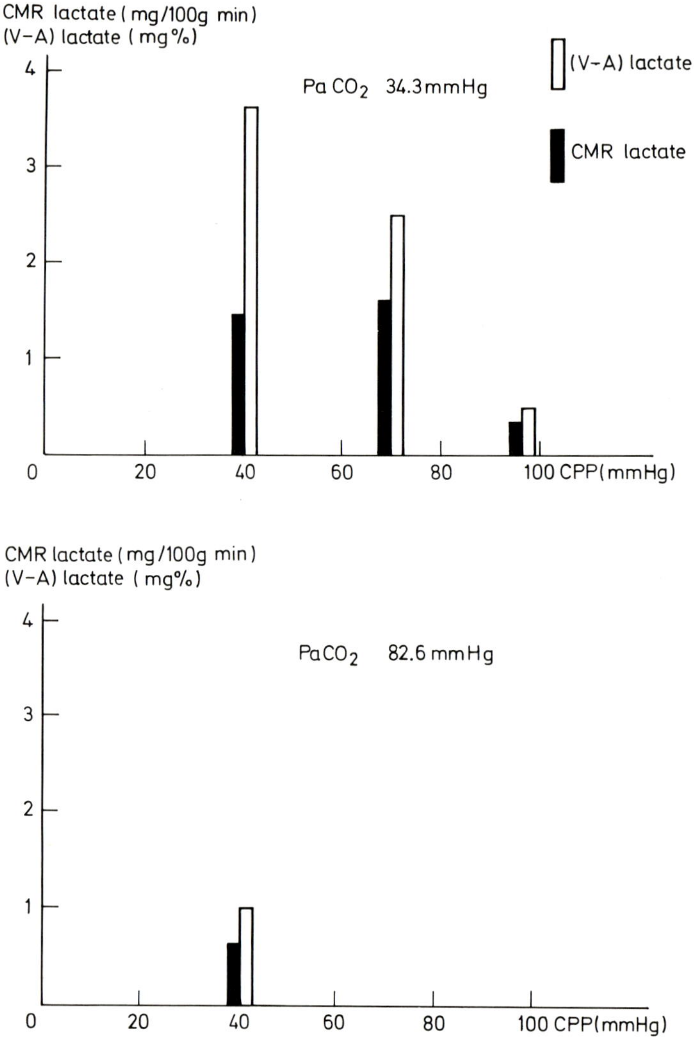

Fig. 3. (see text)

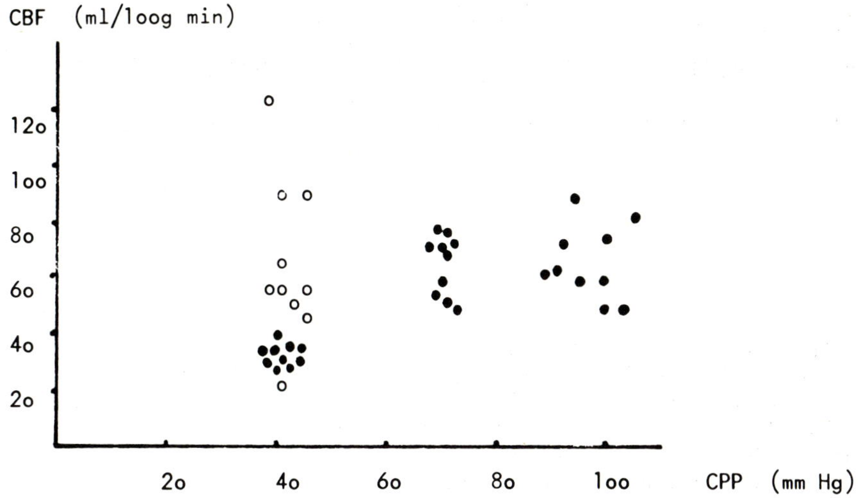

Fig. 4. Closed circles represent CBF-values under normocapnic conditions; open circles reflect values in hypercapnia (for details see text)

Regional Cerebral Blood Flow and Regional Cerebrovascular Reactivity Following Local Brain Injury

T. WALLENFANG, R. SCHUBERT, J. GROTE, W. SCHAAF, and H. J. REULEN

Pathophysiological concepts on the mechanism of changes occurring in the damaged brain hemisphere following head injuries are still quite limited. Therefore the present series of experiments were undertaken to examine the changes of the regional cerebral blood flow and its regulatory mechanism following a cold induced edema. At the same time we investigated the influence of a different arterial PO_2 upon the cerebrovascular reactivity of injured and undamaged brain areas, as well as the influence of hypercapnia and hypocapnia on rCBF. Both methods were applied therapeutically during the last years.

Method

A local cold injury as described by KLATZO was inflicted to the right frontal cortex of 56 cats under Nembutal anesthesia (40 mg/kg b.w.). Twenty-four hours after the induction of the lesion 4 groups of 10 animals were either normoventilated, hypoventilated, moderately or severely hyperventilated. At the end of the experiments rCBF was measured by the ^{85}Krypton clearance in the following areas (Fig. 1):

1. the lesion proper
2. the cortex immediately adjacent to the lesion
3. one cortical area remote from the lesion
4. the contralateral hemisphere, which served as control

In a 5th group of 16 animals under normocapnic conditions rCBF was measured over the area adjacent to the lesion and over the undamaged hemisphere while PaO_2 was gradually lowered from 100 mmHg to 25 mmHg. Following the above measurements, the brain was instantaneously frozen with liquid nitrogen. The water and metabolic contents were determined in the areas corresponding to the CBF measurements.

Results

The changes in regional cerebral blood flow in the neighbourhood of a brain lesion under normoxic normocapnia conditions are demonstrated in figure 2.

The abscissa shows the difference of the water contents between the uninjured control hemisphere and the single areas of the injured hemisphere. The ordinate shows in the same way the difference between the cerebral blood flow of the uninjured hemisphere and the single areas of the injured hemisphere. The point of intersection of abscissa and ordinate corresponds to the control values of the uninjured hemisphere.

The closed circles correspond to the lesion, the triangles to the areas adjacent to the lesion and the open circles to the areas remote from the lesion. Thus, an inhomogenous circulatory pattern can be observed around the brain lesion. Independent of the distance from the lesion 4 different types of flow can be differentiated.

1. normal areas (control values)
2. hyperemic non-edematous areas
3. ischemic non-edematous areas
4. ischemic edematous areas

In the latter areas a close correlation between the severity of local edema and the decrease in local blood flow can be established. i.e. an increasing amount of local brain edema causes progressive reduction of local circulation.

Probably the hyperemia results from a vasodilatation caused by the spreading lactacidosis, which accumulates in the lesion area. Fig. 3 demonstrates the relation between the changes in regional cerebral blood flow and the local brain metabolism, i.e. the local lactate content respectively the local L/P ratio as well as ATP and phosphocreatine.

Thus, a reduction of about 62 % in CBF at the lesion results in a significant decrease in phosphocreatine and ATP concentrations.

A CBF reduction of about 24 % in the remote areas and of about 33 % in the adjacent areas does not cause any significant decrease of these energy-rich phosphates, although the lactate concentration increases progressively due to tissue hypoxia. In accordance with the stability of both compounds, phosphocreatin diminished earlier than ATP due to tissue hypoxia. The increased tissue pressure and the concomitant tissue lactacidosis apparently impairs blood flow regulation in these edematous areas.

The hyperemic non-edematous areas, the vessels of which are already maximally dilated by the tissue lactacidosis, have lost any capacity of vasodilatation to a gradual reduction in PaO_2. These areas, at the limit of their compensation, show a significant decrease in blood flow - an intracerebral steal. Thus, a reduction in PaO_2 soon results in a significantly deficient blood flow. Studies have been performed on the influence of gradually lowering PaO_2 from 100 to 25 mmHg on the regional cerebral blood flow in the uninjured and injured hemisphere (Fig. 4). In the control hemisphere rCBF remains constant until PaO_2 has decreased below 40-50 mmHg. A reduction below this level induces a marked increase of rCBF. These results are in agreement with earlier findings reported by GROTE.

The edematous areas, the blood flow of which was already diminished as compared to the control hemisphere, show a lower and earlier increase in blood flow. When PaO_2 was lowered below 40-30 mmHg we observed a tendency of blood flow to decrease in these edematous areas.

The results of these investigations on moderate and severe hypocapnia respectively hypercapnia and their influence on rCBF is demonstrated in figure 5. The abscissa shows the different $PaCO_2$, the ordinate the corresponding rCBF values.

Under normoxic normocapnia a progressive reduction of rCBF from the remote and the adjacent area toward the lesion was measured as compared to the control hemisphere. Under moderate hypocapnia the cerebral blood flow diminishes in the uninjured hemisphere paralleling the decrease of $PaCO_2$ from 30 to 16 mmHg. In comparison to normoxic normocapnic conditions, no remarkable change in CBF is found under moderate hypocapnia in the lesion area, while rCBF is significantly increased in the adjacent and remote areas. This is known as the so called "inverse steal syndrome". The decrease in $PaCO_2$ results in a vasoconstriction of the uninjured hemisphere and induces a redistribution of blood flow from the healthy toward the affected brain areas. Paralleling the increase in CBF brain edema progressively diminishes.

Under severe hypocapnia, i.e., a decrease in $PaCO_2$ from 30 to 11,5 mmHg, rCBF diminishes in all areas. This controlled ventilation undoubtedly has no clinical importance in treatment of patients.

The rCBF values during hypercapnia diminish in all areas of the injured hemisphere. The well known increase in rCBF in response to CO_2 administration the uninjured hemisphere was observed only in 4 cats. In the other 6 animals rCBF decreased. Such a paradoxical CO_2-reaction of the brain vessels was also described by ROSSANDA et al., FIESCHI et al. in cases of acute brain injury.

In summary, in the neighbourhood of a lesion of the brain an inhomogenous circulatory pattern exists. Independent of the distance from the lesion, 4 types of flow reactions can be differentiated: areas with normal blood flow, hyperemic and ischemic non-edematous areas and, finally, ischemic edematous areas. The areas of the injured hemisphere failed to show the PaO_2 triggered blood flow regulation. A beneficial effect on the damaged brain may only be obtained from the moderate hypocapnia. A lowering of about 10 mmHg in $PaCO_2$ produces hemodynamic alterations resulting in a redistribution of blood flow from the healthy toward the diseased areas of the brain.

REFERENCES

1. BROCK, M., A.HADJIDIMOS, J.P.DERUAZ, F.FISCHER, H.DIETZ, K.KOHLMEYER, W.PÖLL and K.SCHÜRMANN: The effects of hyperventilation of regional cerebral blood flow. On the vole of changes in intracranial pressure and tissue perfusion pressure for shifts in rCBF distribution. In: J.F.Toole, J.Moossy and R.Janeway (eds.) Cerebral Vascular Diseases, N.Y. Grune and Stratton, 1970

2. EKLÖF, B., V.McMILLAN and B.K.SIESJÖ: The effect of ischemia upon the energy state of the brain. In: Cerebral Blood Flow and Intracranial Pressure (eds.) Fieschi, C., Siena, S.Karger Verlag

3. FIESCHI, C., A.BEDUSCHI, A.AGNOLI, N.BATTISTINI, M.COLLICE, M.PRENCIPE and M.RISSO: Regional Cerebral Blood Flow and Intracranial Pressure (ed.) Fieschi, C., Siena, S.Karger Verlag

4. FREI, H.J., T.WALLENFANG, W.PÖLL, H.J.REULEN, R.SCHUBERT and M.BROCK: Regional cerebral blood flow and regional metabolism in cold induced edema. Acta Neurochirurgica (in press)

5. FREI, H.J., W.PÖLL, H.J.REULEN, M.BROCK and K.SCHÜRMANN: Regional energy metabolism, tissue lactate content and rCBF in cold injury edema. In: R.W.R. RUSSEL (ed.) Brain and Blood Flow, Pitman Medical and Scientific Publishing Co. Ltd., London 1971

6. GROTE, J., H.KREUSCHER, R.SCHUBERT and H.J.RUSS: New studies on the influence of PaO_2 and $PaCO_2$ on regional and total cerebral blood flow. 6th Europ. Conf. Microcirculation, Aalborg 1970, pp 294-297 (Karger, Basel, 1971)

7. INGVAR, D.H. and N.A.LASSEN: Regional blood flow of the cerebral cortex determined by ^{85}Krypton. Acta Physiol. scand. 54, 325-338 (1962)

8. KLATZO, I., A.PIVAUX and E.LASKOWSKI: The relationship between edema, blood brain barrier and tissue elements in local brain injury. J.of Neuropath. Exp.Neurol. 17, 548-564 (1968)

9. KLATZO, I., H.WISNIEWSKI, O.STEINWALL, and E.STREICHER: Dynamics of cold injury edema. In: I.Klatzo and F.Seitelberg (eds.) Brain edema, Springer Verlag, New York 1967

lo. LASSEN, N.A.: The luxury perfusion syndrome and its possible relation to acute metabolic acidosis locali zed with brain. The Lancet 2, 1113-1115 (1966)

11. ROSSANDA, M., L.BOSELLI, A.CASTELLI, C.CORONA, T.ERMINIO, M.NARDINI, P.PORTA and C.VILLA: Effects of changes in $PaCO_2$ on rCBF, cerebral oxygenation and EEG in severe brain injuries. In: Cerebral Blood Flow and Intracranial Pressure (ed.) Fieschi, C., Siena, S.Karger Verlag

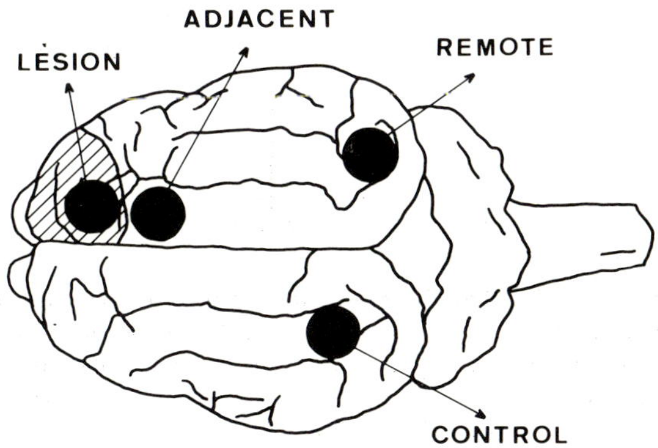

Fig. 1. Schematic representation of the areas for rCBF, water and metabolite content determinations. The shaded area indicates the site of the freezing lesion

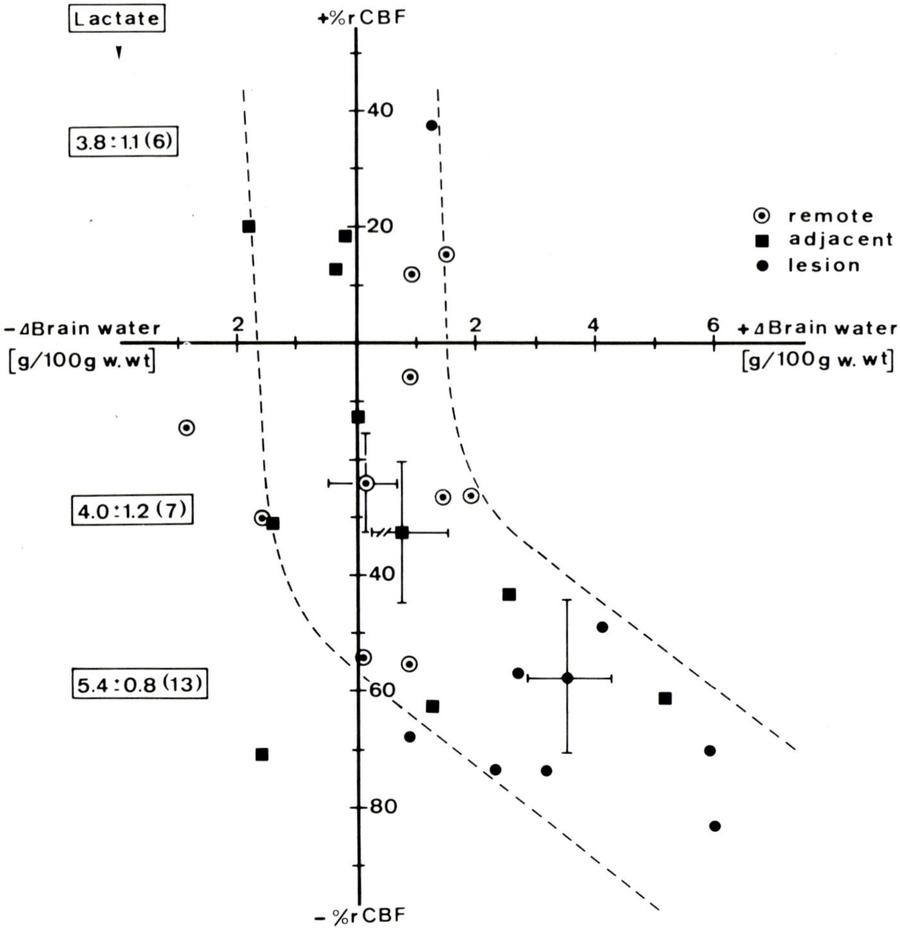

Fig. 2. Changes in regional cerebral blood flow in relation to the local water content. ΔH_2O is expressed as the change in local water content (g/100 g w. wt) of the respective tissue area compared to the value of the contralateral hemisphere in the same animal. rCBF is expressed as the percentage change of the respective tissue area from the value of the contralateral hemisphere of the same animal

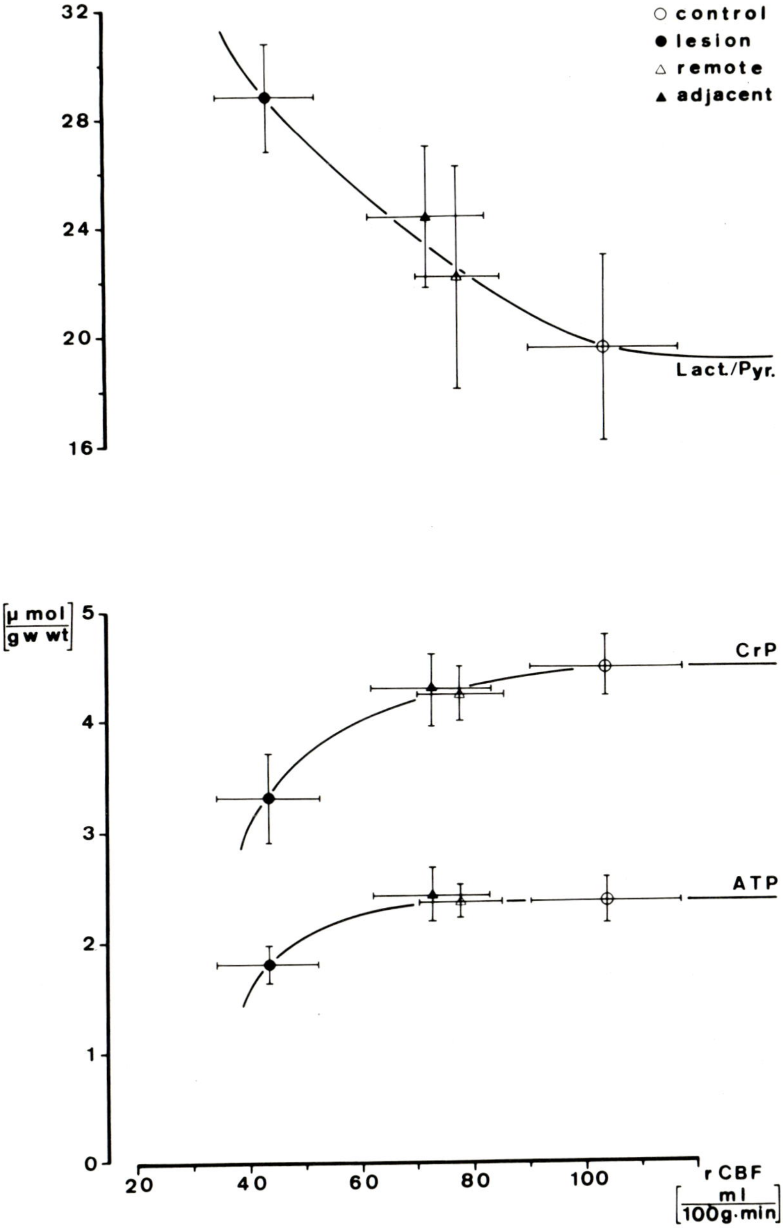

Fig. 3. Local brain tissue contents of phosphocreatine, ATP and the lactate/pyruvate ratio (μ mol/g w.wt) related to the regional cerebral blood flow (ml/100 g x min) in the contralateral, remote, adjacent and lesion area

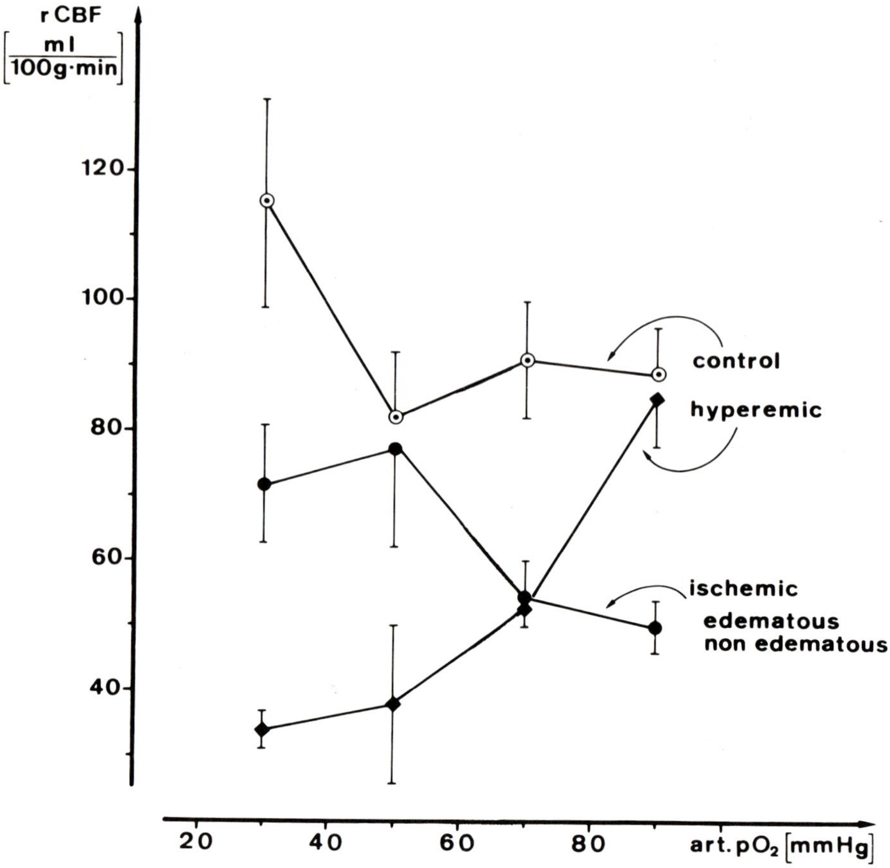

Fig. 4. Changes of regional cerebral blood flow (ml/100 g x min) in the uninjured and injured hemisphere in relation to a gradually lowered PaO_2 from 100 to 25 mmHg

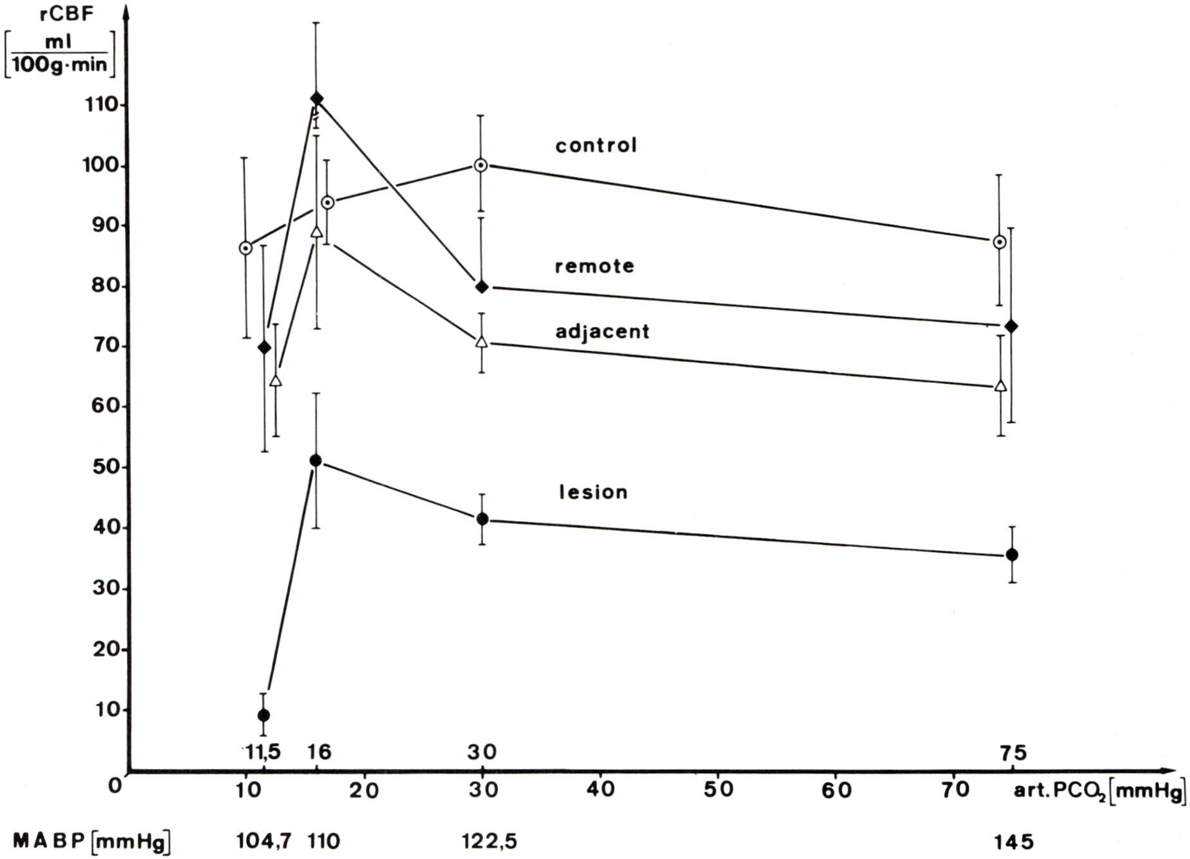

Fig. 5. Changes of regional cerebral blood flow (ml/100 g x min) in the contralateral, remote, adjacent and lesion areas during normoventilation, moderate and pronounced hyperventilation as well as hypoventilation

Cerebrovascular Autoregulation After Acute Brain Injury with Particular Reference to Changes in Intra-Ventricular Pressure

J. OVERGAARD and A. TWEED

Arterial hypertension (HT) has been shown to promote the formation and spread of cerebral edema in animal models (1, 2, 3), but the effect of HT on intracranial pressures (ICP) in patients with acute brain injuries and impaired autoregulation has not been clearly established.

We have continuously monitored mean intraventricular pressure (MIVP) during periods of induced transient arterial HT (during testing of autoregulation) in 28 rCBF studies done at times ranging from 2 hours to over 30 days after acute brain injuries. rCBF was measured by the intra-arterial Xenon method with 35 channel recording and calculated from the initial slope (4). Mean global flow ($CBF_{init.}$) was measured from the continuously recorded sum of the 35 channels. Autoregulation was tested in each study by a slow intra-venous infusion of angiotensin to produce a transient (3-5 minutes) increase of MABP of between 25-75 torr. Global or major focal impairment of autoregulation was determined from the increase in $CBF_{init.}$ or $rCBF_{init.}$ during HT as described by OLESEN (5).

Results

Changes in MIVP during transient HT are described in 4 groups of patients as follows:

Group 1 was 8 patients with intact autoregulation and MIVP ranging from 6-34 torr. No change in MIVP was seen during HT, even with rapidly rising BP. We conclude that normal autoregulation responds rapidly to rising BP so that CBF and intracranial blood volume are maintained constant, and ICP, even when moderately elevated, is unaffected.

Group 2 was 8 patients with impaired autoregulation but with resting MIVP controlled to levels less than 25 torr (av· 15, 9 torr). A small but inconsistent rise in MIVP was seen during HT in this group (increase 3, 8 torr). It appears that these patients maintained some margin for volume compensation so that they were able to accomodate a small increase in intracranial blood volume.

Group 3 was 7 patients with severely impaired autoregulation and resting MIVP elevated above 25 torr (av. 48 torr). In this group a rise in BP was consistently accompanied by a significant rise in MIVP, the change in MIVP being coincident in time and proportional in amplitude to the change in MABP. The proportional relationship MIVP/MABP ranged from 0, 12 to 0, 69 (av. 0, 49). We presume that intracranial volume reserves were exhausted in these patients and they were unable to compensate for a small increase in blood volume. We suggest, therefore, that this response represents vasocongestive ICP elevation.

One patient in group 3 had an MICP which rose progressively during HT and persisted at the elevated level after reduction of BP and despite vigorous hyperventilation, but was reduced to the resting level after CSF drainage. We believe this represents edema formation provoked by the episode of HT.

Group 4 was 5 patients who had autoregulation tested during hypercapnia ($PaCO_2$ 45-70 torr). Resting MIVP was moderately elevated (av. 25,8 torr) and rose during HT in a manner similar to that of group 3 in 4 of the 5 patients.

Summary

1. In patients with impaired autoregulation after acute brain injury HT may provoke vasocongestive or edematous elevation of ICP.

2. Control of MIVP to less than 25 torr prevents the vasocongestive response, but it is uncertain whether it prevents edema formation.

3. Direct measurement of ICP and observation of the relationship between ICP and BP are essential features in the care of these patients.

4. Spontaneous episodes of HT should be anticipated and preventative measures employed. Since spontaneous HT is often related to elevation of ICP, CSF acidosis, hypoxia, hypercapnia or restlessness, measures such as control of ICP, hyperventilation, and sedation should be considered in preference to hypotensive drug therapy.

REFERENCES

1. MARSHALL, W.J.S., J.L.F.JACKSON and T.W.LANGFITT: Brain swelling caused by trauma and arterial hypertension - hemodynamic aspects. Arch. Neurol. 21, 545-553 (1969)

2. MEINIG, G., H.J.REULEN, A.HADJIDIMOS, C.SIEMON, D.BARTKO and K.SCHÜRMANN: Induction of filtration edema by extreme reduction of cerebrovascular resistance associated with hypertension. European Neurology 8, 97-103 (1972)

3. KLATZO, I.: Pathophysiological aspects on brain edema. In: Steroids and brain edema. (eds.) H.J.Reulen and K.Schürmann. Springer Verlag 1972

4. OLESEN, J., O.PAULSON and N.A.LASSEN: Regional cerebral blood flow in man determined by the initial slope of the clearance of intra-arterially injected ^{133}Xe. Stroke 2, 519-540 (1971)

5. OLESEN, J.: Quantitative evaluation of normal and pathologic cerebral blood flow regulation to perfusion pressure. Arch.Neurol. 28, 143-149 (1973)

Desintegration of Polysynaptic Vegetative Control of the Mesencephalic Reticular Formation After Brain Edema in Animal Experiments

E. MARKAKIS, W. WINKELMUELLER, and A. SPRING

Three methods have mainly been used in order to localize the vegetative centers in brain, especially those with respiratory and cardiovascular function:

1. lesions and transections of the brainstem, which provide only a rough (9, 14) anatomic-functional study, 2. electrostimulation of brainstem areas, allowing a more exact localization of the vegetative centers and 3. recording of the neuronal activity by means of microelectrodes implanted into the brainstem.

In this way the central cardiovascular regulation was defined in a large number of superposed centers, beginning with the pontomedullar formatio reticularis, up to mesodiencephalic centers of the formatio reticularis with bulbo-thalamic and bulbo-hypothalamic projection pathways and ending at the cerebral cortex (3, 12, 13, 14, 19).

The respiratory centers in brainstem were localized especially as:

a) a pneumotaxic center in the upper pons (inspiratory-inhibitory), b) an apneustic center in the lower pons (inspiratory-facilitatory) and c) a primitive rhythmic center in the medulla (4, 9, 17, 19, 21). By means of electrostimulation a respiratory-expiratory center was defined in the dorsal part and a respiratory-inspiratory center in the ventral part of the floor of the fourth ventricle (2, 6, 9, 16, 18).

The way in which all these centers influence each other is not yet clear.

Own previous studies (22) of the basal mesencephalic area have shown that electrostimulation in the ventromedian segment cause an increase in vigilance combined with a marked motoric and electrocorticographic activation.

The question arises if, by electrostimulating these mesencephalic regions, the changes of vigilance correlate with changes of vegetative functions (especially of blood pressure and respiration) and if the functional pattern of reaction is modified during the increased intracranial pressure.

In a series of animal experiments (30 spontaneous breathing, adult cats of both sexes in light anesthesia) the ECoG, intracranial pressure, blood pressure, ECG, respiratory frequence and pattern, aortic and brain pulsations were recorded.

By means of a bipolar electrode, stereotactically implanted into the left mesencephalic reticular formation, we registrated the stimulation effects in different depths and the changes in vegetative functions, especially in respiration and blood pressure at normal intracranial pressures (100 Hz stimuli for 20 sec.).

As shown in figure 1 an initial depression of respiration followed by a deeper and increased respiratory rate and simultaneously an instant phasic rise of blood pressure was recorded at a depth of 21 to 22 mm.

We also applied 0,25-1 Hz and 8-12 Hz low-frequency stimuli and recorded in the frontal ECoG (area 6) the specific (field potential) and unspecific (recruiting-spindling) responses.

Figure 2 illustrates the reaction of respiration and cardiovascular activity after a high-frequency stimulus has been repeatedly applied under normal intracranial pressure conditions (the period of a 100 Hz stimulus for 20 sec. is seen in the grey field).

As shown in figure 3, brain edema and increase in intracranial pressure was caused by oil embolisation through the right lingual artery.

In nearly all the cases we observed a postembolic ECoG depression, which, however, could be reversible (figure 4) and recorded not only on the right hemisphere, because of the rich anastomoses of the cranial vessels.

During increasing the intracranial pressure we repeated the low- and high-frequency stimulations (figure 5).

At a level of 40-50 mmHg we recorded the reversal of the respiratory brain pulse amplitudes - larger amplitudes during the inspiratory phase (15).

At the same time it was possible to induce respiration by 100 Hz stimuli. The blood pressure regulation seemed to be fixed at an autonomic level and was no longer influenced by mesencephalic stimulations.

In the same phase (figure 6) we observed that following low-frequency stimuli an inhibition of the unspecific ECoG responses (recruiting) took place, whereas the specific responses (field potential) were further recorded.

The inhibition of the unspecific responses in ECoG, appearing at a level of ICP about 40-50 mmHg, points towards a breakdown of polysynaptic connections. As the functional response of blood pressure centers following high-frequency stimuli simultaneously disappears, we assume that the cardiovascular regulation is modulated in mesencephalic areas by polysynaptic connections. Blood pressure is now regulated by an autonomic pontomedullar generator and can no longer be influenced by midbrain stimulation.

On the other hand the specific ECoG responses and functional reaction in respiration following midbrain stimulation remain constant, showing the oligosynaptic pathways are still intact.

The reversal of the respiratory changes in brain pulsations seems to be a sign of the mesencephalic desintegration of cardiovascular and respiratory regulation.

We thus conclude that midbrain stimulation causes a general activation of the motoricity, vigilance and vegetative reactions. At high intracranial pressures (above 40 to 50 mmHg) an interruption of the polysynaptic neuronal connections takes place, which clinically is seen as the desintegration of the vegetative functions and the disturbance of consciousness.

REFERENCES

1. BAUMGARTEN, R. von, A. von BAUMGARTEN and K.-P. SCHAEFER: Beitrag zur Lokalisationsfrage bulboretikulärer respiratorischer Neurone der Katze. Pflügers Arch. ges. Physiol. 264, 217-227 (1957)

2. BAXTER, D.W. and J. OLSZEWSKI: Respiratory responses evoked by electrical stimulation of pons and mesencephalon. J. Neurophysiol. 18, 276-287 (1955)

3. BITTMAN, E. and N. RAICIULESCU: Summation and reciprocal innervation-like phenomena in central cardiovascular control. Symposium: central rhythmic and regulation, Berlin, July 13-16 th (1972)

4. BRECKENRIDGE, C.G. and H.E. HOFF: Adrenaline apnea in the medullary animal. Am. J. Physiol. 160, 385-394 (1950)

5. BROCK, M., J. BECK, E. MARKAKIS and H. DIETZ: Intracranial pressure gradients associated with experimental cerebral embolism. Stroke 3, 123-130 (1972)

6. BROOKHART, J.M.: Respiratory effects of localized faradic stimulation of medulla oblongata. Am. J. Physiol. 129, 709-723 (1940)

7. COHEN, M.I. and S.C. WANG: Respiratory neuronal activity in pons of cat. J. Neurophysiol. 22, 33-50 (1959)

8. COHEN, M.I.: Discharge patterns of brain-stem respiratory neurons during Hering-Breuer reflex evoked by lung inflation. J. Neurophysiol. 32, 356-374 (1969)

9. COHEN, M.I.: How respiratory rhythm originates: evidence from discharge patterns of brainstem respiratory neurons. Breathing: J. & A. Churcill, London 1970, pp. 125-150

10. DIRKEN, M.N.J. and S. WOLDRING: Unit activity in bulbar respiratory centre. J. Neurophysiol. 14, 211-226 (1951)

11. GESELL, R., J. BRICKER and C. MAGEE: Structural and functional organisation of central mechanism controlling breathing. Am. J. Physiol. 117, 423-452 (1936)

12. HONEYSECK, G., W. JAENIG, F. KIRCHNER and V. THAEMER: The activity of vasomotor and vasodilatator single units in the hind limb of cat upon stimulation of the defence area. Symposium: central rhythmic and regulation, Berlin, July 13-16 th 1972

13. KIM, Y.K. and H. HEIDRICH: Stereotaxic hypothalamotomy in Raynaud's disease. Symposium: central rhythmic and regulation, Berlin, July 13-16 th 1972

14. LANGHORST, P.: Concept of functional organisation of the brainstem "cardiovascular center". Symposium: central rhythmic and regulation, Berlin, July 13-16 th 1972

15. MARKAKIS, E., M. BROCK and H. DIETZ: Respiratory changes of brain pulsations during intracranial hypertension. 6th Annual Meeting of the European Society for Clinical Investigation, Scheveningen, April 27-29 th 1972

16. PITTS, R.F., H.W. MAGOUN and S.W. RANSON: Localization of medullary respiratory centres in cat. Am. J. Physiol. 126, 673-688 (1939)

17. PITTS, R.F., H.W.MAGOUN and S.W.RANSON: Origin of respiratory rhythmicity. Am.J.Physiol. 127, 654-670 (1939)

18. RANSON, W.W. and H.W.MAGOUN: Respiratory and pupillary reactions induced by electrical stimulation of hypothalamus. Arch.Neurol.Psychiat. 29, 1179-1194 (1933)

19. RANSON, S.W.: Anatomy of the nervous system. W.B.Saunders Co, Philadelphia & London, 1953

20. SALMOIRAGHI, G.C. and B.D.BURNS: Localisation and patterns of discharge of respiratory neurons in brain-stem of cat. J.Neurophysiol. 23, 2-13 (1960)

21. TANG, P.C.: Localization of the pneumotaxic center in the cat. Am.J. Physiol. 172, 645-652 (1953)

22. WINKELMUELLER, W.: Wirkung von Reizeffekten und Auschaltungen der Substantia nigra auf das motorische Verhalten der freibeweglichen Katze. Acta Neurochir. 24, 269-303 (1971)

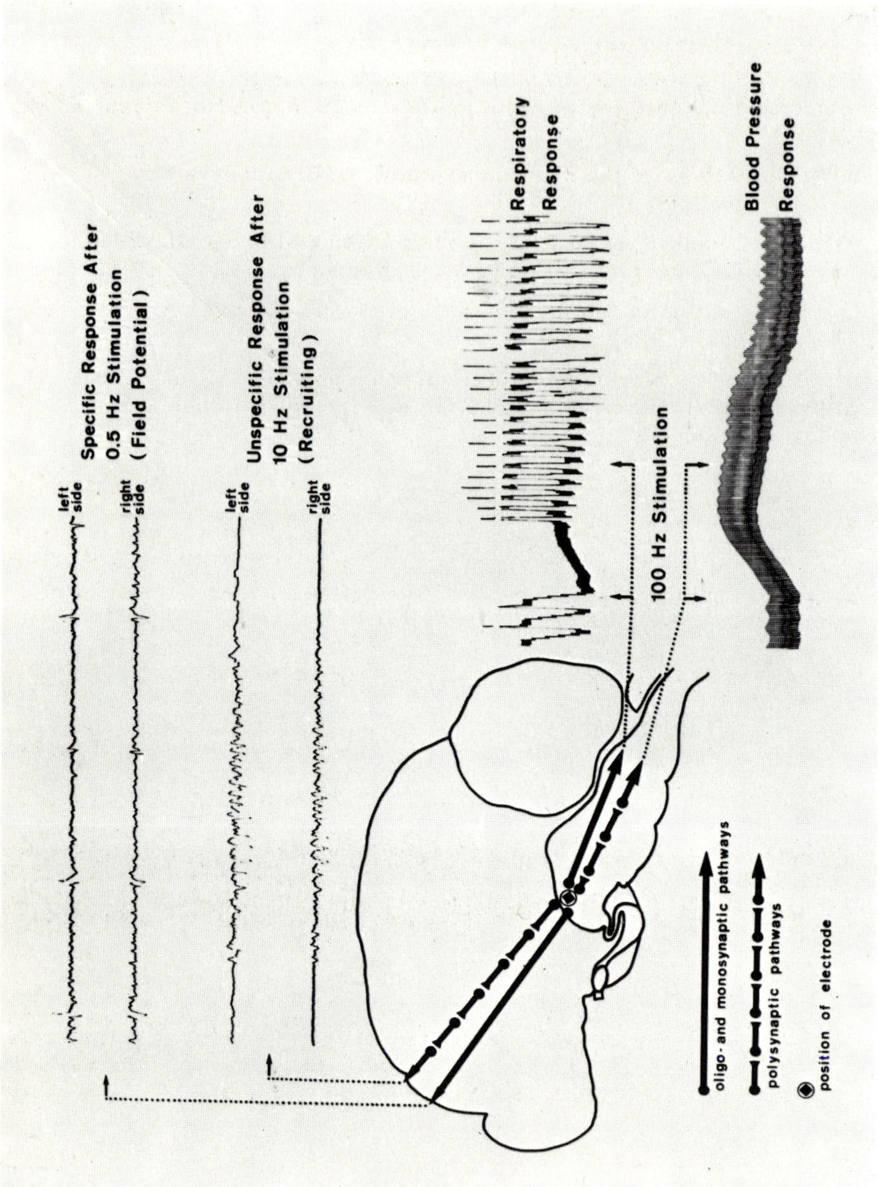

Fig. 1. Electrocorticographic and functional responses following low-and high-frequency midbrain stimulations

Fig. 2. Respiratory and cardiovascular response following a 100 Hz stimulus ▶ (see p. 191 above)

Fig. 3. ICP increase following oil embolisation of the brain (see p. 191 below) ▶

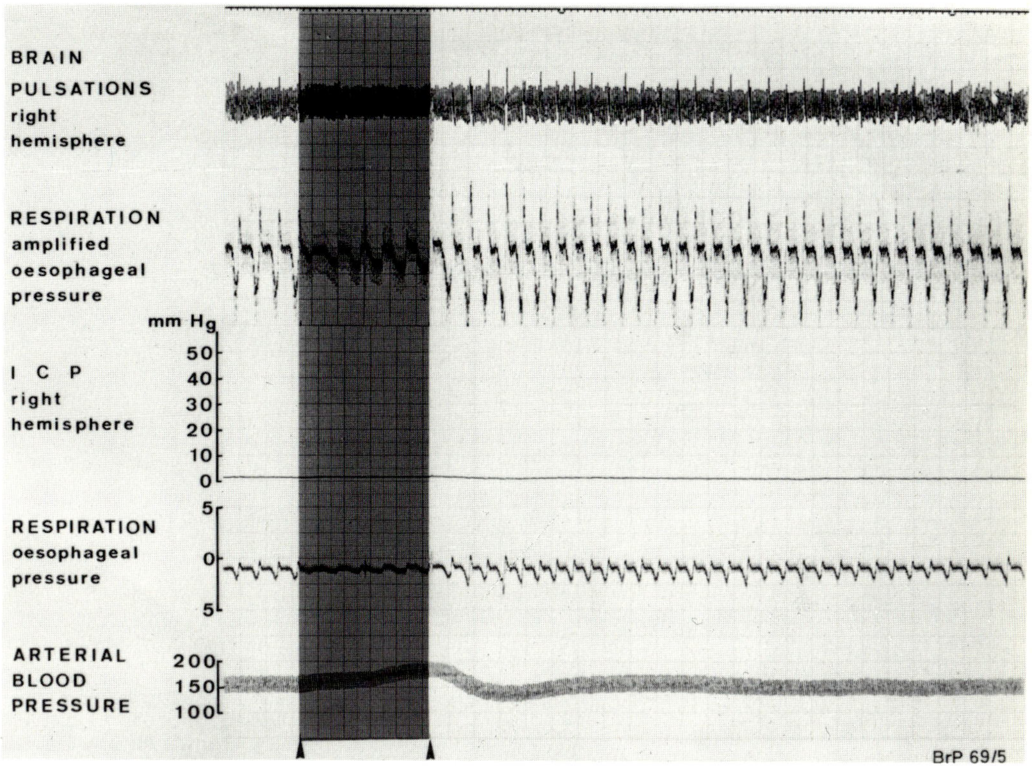
BRAIN
PULSATIONS
right
hemisphere
RESPIRATION
amplified
oesophageal
pressure
mm Hg
I C P
right
hemisphere
50
40
30
20
10
0
RESPIRATION
oesophageal
pressure
5
0
5
ARTERIAL
BLOOD
PRESSURE
200
150
100
BrP 69/5

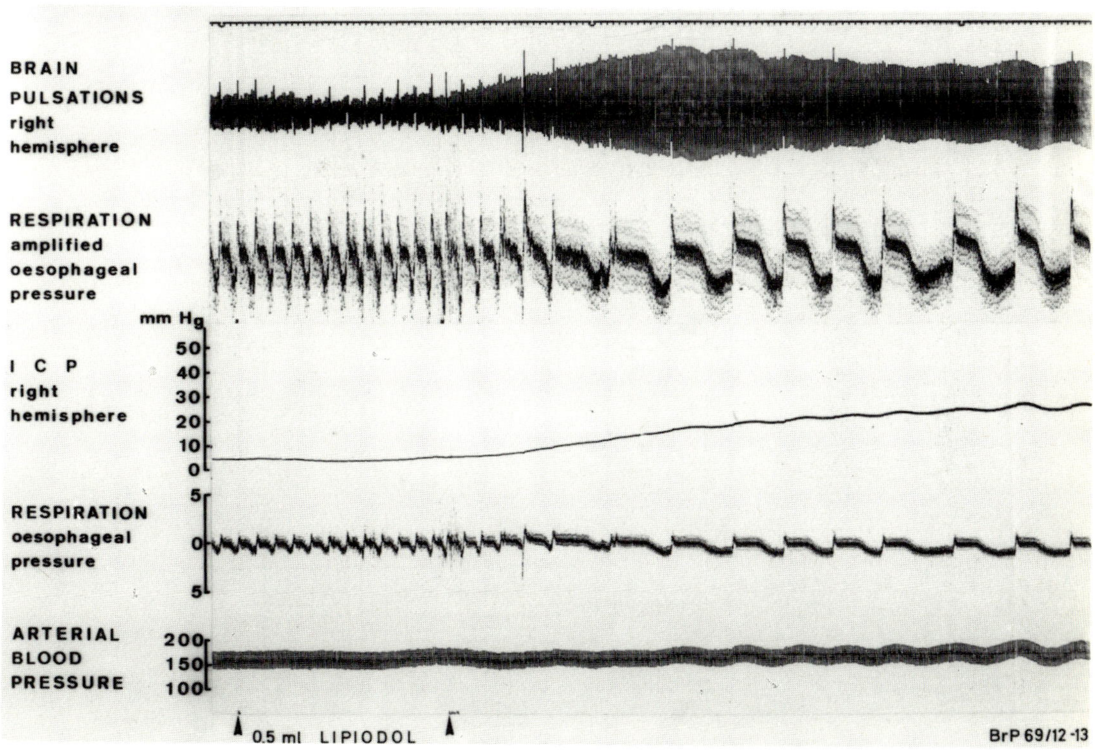
BRAIN
PULSATIONS
right
hemisphere
RESPIRATION
amplified
oesophageal
pressure
mm Hg
I C P
right
hemisphere
50
40
30
20
10
0
RESPIRATION
oesophageal
pressure
5
0
5
ARTERIAL
BLOOD
PRESSURE
200
150
100
0.5 ml LIPIODOL
BrP 69/12-13

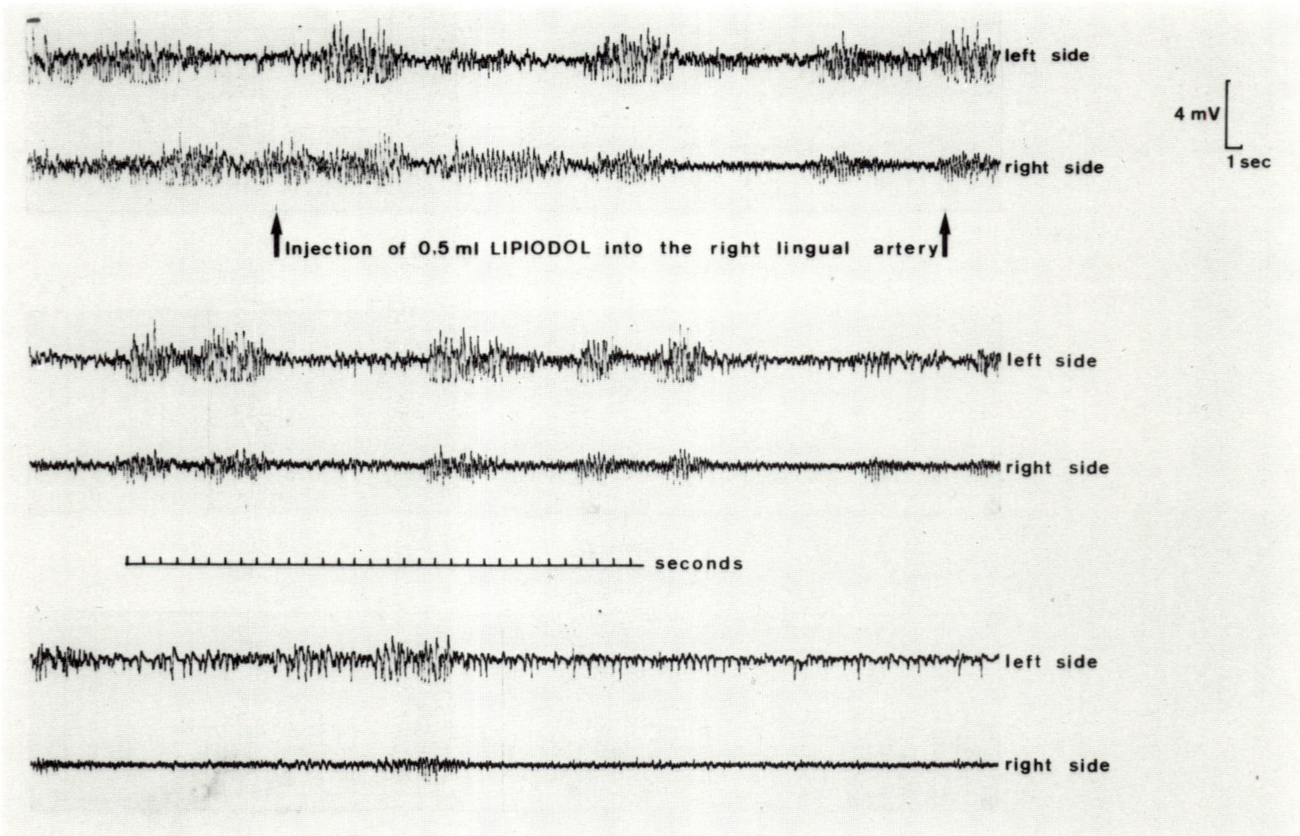

Fig. 4. Depression of ECoG (area 6) following oil embolisation through the right lingual artery

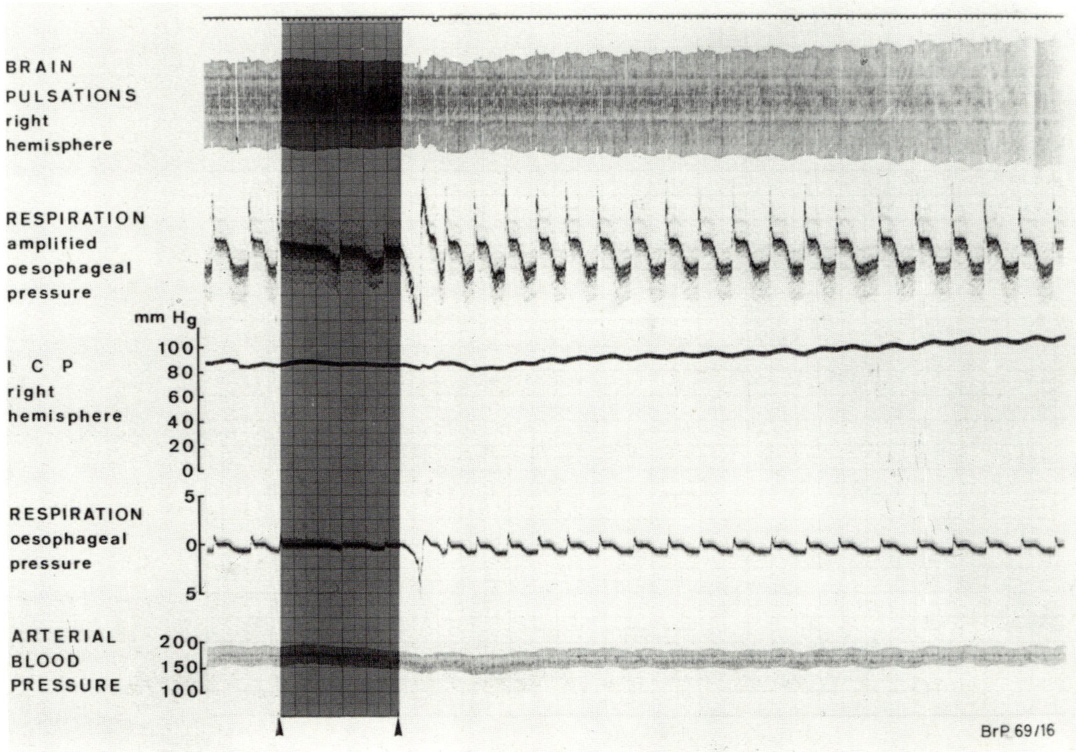

Fig. 5. Desintegration of respiratory and cardiovascular response at high ICP

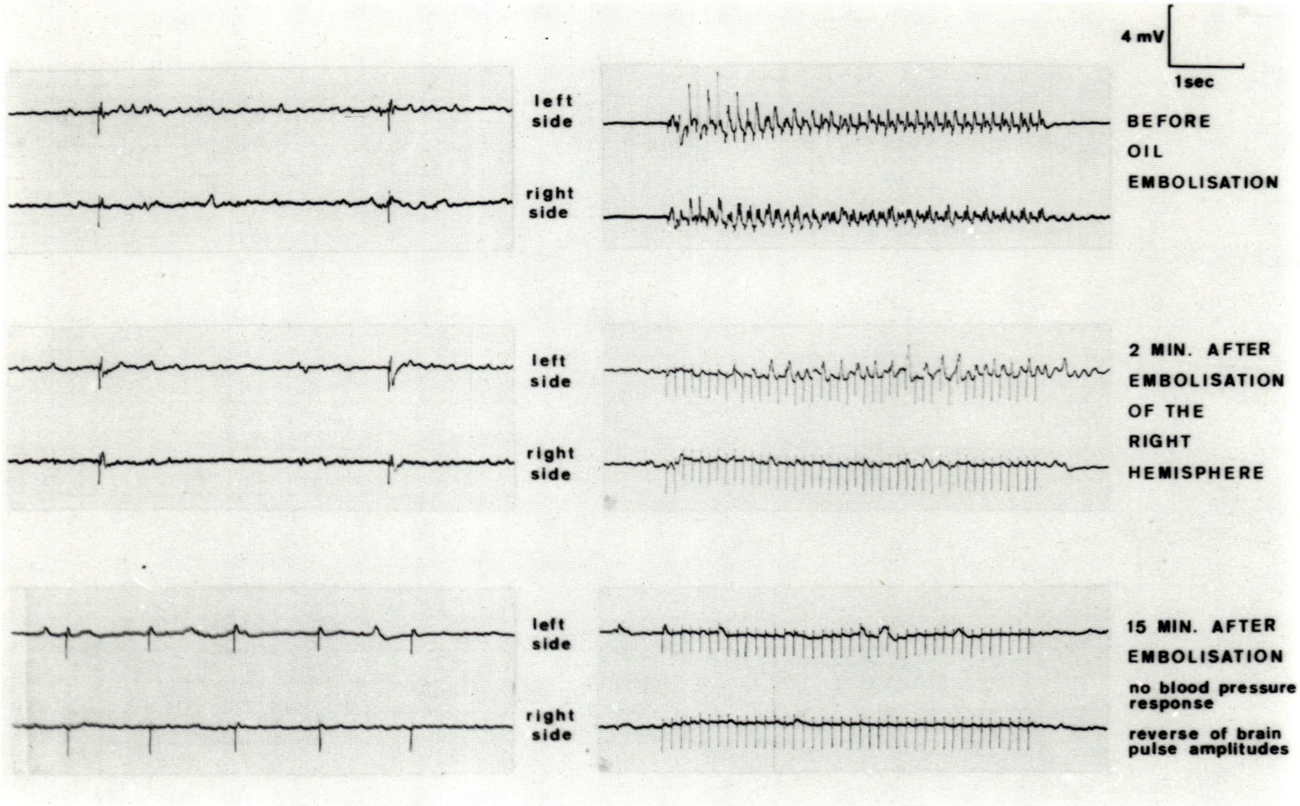

Fig. 6. Inhibition of the unspecific responses following brain edema (ICP:60 mmHg)

The Influence of Hypercapnia and Hypoxia on Intracranial Pressure and on CSF Electrolyte Concentrations

P. MARX, G. WEINERT, P. PFIESTER, and H. KUHN

Hypercapnia has been shown to increase intracranial pressure (ICP) by augmentation of cerebral blood volume. Hypoxia also increases ICP, the mechanisms by which this pressure increase occurs being at least twofold: vasodilatation and cerebral edema. However, it is as yet unknown whether slight and shortlasting hypoxia may also disturb cerebral electrolyte transport mechanisms, thus causing cerebral edema, and whether such disturbances may be reflected in cerebrospinal fluid (CSF) electrolyte concentrations.

The following investigation has been designed to show the influence of hypercapnia and hypoxia on CSF displacement, intracranial pressure and CSF electrolyte concentrations. Mongrel dogs were paralysed with succinylcholine under neuroleptanalgesia. Artificial ventilation was adjusted so that arterial pO_2, pCO_2 and pH were within normal limits. Ventricular cisternal perfusion (PAPPENHEIMER et al.) was established by puncturing the right lateral ventricle through a small burrhole by a specially constructed needle tightly fixed to the calvarium in order to avoid fluid losses. An ELLIOTT's-B-solution (pH = 7, 4) was pumped through this needle at a speed of 0, 1 ml/min and ICP was recorded using a simple manometer. The cisterna magna was punctured percutaneously and the outflow system adjusted so that intraventricular pressure became less than -10 mmHg during steady state. (Na^+) and (K^+) in the effluent fluid were measured three times in each 20 minute sample by flame photometry.

The perfusion system came to a steady state approximately after three hours. Starting at the fourth hour of perfusion, 5% CO_2 were added to the inspiratory gas mixture for five minutes. After restoring steady state conditions hypoxia was induced at the beginning of the fifth hour by reducing O_2 in the inspiratory gas mixture to 10% for ten minutes. During this period all animals showed progressive slowing of EEG.

For statistical analysis the FRIEDMAN-test was chosen which showed significant differences both for intracranial pressure and CSF (Na^+) and (K^+) at a level of α = 0, 005. Two minutes after starting 5% CO_2 inhalation intracranial pressure rapidly rose and increased by 5, 4 mmHg at the fifth minute of hypercapnia indicating well preserved reactivity of the cerebral vasculature to CO_2 (Fig. 1). After restoring normal gas mixtures ICP fell to steady state values within 15 minutes.

A very similar curve was obtained during and after hypoxia, the quantitative differences being due mainly to the longer exposure time to hypoxia as compared with the hypercapnic period (Fig. 2).

The ICP changes occurred although cisternal outflow increased from 0, 161 ml/min during steady state up to 0, 427 ml/min during hypoxia (Fig. 3), the total outflow increment during hypoxia amounting to 1, 52 ml. This seems to be a rather small fluid volume which - as indicated by the ICP rise - cannot be equal to the intracranial volume increment during hypoxia. Nevertheless it permits an interesting comparison to the CSF absorption rate which, using the regression lines of BERING and SATO, can be calculated to be 0, 01 ml/min at the highest ICP during hypoxia. This means that intracranial volume increase during hypoxia is many times larger than the possible CSF absorption at the same time. Hypoxia therefore must increase intracranial pressure and the same applies to hypercapnia.

The finding that the increase in intracranial volume during hypercapnia and hypoxia cannot be compensated for by increased cisternal outflow in our experiments can not be explained by obstruction of the cisternal outflow system, since the outflowing fluid showed free respiratory movements. We therefore believe that CSF pathways have been obstructed most likely at the tentorial aperture due to rapidly rising pressure differentials between supra- and infratentorial cavity. Such pressure differentials during hypercapnia have recently been reported by DORSCH and SYMON in the monkey.

Both, outflow (Na^+) and (K^+) increased during and after hypercapnia (Fig. 4). This increase is lasting longer than the entire hypercapnic period, probably because of the very slow perfusion speed of 0, 1 ml/min. The rise in (K^+) cannot be explained by a higher rate of addition of subarachnoid or ventricular fluid to the perfusion fluid during hypercapnia, since (K^+) was 0, 7 mval/l lower in the original CSF than in the ELLIOTT's-B-solution. A similar increase in CSF (K^+) during respiratory acidosis has been observed by CAMERON and might be attributed to a pH dependant exchange of K^+ between intracellular and extracellular compartments of the brain tissue. Since (Na^+) in the original CSF was 10 mval/l higher than in the ELLIOTT's-B-solution, the observed increase in outflow (Na^+) should mainly be due to increased admixture of ventricular and subarachnoid fluid to the perfusion fluid during hypercapnia.

Outflow (K^+) also increased during and after hypoxia, whereas (Na^+) remained low in the same 20 minutes sample. However, (Na^+) inreased during the next 20 minutes. 50 minutes after restoring normal gas mixtures (Na^+) almost came back to steady state level. (K^+), although also coming down, was still considerably higher than before onset of hypoxia. These findings should be compared with results, obtained by GOTOH and MEYER, MEYER and KANDA and WEST and MATSEN, who showed a decrease in CSF (K^+) during ischemic hypoxia. Our results only differ slightly with respect to the changes in (Na^+) which might be due to the fact that both, degree and duration of hypoxia in our experiments were much smaller, so that all animals survived without neurological deficits. However, the fact that CSF (Na^+) did not increase during and immediately after hypoxia, as this was seen during hypercapnia, might be interpreted as an early indication of disturbed active ion transport mechanisms as shown by others. These disturbances might be expected to cause intracellular Na^+ and water accumulation, i. e. brain edema.

In conclusion, since both, hypercapnia and hypoxia increase intracranial contents much faster than can be compensated for by an increase in CSF-absorption, special care should be given to ventilatory disturbances in patients with increased intracranial pressure. CSF electrolyte concentrations change during hypercapnia due to a pH effect on intra-extracellular-cation distribution in the brain. The recorded changes in CSF (Na^+) and (K^+) during hypoxia might be related both to a pH effect and to inhibition of active ion transport mechanisms.

REFERENCES

1. BERING, E.A. and O.SATO: Hydrocephalus: Changes in Formation and Absorption of Cerebrospinal Fluid Within the Cerebral Ventricles. J.Neurosurg. 20, 1050-1063 (1963)

2. CAMERON, I.R.: in: B.K.Siesjö and S.C.Sørensen: Ionic homeostasis of the brain. Munksgaard 1971

3. DORSCH, N.W.C. and L.SYMON: in: M.Brock and H.Dietz: Intracranial pressure, Berlin 1972

4. ELLIOTT, K.A. and H.H.JASPER: Physiological salt solutions for brain surgery. Studies of local pH and pial vessel reactions to buffered and unbuffered isotonic solutions. J.Neurosurg. 6, 140-152 (1949)

5. GOTOH, F. et al.: Neurochem. 9, 81-97 (1962)

6. MEYER, J.S. et al.: Neurology 21, 889-895 (1971)

7. PAPPENHEIMER, J.R. et al.: Amer.J.Physiol. 203, 763-774 (1962)

8. WEST, C.R. and F.A.MATSEN: Effects of experimental ischemia on electrolytes of cortical cerebrospinal fluid and on brain water. J.Neurosurg. 36, 687-699 (1972)

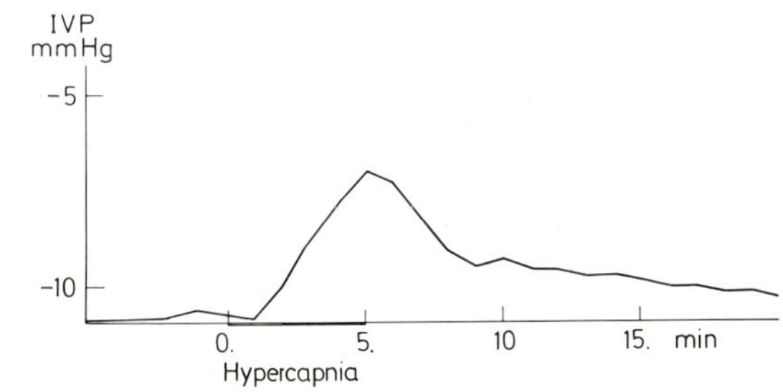

Fig. 1. The influence of hypercapnia on intraventricular pressure during ventricular-cisternal-perfusion

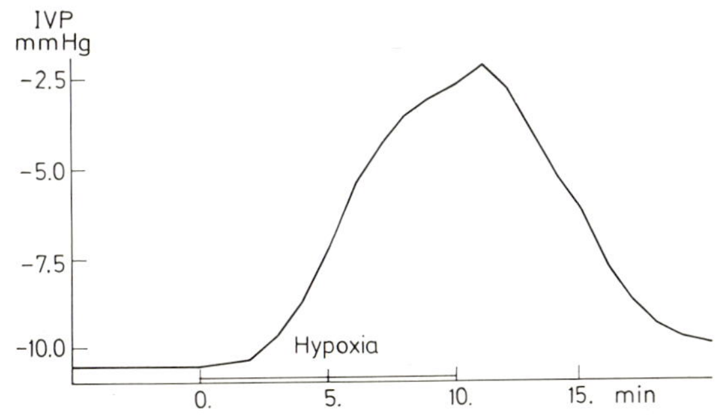

Fig. 2. The influence of hypoxia on intraventricular pressure during ventricular-cisternal-perfusion

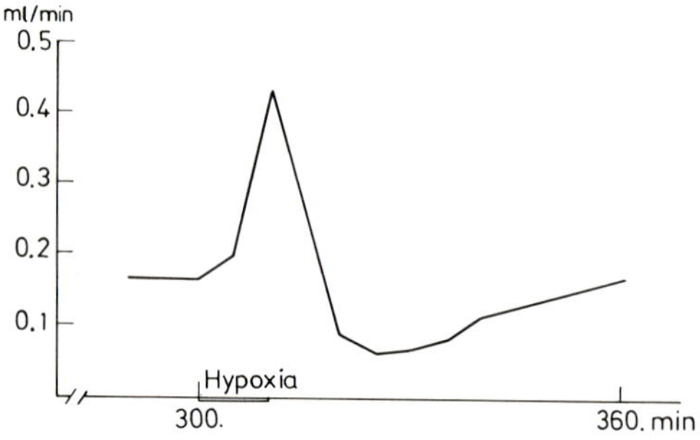

Fig. 3. The effect of hypoxia on CSF outflow during ventricular-cisternal-perfusion

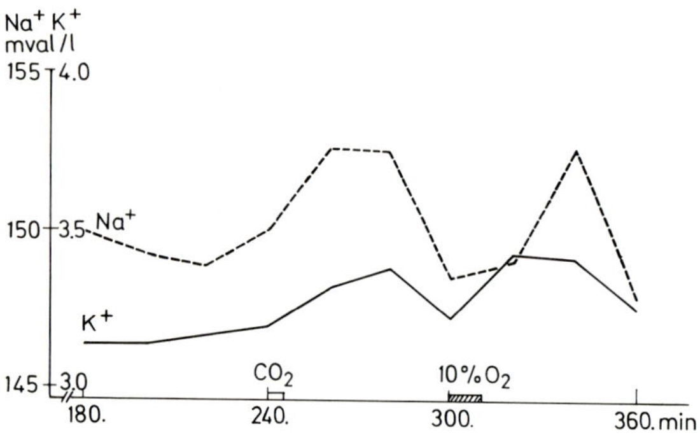

Fig. 4. The influence of hypercapnia and hypoxia upon $(Na^+)_O$ and $(K^+)_O$ during ventricular-cisternal-perfusion

Dissociation of rCBF from Perfusion Pressure in Early State of Cerebral Death (Abstract)

A. TWEED and J. OVERGAARD

Death from traumatic brain injury has usually been found to occur when intracranial pressure rises to near the level of systemic blood pressure, with arrest of cerebral circulation and subsequent respiratory arrest. The ability of the human cerebral circulation to recover after a period of total ischemia is not known, though CBF and functional brain recovery do occur in certain situations: after cardiac arrest of only a few minutes duration, and after prolonged circulatory arrest during deep hypothermia and anesthesia. With animal experiments both hyperemia and "no reflow" after total cerebral ischemia have been reported.

We have studied two young patients within 4 hours of severe, traumatic brain injury. Both were deeply comatose, though not "brain dead", since spontaneous respiration and brain stem reflexes remained. There is good evidence that an indeterminate period of severe intracranial hypertension preceded the investigation in both patients. Regional CBF was measured by the intra-arterial Xenon washout method, mean arterial blood pressure (MABP) was recorded from the carotid artery catheter, and intraventricular pressure (IVP) from a catheter in the lateral ventricle. Position of the ventricular catheters was confirmed by the presence of arterial pulsations and by subsequent injection of radiopaque dye into the ventricles.

IVP was less than 20 torr at the time of CBF measurement in both patients, and rCBF was near zero despite a cerebral perfusion pressure greater than 100 torr. (CPP = MABP - IVP). The absence of cerebral perfusion and correct placement of the arterial catheter were confirmed by cerebral angiography.

The extremely high cerebrovascular resistance in these cases, more than 10 times normal, was an unexpected finding and much higher than any values previously reported in humans. The physiologic and clinical implications of this phenomenon in the series of cerebral death will be discussed.

Chapter IV.

Diagnosis of Cerebello-Pontine Angle Tumors

Microtopography of the Cerebellopontine Angle and Early Otologic Diagnosis of Cerebellopontine Angle Tumors (Abstract)

W. E. HITSELBERGER and W. F. HOUSE

There has been an amazing increase in the number of acoustic tumors that have come to operation. This is primarily the result of much improved diagnostic techniques. Foremost in this area has been the development of positive contrast material making use of Iophendylate as a contrast substance. This has allowed the early radiologic diagnosis of many cerebellopontine angle tumors before they have reached the size that causes increased intracranial pressure.

Additionally, other advances have been made in the audiologic diagnostic capability. The recognition of the early high tone sensory neural hearing loss in these patients has been extremely important. Refinements in measuring vestibular function have made it possible to pick up even small changes in balance impairment that are related to malfunction of the semicircular canals.

Neurologically the changes associated with a small acoustic neuroma or other cerebellopontine angle tumor are much more subtile than the full blown neurologic picture - an awareness of the many functions of the 5th and 7th nerves especially has allowed these parameters to be tested.

There have been many changes in other aspects of these tumors as well, including the recognition that acoustic tumors are not necessarily associated with elevation of the cerebrospinal fluid protein. Additionally, tumors may be present without changes being seen in the internal auditory canals. The recognition of abnormalities produced by other cerebellopontine angle tumors which can be mistaken for acoustic neuromas has been very important.

This paper will attempt to correlate the above discussion in such a way as to make it practical to the otolaryngologist and neurosurgeon who are confronted with these problems. Hopefully we will be able to point out some of the important aspects in diagnosis that will increase our awareness of the early diagnosis of this tumor.

Neuroradiological Diagnosis of Cerebellopontine Angle Tumors

S. Wende

The neuroradiological diagnosis for the demonstration of a cerebellopontine angle tumor should be initiated by a special examination of both petrous bones (representation of the pyramids in STENVER's projection, in frontal projection, in TOWNE projection , in axial projection). Furthermore, tomography is necessary in order to visualize fine bone structures of the internal auditory canal.

The classical symptom of the acoustic neurinoma is the dilatation of the internal auditory canal which, however, should not be considered as pathognomonic, for it can also occur in general intracranial pressure increase. There are different answers to the question as to when a dilatation of the internal auditory canal is to be diagnosed. LINDGREN considered a side difference of 2-3 mm as still normal. GRAF, however, never obtained a side difference over 1, 5 mm in his comprehensive histological and radiological studies. According to MAYER, a side difference over 1 mm should already be considered as pathological.

Pathological changes of the petrous bone do not allow any conclusion about the tumor size. Extensive destructions indeed are always caused by a large mass, however, a slight defect appears not only in small but also in large tumors, since the intracranial neoplasm develops in the direction of least resistence. Thus, the question of the tumor size cannot be answered by routine neuroradiological diagnosis.

Another outpatient examination method is the radioisotope diagnosis. Following intravenous injection of 99 m technetium cerebral scintigraphy is carried out (2 1/2 hrs post injectionem). In tumors which already exceeded the internal auditory canal in the majority of the cases a radioisotope uptake in the cerebellopontine angle region is present. This radioisotope method however fails to diagnose very small tumors still lying in the internal auditory canal.

There is only one method for definite confirmation of cerebellopontine angle tumor and its extent: representation of the cisterns by means of positive or negative contrast medium. This contrast examination applied to an exact examination technique enables a distinct diagnosis. Thus, the tumor can be identified before having surpassed the internal auditory canal.

Pneumo-encephalo-cisternography

In small tumors the ventricles can show normal position and form, therefore the picture of the cisterns plays a decisive role. Most important for the diagnosis of the cerebellopontine angle tumor are the pontocerebellar cistern, the medullary cistern and the ambient cistern. In case of a small tumor the pontocerebellar cistern is enlarged as a sign of the liquor blocking. The tumor can be completely surrounded by air, then the picture of the cisterns (tomography) represents the actual extent of the mass. Larger neoplasms show more pronounced changes, also the pons is deformed and its lateral surface appears to be flattened. The cistern is medially dilated and shows laterally a concave outline. The cistern can also be withdrawn from the margin of the petrous bone. Simultaneously very often a flattening of the cistern on the opposite side caused by pressure occurs. In all these cases also a deformity of the ambient cistern is present which is significantly dilated on the tumor side and can appear to be resected in its lower outline. Large tumors cause also changes in the region of the 4th ventricle which in pneumoencephalography should always be visualised too.

The diagnosis of the cerebellopontine angle tumor by pneumoencephalography yields satisfactory information about tumors which already exceeded the internal auditory canal extending into the intracranial region. Thus, the tumor must have reached certain size to become visualised in the pneumoencephalogram. At this stage the patient shows already pronounced neurological deficiency symptoms.

It is desirable to recognize the cerebellopontine angle tumor in its earliest possible stage before having exceeded the internal auditory canal and before the appearance of neurological deficiency symptoms. Relating to this cisternography with positive contrast medium (Duroliopaque and Pantopaque) has led to significant progress which is of crucial relevance for the recognition of cerebellopontine angle tumors.

Roentgenograms of Duroliopaque-cisternography demonstrate the contrast spilling into the internal auditory canal on both sides. In the majority of cases the falciform crest is identifiable, also in the medial part of the pontocerebellar cistern the trigeminal nerve can be visualised as an outlined contrast filling defect. Furthermore, representation of the terminal segment of the facial nerve and cochlear nerve is possible.

If pathological changes are present Duroliopaque does not completely enter the internal auditory canal. Then a smoothly outlined crescentic contrast filling defect appears in the region of the internal acoustic meatus. The tumor can be completely encircled by contrast medium, in larger tumors the contrast medium outlines only one side of the mass.

A pathological finding in the Duroliopaque cisternogram is obtained if arachnoidal adhesions or swellings in the region of the 8th cerebral nerve occur. Here, however, the contrast medium appears to be irregular and does not show the typical tumor configuration.

Which method should be preferred ? If a small tumor in the region of the stato-acoustic nerve is suspected (only otological, no neurological deficits) cisternography with Duroliopaque should be carried out. If, however, in addition significant neurological symptoms are also present pneumoencephalography is preferable, since this examination method enables additional demonstration of changes of the cerebellum and midbrain. Both examination methods complement each other. For the early diagnosis of a cerebellopontine angle tumor cisternography with positive contrast medium is the method of choice.

Another reliable examination method is the representation of the internal auditory artery by means of the magnification angiogram. In order to recognise pathological changes of these small vessels in case of acoustic neurinomas or hypacousis we started practising magnification angiography in frontal projection one year ago. These examinations are performed by means of a 0, 1 mm focal spot tube with a magnification factor of 3.

The internal auditory artery is optimally recognisable in its total extent. Displacements or occlusions are clearly identifiable, also fine tumor vessels are easily demonstrable.

In conclusion, the radiological procedure shall be described as it is carried out in our department in each case of a suspected cerebellopontine angle tumor: the presence only of otological deficiency symptoms requires standard diagnosis with tomography of the pyramid region. Subsequently cisternography with positive contrast medium and finally magnification angiography of the internal auditory artery are necessary.

If, however, additionally to the otological deficiency symptoms also neurological changes occur following standard diagnosis with additional tomography cerebral scintigraphy should be carried out. Magnification angiography of the internal auditory artery is third-ranked and finally - if still necessary - pneumoencephalography is indicated.

REFERENCES

1. WENDE, S. and B. LÜDECKE: Technique and value of gas and pantopaque cisternography in the diagnosis of cerebellopontine angle tumors. Neuroradiology 2, 24-29 (1971)

2. WENDE, W. and N. NAKAYAMA: Die neuroradiologische Diagnostik des Kleinhirnbrückenwinkel-Tumors. Ż. Neurol. 203, 1-12 (1972)

▶

Fig. 1. Gas-cisternography. Indentation of right cerebellopontine cistern by a cerebellopontine angle tumor

Fig. 2. Pantopaque-cisternogram. Localized filling defect due to a tumor ▶

Fig.1

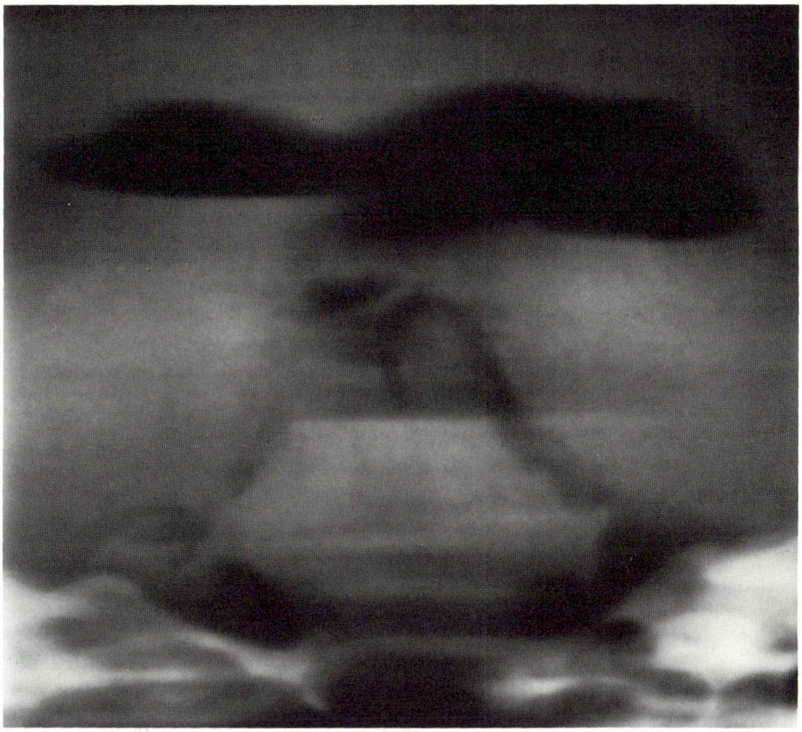

Fig.2

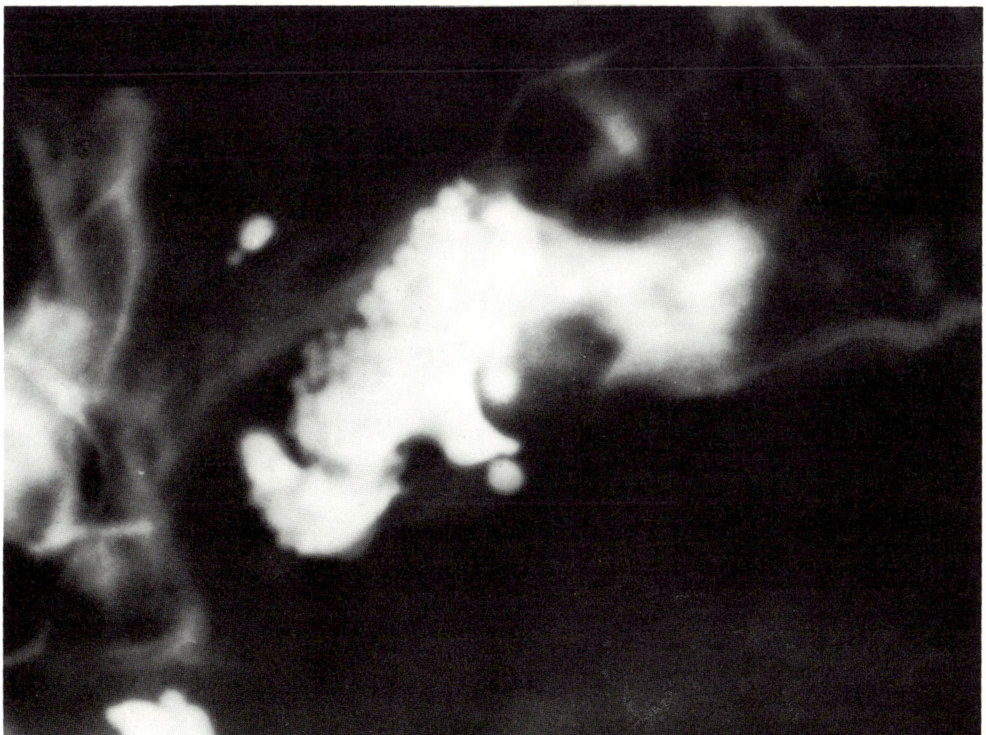

Anomalies of the Arteries of the Caudal Brain Stem and the Cerebellopontine Angle

E. HALVES

The cerebral arteries of 35 human brains were injected post mortally with a mixture of barium sulfate, gelatine and malachite green. The specimens were studied radiologically and macroscopically. By ligature of the Aa. communicantes posteriores the arterial vascular system of the posterior fossa could be demonstrated selectively.
This report deals with:

1. Neurovascular correlations
2. Arterial anastomoses
3. Malformations

1. Variants in the development of the anterior inferior cerebellar artery (AICA) and the internal auditory artery (IAA) and the topographical situation resulting from it in the cerebellopontine angle.

The posterior inferior cerebellar artery (PICA) will take over the circulation area of the AICA if its caliber is reduced, except for the cerebellar flake (Fig. 6). One may often find a small branch of the AICA reaching the flake while its trunk competes with the circulation area of the PICA. A very characteristical course of the AICA consists in a looping around the VII. and VIII. cranial nerves at the internal auditory meatus as well as a close contact to the abducens nerve notching it sometimes at its root.

The point of origin of the IAA will be found most commonly at the lateral third of the AICA during its course through the cerebellopontine angle - especially when it crosses the VII. and VIII. cranial nerves or at the top of the loop in or at the internal auditory meatus.

2. Anastomoses of the arteries of the caudal brain stem. The most extensive anastomoses connect the superior and the inferior arterial group. These will be generally small arterial branches or a network of arterioles on the surface of the cerebellum. You can often find a bigger branch of the artery of the upper worm anastomosing with an arterial branch of the lower worm artery (from PICA) whereas contralateral anastomoses will be commonly small. A linkage of the inferior arterial group among one another is not so important except a contralateral connection across the lower worm and the roof of the IV. ventricle (Fig. 1).

3. Neurovascular malformations of the caudal brain stem. Figure 2 shows a formation of a vascular circle by the right vertebral artery. Part of the root of the hypoglossal nerve is surrounded by this arterial circle. There is another circular lateral anastomosis between the vertebral and basilar artery on the same side.

Those malformations represent a transitory stage of embryological development demonstrated in figure 3. It illustrates the stage of caudal cerebral arteries seen at the 30th day of the embryological development (i. e. fetal length of ca. 6 mm). The vertebral artery comes into existence developing from rostral to caudal. Parallel with it there is still the so called "primitive lateral channel" while the segmental connections to the carotid artery and to the aorta are regressing. False regulation in regression and development of the vertebral artery during the following developmental phase will lead to abnormal courses or arterial circles around the root of the hypoglossal nerve.

Figure 4 demonstrates a similar malformation of the left vertebral artery surrounding parts of the root of the XII. cranial nerve. Radiologically it appears like a vascular island (Fig. 5). Persistence of primitive arterial channels may also lead to partial duplication of the vertebral artery or large caliber circular anastomosis between PICA and the vertebral artery (Fig. 6). The vertebral artery's caliber rostral of the anastomosis may be reduced as demonstrated so that it continues as PICA chiefly. In this case there is typical reciprocal caliber or the AICA extending to the flake exclusively - but even here it gives off IAA in the cerebellopontine angle.

The arterial variants reported are caused almost exclusively by disontogenesis. They had not caused any clinical signs. They may gain practical importance during posterior fossa surgery because of altered topography and circulation.

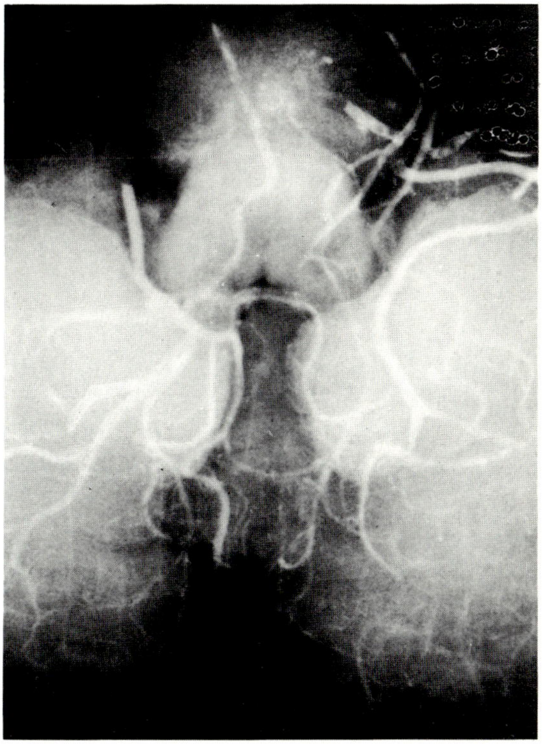

Fig. 1. Postmortal arteriogram demonstrating contralateral anastomosis across the lower worm and the roof of the IV. ventricle

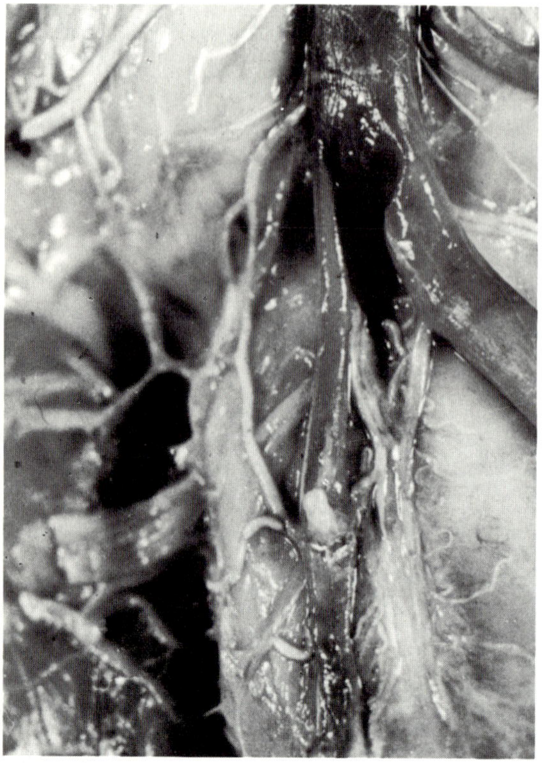

Fig. 2. Vascular circle of the right vertebral artery surrounding part of the hypoglossal nerve root. Lateral anastomosis between vertebral and basilar artery

Fig. 3. Development of the vertebral artery and its branches, (fetal length of 6 mm corresponding to the 30th day of the embryological development)

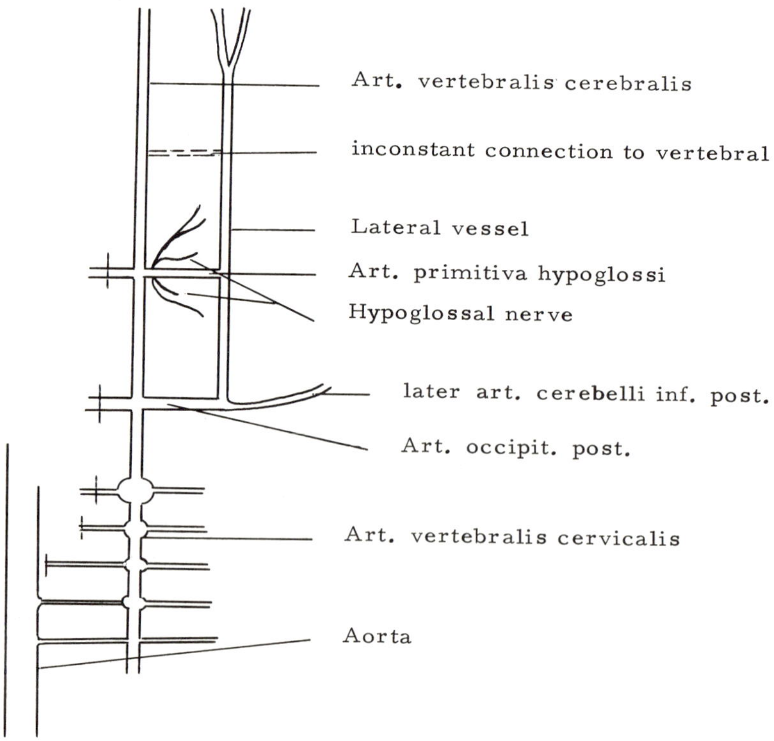

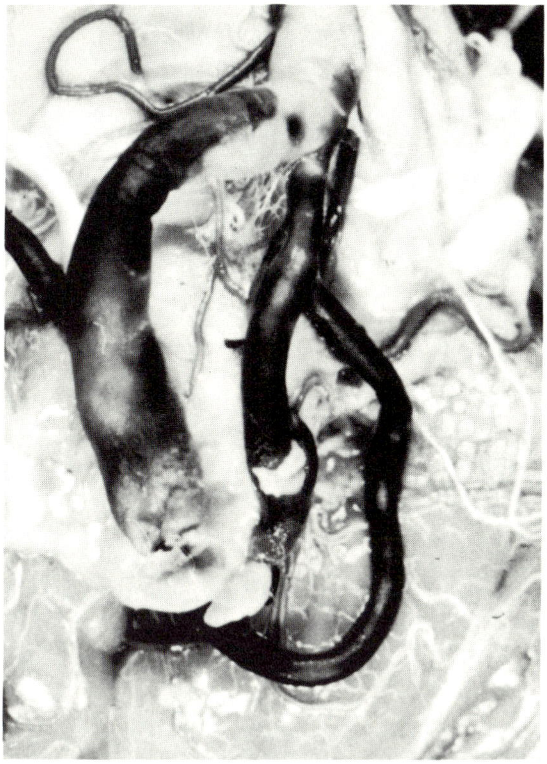

Fig. 4. Part of the hypoglossal nerve root penetrating the left vertebral artery

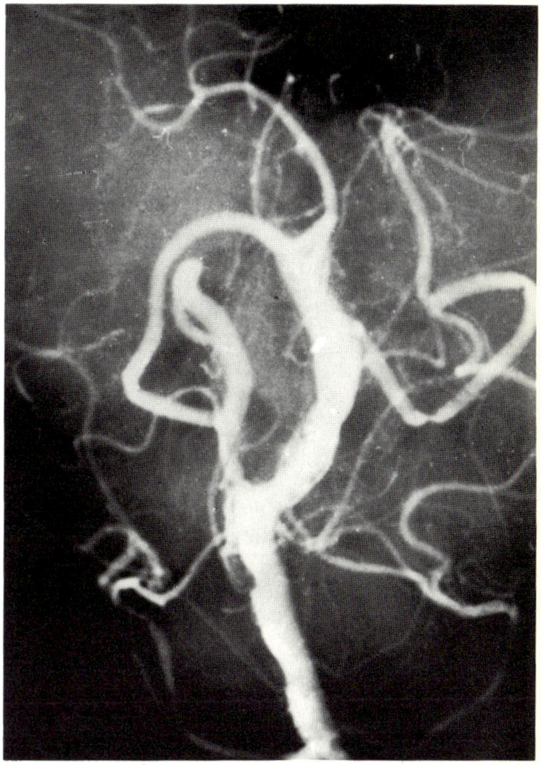

Fig. 5. X-ray picture of Fig. 4

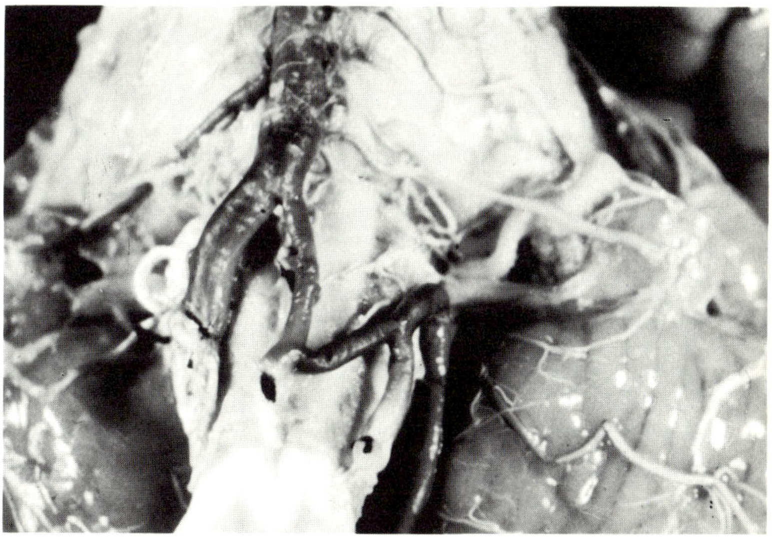

Fig. 6. Partial duplications of the left vertebral artery - or large caliber anastomosis with the PICA

The Diagonal Distribution of Spontaneous Nystagmus

P. C. POTTHOFF

Nystagmus is - still - one of the most frequent concomitant symptoms in cerebellopontine angle lesions. Until now, different (6, 7, 8) and own statistics (2) record gaze nystagmus in up to 95 percent, and spontaneous nystagmus in up to 80 percent of cases. It is to be expected, however, that newer methods of early diagnosis in cerebellopontine angle tumors (HITSELBERGER and HOUSE, this congress (1)) will lead to such an early detection of brain-stem for lesion in the cerebellopontine angle, that nystagmus may not be a concomitant symptom in some cases, and that its frequency will become less in future statistics.

Nystagmus - under these aspects - cannot be considered an early symptom in cerebellopontine angle tumors. This does not, however, alter the importance of the caloric test as an early investigation method in these lesions.

Predominant tumor remains the acoustic neurinoma in more than 80 percent of patients, followed by an average of 4 percent each for meningiomas, cholesteatoma resp. epidermoids, and vascular malformations (angioma, angioblastoma) (unpublished statistics, POTTHOFF and KOERWER, of 181 surgically proven angle lesions: 149 acoustic neurinomas, 8 meningiomas, 6 cholesteatomas resp. epidermoids, 7 vascular malformations). The same arguments for early diagnosis - as described above (HITSELBERGER and HOUSE (1)) - hold true for the expectance that the statistical frequency of acoustic neurinomas will become higher in future collectives.

Early nystagmus findings in smaller cerebellopontine angle tumors (less than 2 cm diameter) - minor signs of mainly contralateral spontaneous and/or gaze nystagmus, and decrease of ipsilateral caloric response in acoustic neurinomas - are, even today, not often seen by the neurosurgeon. In contrast to ENT-investigations giving differentiated nystagmus gradings in cerebellopontine angle lesions (6, 7, 8), the neurosurgeon, as a rule, is still confronted with late nystagmus symptoms only.

This stage of late, or rather terminal nystagmus in cerebellopontine angle lesions shows two characteristics to be demonstrated here. These characteristics emerge preoperatively in larger cerebellopontine angle tumors as well as postoperatively after extensive cerebellopontine angle surgery. They are

1. BRUNS-gaze nystagmus and
2. the diagonal distribution of spontaneons nystagmus.

(While BRUNS-gaze nystagmus has been well known for a long time, the diagonal distribution of spontaneous nystagmus has been assessed for the first time in 1965 by POTTHOFF, PÜRCKHAUER and KORNHUBER (2) in a group of 16 operated larger acoustic neurinomas.)

BRUNS-gaze nystagmus consists of ipsilateral slow and coarse, contralateral rapid and fine gaze nystagmus (lateral compartments, Fig. 1).

The diagonal distribution of spontaneous nystagmus shows the following characteristics of "diagonal distribution" between upward and downward gaze in straight forward direction: On upward gaze the contralateral spontaneous nystagmus increases, on downward gaze it decreases or even reverses to ispsilateral nystagmus in exemplary cases (medial compartments, Fig. 1). Rotatory components are frequent; they should not be mistaken for vertical or oblique nystagmus.

The incidence of both characteristics in our preoperative observations of - usually larger - cerebellopontine angle tumors has been about 70 percent in recent years (17 out of 25 patients).

Two individual examples are given (Fig. 2 and 3).

Neither BRUNS-gaze nystagmus nor the diagonal distribution of spontaneous nystagmus are specific for the etiology of the lesion; they may also be observed in vascular lesions (infarction of the brain stem). Therefore this nystagmus syndrome does also not allow to determine if the lesion lies inside or outside the brain stem.

This nystagmus syndrome is, however, specific for

1. localisation of the lesion at the level of the cerebellopontine angle
2. lateralisation of the lesion
3. its phenomenology

1. The localisation value - especially of the diagonal distribution - is confirmed by our nystagmus investigation of 41 operated cerebellar tumors (5). In that group only 3 cases showed a diagonal distribution of spontaneous nystagmus: Two patients after repeated lateral cerebellar operation for hemangioblastoma resp. cerebellar astrocytoma, one patient after lateral teratoma operation, all three cases with corresponding extension of the lesion towards the brain stem at the cerebellopontine angle. - Case 2, in Fig. 3 of this publication, gives additional evidence. In spite of the fact that this very large meningioma reached far supratentorally, its nystagmus syndrome still preserved the above characteristics of an extensive lesion at the cerebellopontine angle from where the tumor protruded. -
2. The lateralisation of a cerebellopontine angle lesion is specified in this nystagmus syndrome by the following rule: The lesion is contralateral to the direction of spontaneous nystagmus on upward gaze in the "diagonal distribution" and contralateral to the fine and rapid, ipsilateral to the slow and coarse component of BRUNS-gaze nystagmus.

The nystagmus syndrome of the diagonal distribution of spontaneous nystagmus and BRUNS-gaze nystagmus, therefore, is one of the very few specific nystagmus features in the brain stem. Among these, retraction and convergence nystagmus in bilateral upper aqueductal lesions affecting the pretectal areas (3, 4), the above nystagmus syndrome at the cerebellopontine angle, and - possibly, and not to be discussed here - a further nystagmus syndrome in occluding lesions of the lower fourth ventricle, have to be named (Fig. 4).

REFERENCES

1. HITSELBERGER, W. E. and W. F. HOUSE: Microtopography of the cerebellopontine angle and early diagnosis of cerebellopontine angle tumors. (this congress)
2. POTTHOFF, P. C., K. PÜRCKHAUER and H. H. KORNHUBER: Nystagmographie, Diagnose und Verlauf bei Kleinhirnbrückenwinkeltumoren. Dtsch. Z. Nervenheilk. 187, 497-502 (1965)
3. POTTHOFF, P. C.: Das Koerber-Salus-Elschnig-Syndrom. Dtsch. Med. Wschr. 94, 381-385 (1969)
4. POTTHOFF, P. C.: Koerber-Salus-Elschnig - Upper Sylvanian Digest 4, 9, 16-17 (1969)
5. POTTHOFF, P. C. and M. HAUSTEIN: Nystagmus und Elektronystagmogramm nach Kleinhirntumoroperationen. Neurochirurgia (Stuttg.) 13, 174-188 (1970)
6. SAKATA, E., K. TOKOMASU and A. KOMATSUZAKI: Die diagnostische Bedeutung des Spontan- und Provokationsnystagmus beim Acusticustumor. HNO (Berl.) 11, 310-316 (1963)
7. STENGER, H. H.: Nystagmustypen bei Kleinhirnbrückenwinkeltumoren. HNO (Berl.) 7, 33-38 (1958)
8. TOMITS, G. and J. HULLAY: Der Nystagmus bei Brückenwinkeltumoren. Acta otolaryng. (Stockh.) 56, 612-616 (1963)

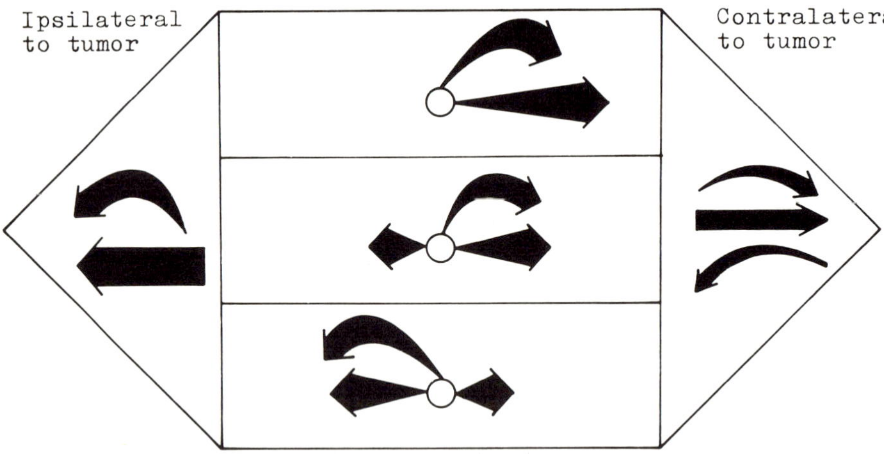

Fig. 1. The "diagonal distribution of spontaneous nystagmus" (medial compartments): On upward gaze increase of contralateral spontaneous nystagmus, on downward gaze decrease or abolition of the contralateral spontaneous nystagmus or reversal to ipsilateral spontaneous nystagmus. BRUNS-gaze nystagmus (lateral compartment): see text

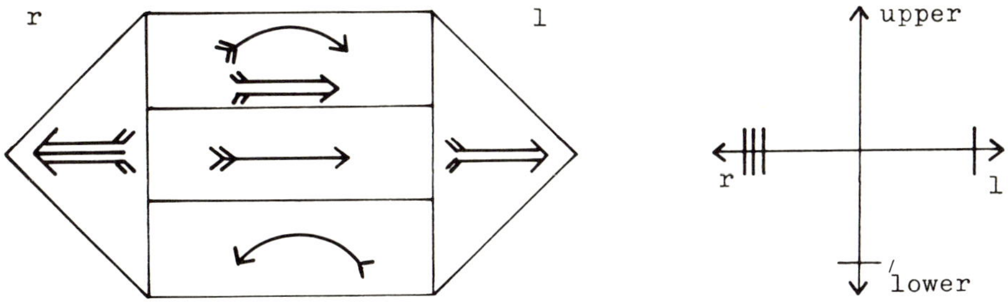

E. A., w, 54 : Meningioma right KBW
(preoperative) (~10 x 4 x 5 cm)

Fig. 2. Case 1 Acoustic neurinoma, left side: Spontaneous nystagmus directed to the contralateral right side, increasing on upward gaze, on downward gaze reversing to the left = Diagonal distribution of spontaneous nystagmus. (BRUNS-gaze nystagmus coarse to the ipsilateral left side, less coarse and of higher frequency to the right. - The crossed arrows indicate optokinetic nystagmus, widely impaired to the right and left side.)

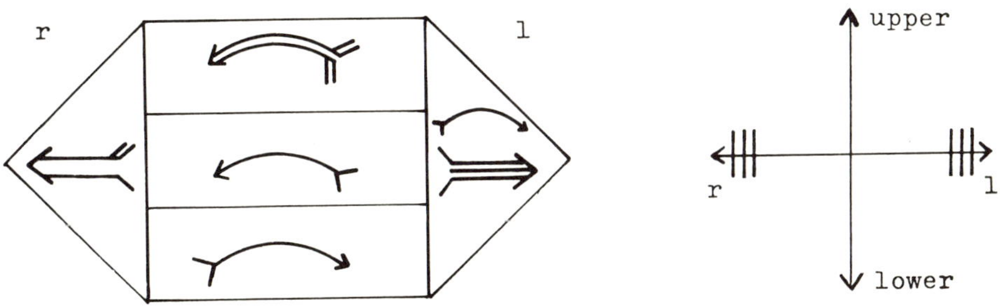

N.A., m, 51 : AN left KBW
(preoperative) (~3 cm ø)

Fig. 3. Case 2 Meningioma, right side: Spontaneous nystagmus directed to the contralateral left side, increasing on upward gaze, reversing on downward gaze to the ipsilateral right side = Diagonal distribution of spontaneous nystagmus (BRUNS-gaze nystagmus more pronounced to the right tumor side than to the contralateral left side. - The crossed arrows indicate optokinetic nystagmus, widely reduced to the right side, moderately impaired to the left side and downwards.)

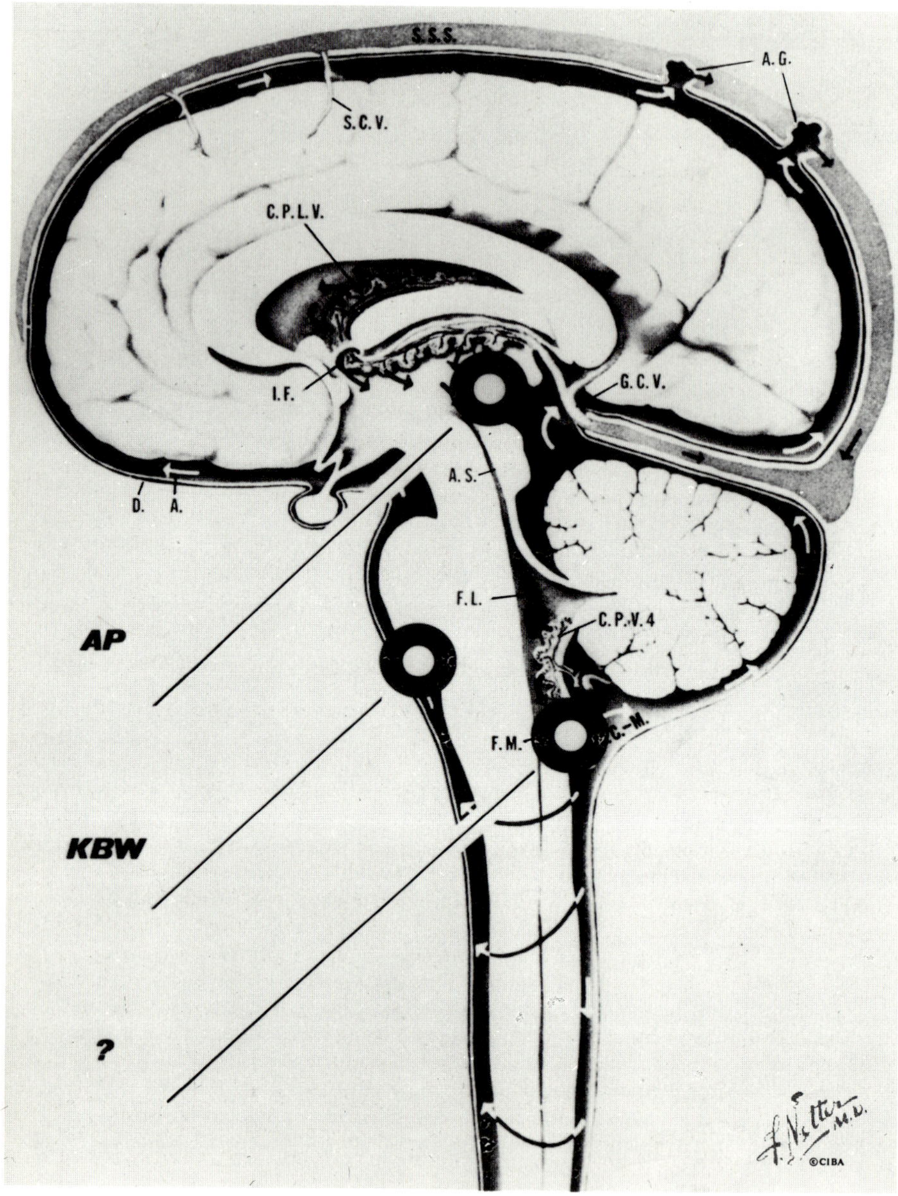

Fig. 4. Anatomy of specific nystagmus syndromes in the brain stem
AP = pretectal area
KBW = cerebellopontine angle
? = questionable nystagmus syndrome in occluding lesions of the lower fourth ventricle (see text)

("Copyright the CIBA Collection of Medical Illustration by Frank H. Netter, M.D.")

The Value of Petrous Bone Exposures in STENVERS' Position and of Brain Scanning in the Diagnosis of Tumors of the Cerebellopontine Angle Region

H. STEINHOFF and V. OLTENAU-NERBE

Tumors of the cerebellopontine angle cause pathological changes in the petrous bone in a high percentage of cases, which usually can be best recognized by X-ray examination in STENVERS' view. The most frequent alteration in the petrous bone, as caused by acoustic neurinomas, is the enlargement of the internal auditory canal (IAC). For the early recognition of a pathological enlargement it is important to know the physiological variations of the internal auditory canal. In the literature different opinions are presented. Among others, CRABTREE (5) reported that a difference of 1 mm in diameter of the IAC between the two sides is to be considered as pathologic whereas CAMP and CILLEY (4) state that physiological variations between the two sides may be as great as 2.5 mm. The opinions concerning the upper margin of the physiological diameter of the IAC differ from 7 mm (9) to 11 mm (4).

Statistical evaluation of physiological variations of the internal auditory canal

Our own evaluation, based on 40 proved unilateral acoustic neurinomas and a group of 100 normal patients, led to the following results: 39 of the acoustic neurinomas, nearly 98 %, showed differences in diameter (Table I). In the normal group differences in diameter were found in 15 %, the largest being 1.5 mm. In 28 cases of acoustic neurinomas (70%) the difference was 2.0 mm or more, 4 cases (10%) showed a difference of 1 mm and in 8 cases (20%) there was a difference of 0.5 mm or none. Due to the statistical analysis using the t-test (STUDENT) a difference in diameter of 2.0 mm is significantly pathologic. The same result has been reported by HOUSE et al. (13) and by APPEL et al. (1). There is no question that a difference in diameter of only 1 mm, accompanied by additional erosions in the petrous bone, is also to be considered as pathologic.

In the normal group the diameter of the IAC varied from 3.0 to 9.0 mm (Table Ia). In 77 % of the normal cases the diameter was between 4.0 and 5.0 mm. In the group of 43 acoustic neurinomas (among them 3 cases with acoustic neurinomas on both sides), diameters between 4.0 and 15.0 mm were found. A diameter greater than 5.5 mm occurred in 85 % of the cases in this group. The statistical analysis using the t-test (STUDENT) led to the result that a diameter of 7 mm is significantly pathologic.

Results of X-ray diagnosis in STENVERS' view

Of 62 proved cerebellopontine angle tumors 44 (66%) showed pathological findings in STENVERS' view, tomography with the polytome in STENVERS' position included (Table II). Pathological changes in the petrous bone were more frequent in the group of 43 acoustic neurinomas (79%) than in tumors of other origin (53%). In

Table I. Differences in diameter of the internal auditory canal between the two sides in STENVERS' view, statistical evaluation of 40 proved unilateral acoustic neurinomas and 100 normal patients

	Acoustic neurinomas	Normal group
Number of cases with differences in diameter	39 (98%)	15 (15%)
Average difference in diameter, mm	2.0	1.2
Greatest difference, mm	5.5	1.5
Smallest measurable difference, mm	0.5	0.5
t = 3.087 (STUDENT'S t = 2.21)		

Table Ia. Statistical evaluation of the diameter of the internal auditory canal in 43 proved acoustic neurinomas and a group of 100 normal patients

	Acoustic neurinomas	Normal group
Average diameter, mm	7.1	5.2
Greatest diameter, mm	15.0	9.0 (1%)
Smallest diameter, mm	4.0	3.5
Predominant diameter, mm (% of total number of cases)	> 5.5 (85%)	4.0-5.0 (77%)
t = 4.5 (STUDENT'S t = 1.960)		

the group of acoustic neurinomas a pathological enlargement of the IAC occurred in 72 % whereas this finding was seen in the group of other tumors only in 16 %. Erosions within the internal auditory canal (Fig. 1) were more frequent in the acoustic nerve tumors (33%) than in other tumors (5%). An erosion of the petrous apex was found in the group of acoustic neurinomas in 18 %, but in 44 % of the cases of other tumors. By the use of additional tomography with the polytome in 7 % of all cases more pathological findings could be achieved.

In the group of acoustic nerve tumors there was no correlation between the size of the tumor and the degree of enlargement of the IAC. Of the tumors with a diameter

Table II. Pathological findings in STENVERS' view in 62 proved cerebellopontine angle tumors

Tumorgroup	Enlargement of int. auditory canal (IAC)	Erosion of petrous apex	Erosion of IAC	Total number of pathol. findings
Acoustic neurinomas n = 43	31 (72%)	8 (18%)	14 (33%)	34 (79%)
Cerebellopontine angle tumors (Acoust. n. excluded) n = 19	3 (16%)	8 (44%)	1 (5%)	10 (53%)
Total cases of cerebellopontine angle tumors n = 62	34 (55%)	16 (26%)	15 (24%)	44 (66%)

of more than 3 cm 23 % showed no enlargement of the internal auditory canal at all. On the other hand 67 % of the tumors smaller than 3 or 2 cm in diameter showed a significantly pathological enlargement of the IAC (Fig. 2). In the group of other tumors we can state that a large erosion in the petrous apex was found only in the presence of a large tumor, but that small changes in the petrous apex do not rule out a large tumor in the cerebellopontine angle.

Concerning differential diagnosis our results led to the conclusion that a large ballooning of the IAC is typical for an acoustic neurinoma whereas a large destruction of the petrous apex without enlargement of the IAC should lead one to suspect a tumor of other origin.

Results of brain scanning

Brain scanning with 99m technetium as well as plain X-ray examinations of the skull (including STENVERS' view) are methods without any risk for an ambulatory patient with clinical signs of tumor of the cerebellopontine angle. The question arises as to what extent brain scintigraphy is of additional value in detecting tumors of this region.

Brain scanning was performed on 41 patients with proved tumors of the cerebellopontine angle including 27 acoustic neurinomas. The results of scintiscanning were compared with those obtained by X-ray examination in STENVERS' view, tomography excluded.

Of the 41 tumors 61 % showed positive results in the brain scan and 64 % showed pathological changes in STENVERS' view (Table III). In the group of 27 acoustic nerve tumors the percentage of pathological findings was higher by means of skull exposures in STENVERS' position (78%) than by brain scanning (59%).

Table III. Results of scintigraphy and X-ray examination in STENVERS' view in the diagnosis of tumors in the cerebellopontine angle region

Tumorgroup	Scintigraphy				STENVERS' View			
	n	pos.	susp.	neg.	n	pos.	susp.	neg.
Cerebellopontine angle tumors, total	41	25 (61%)	6 (15%)	10 (24%)	39	25 (64%)	2 (5%)	12 (31%)
Acoustic neurinomas	27	16 (59%)	4 (15%)	7 (26%)	27	21 (78%)	0	6 (22%)
Cerebellopontine angle tumors (Acoust. n. excluded)	14	9 (64%)	2	3	12	4 (33%)	2	6

The frequency of positive results of brain scanning depends on the size of the tumor in contrast to the pathological results in STENVERS' view, which generally do not necessarily depend on the stage of tumor expansion. That means, that small tumors (< 2 cm in diameter) and tumors smaller than 3 cm in diameter can be detected in a higher percentage by STENVERS' examination than by brain scanning. Of 8 acoustic neurinomas smaller than 2 or 3 cm in diameter, all of them showing positive results in STENVERS' view, only one (greater than 2 cm in diameter) showed a positive result in the brain scan. On the other hand, tumors of more than 3 cm in diameter showed more positive results in the scintigram than in STENVERS' examination. Of 19 acoustic neurinomas of more than 3 cm in diameter 79 % were positive in the brain scan and 68 % were positive in STENVERS' view (Table IV

Table IV. Results of scintigraphy and X-ray examination in STENVERS' view in acoustic neurinomas in relation to the diameter of tumor

Diameter of tumor	n	Scintigraphy			STENVERS' View		
		pos.	susp.	neg.	pos.	susp.	neg.
< 2 cm	4	-	1	3	4	-	-
> 2 cm - 3 cm	4	1	1	2	4	-	-
> 3 cm	19	15 (79%)	1 (5%)	3 (16%)	13 (68%)	-	6 (32%)

Table V. Results of scintigraphy and X-ray examination in STENVERS' view in tumors of the cerebellopontine angle region in relation to the diameter of tumor

Diameter of tumor	n	Scintigraphy			STENVERS' View		
		pos.	susp.	neg.	pos.	susp.	neg.
< 2 cm	4	-	1	3	4	-	-
> 2 cm - 3 cm	5	2	1	2	5	-	-
> 3 cm	30	21 (70 %)	3 (10 %)	6 (20 %)	16 (53 %)	2 (7 %)	12 (40 %)

and Fig. 3). Of all tumors of the cerebellopontine angle region larger than 3 cm in diameter (n = 30) 70 % showed positive results in the scan and only 53 % had pathological changes in STENVERS' view (Table V).

In contrast to plain skull X-ray examination, including STENVERS' projection, brain scintigraphy makes it possible to estimate exactly the size of the tumor in a high percentage of cases.

By the use of both methods the percentage of pathological findings can be improved to 94 % in acoustic neurinomas and to 79 % in the group of the other tumors.

Summary

The results of X-ray examination in STENVERS' projection of 62 proved tumors of the cerebellopontine angle region, tomography with the polytome in STENVERS' position included, are discussed. In 39 tumors the results of STENVERS' examination, tomography excluded, are compared to those of brain scanning.
Brain scanning in addition to X-ray examination in STENVERS' view is of great value especially in the detection of larger tumors. By the use of both methods 94 % of the acoustic neurinomas and 79 % of the tumors of other origin can be detected. In contrast to STENVERS' examination brain scintigraphy enables one in a high percentage of cases to make an exact estimation of the size of the tumor. On the other hand, brain scanning is of no value in the early detection of small tumors of the cerebellopontine angle region, as tumors smaller than 2 cm in diameter are not revealed by this method.

REFERENCES

1. APPEL, L., J. METZGER et B. PERTUISET: Le diagnostic du neurinome de l'acoustique par la radiologie conventionelle, la tomographie et les examens de contrast. J. Belge Radiol. 54, 233, (1971)
2. BAUM, S., B. ROTHBALLER, F. SHIFFMAN and R. F. GIROLAMO: Brain scanning in the diagnosis of acoustic neuromas. J. Neurosurg. 36, 141 (1972)

3. BEST, P.V. and M.C.PATH: Erosion of the petrous temporal bone by neurilemmoma. J. Neurosurg. 28, 445 (1968)

4. CAMP, J.D. and E.I.L.CILLEY: The significance of asymmetry of the pori acustici as an aid in the diagnosis of eight nerve tumors. Amer. J. Roentgenol. 41, 713 (1939)

5. CRABTREE, J.A. and W.F.HOUSE: X-ray diagnosis of acoustic neuromas. Arch. otolaryng. 80, 695 (1964)

6. DRAKE, Ch.G.: Akustikusneurinom. Fortschr. auf d. Geb. d. Neurochir., Referate- u. Vortragssamml. d. Deutsch. Ges. f. Neurochir., Göttingen, 1968

7. FISCHGOLD, H., J.METZGER et G.SALOMON: Les neurinomes du VIII. 1 vol., Garnier éd., Paris, 1961

8. GLASSCOCK, M.E.: History of the diagnosis and treatment of acoustic neuroma. Arch. otolaryng. 88, 578 (1968)

9. GRAF, K.: Die Geschwülste des Ohres und des Kleinhirnbrückenwinkels. G. Thieme Verlag, Stuttgart, 1 vol., 1952

10. HAMBLY, W.H. et al.: The differentialdiagnosis of acoustic neuroma. Arch. otolaryng. 80, 708 (1964)

11. HITSELBERGER, W.E. and W.F.HOUSE: Polytome-pantopaque: a technique for the diagnoses of small acoustic tumors. J. Neurosurg. 29, 214 (1968)

12. HITSELBERGER, W.E., W.EMD and G.Jr.GARDNER: Other tumors of the cerebellopontine angle. Arch. Otolaryng. 88, 712 (1968)

13. HOUSE, W.F. et al.: Acoustic neuroma: monograph II. Arch. Otolaryng. 88, No. 6 (entire issue), 1968

14. JIROUT, J.: Neuroradiologie, VEB-Verlag, Volk u. Gesundheit - Berlin (S. 340), 1966

15. LEONHARD, J.R. and M.L.TALBOT: Asymptomatic acoustic neurilemmoma. Arch. Otolaryng. 91, 117 (1970)

16. LINDGREN, E.: Akustikustumoren. Handbuch d. Neurochir., Bd.II, Springer Verlag, Berlin-Göttingen-Heidelberg (S. 22), 1954

17. MOODY, R.A., J.O.OLSEN, A.GOTTSCHALK and P.B.HOFFER: Brain scans of the posterior fossa. J. Neurosurg. 36, 148 (1972)

18. OLIVECRONA, H.: Acoustic tumors. J. Neurosurg. 26, 6 (1967)

19. PERTUISET, B. et al.: Les neurinomes de l'acoustique développes dans l'angle pontocérébelleux. Neurochir., Tome 16, Suppl. 1 (1970)

20. POOL, L.J., A.PAVA and E.C.GREENFIELD: Acoustic nerve tumors; early diagnosis and treatment. Sec. Ed. Charles C. Thomas, Publ. Springfield, Ill., 1970

21. SHEEHY, J.L.: The neuro-otologic evaluation. Arch. Otolaryng. 88, 592 (1968)

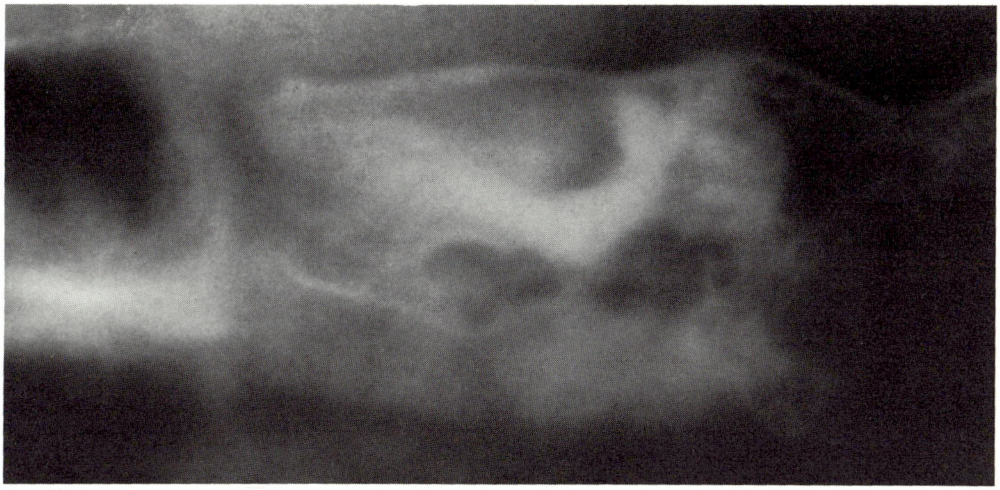

Fig. 1. Right acoustic neurinoma with severe enlargement of the internal auditory canal plus additional erosion in the petrous bone tomography with the polytome in STENVERS' projection

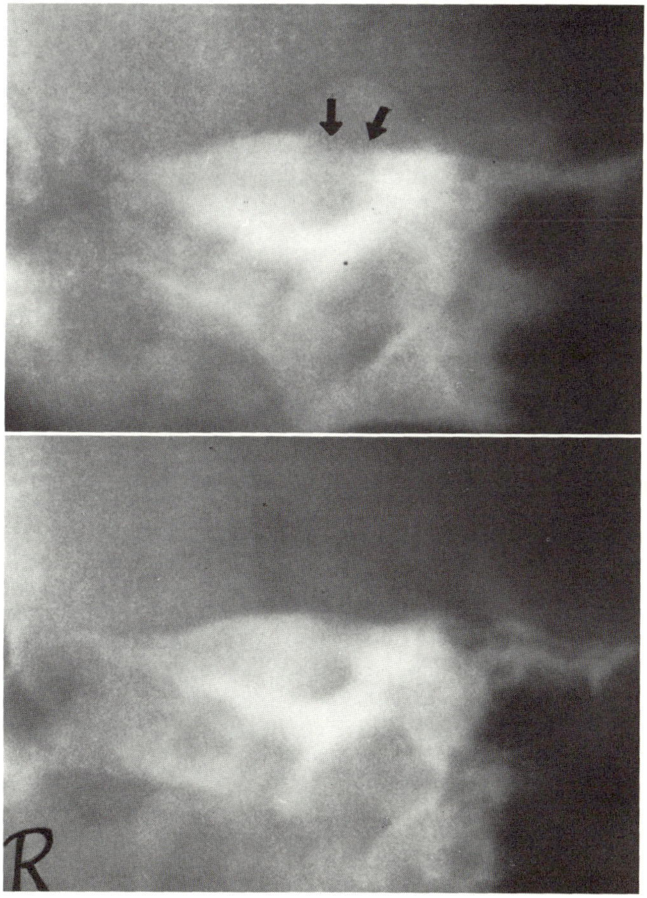

Fig. 2. Acoustic neurinoma of about 2 cm in diameter with severe enlargement of the internal auditory canal; tomography (Polytome) in STENVERS' position

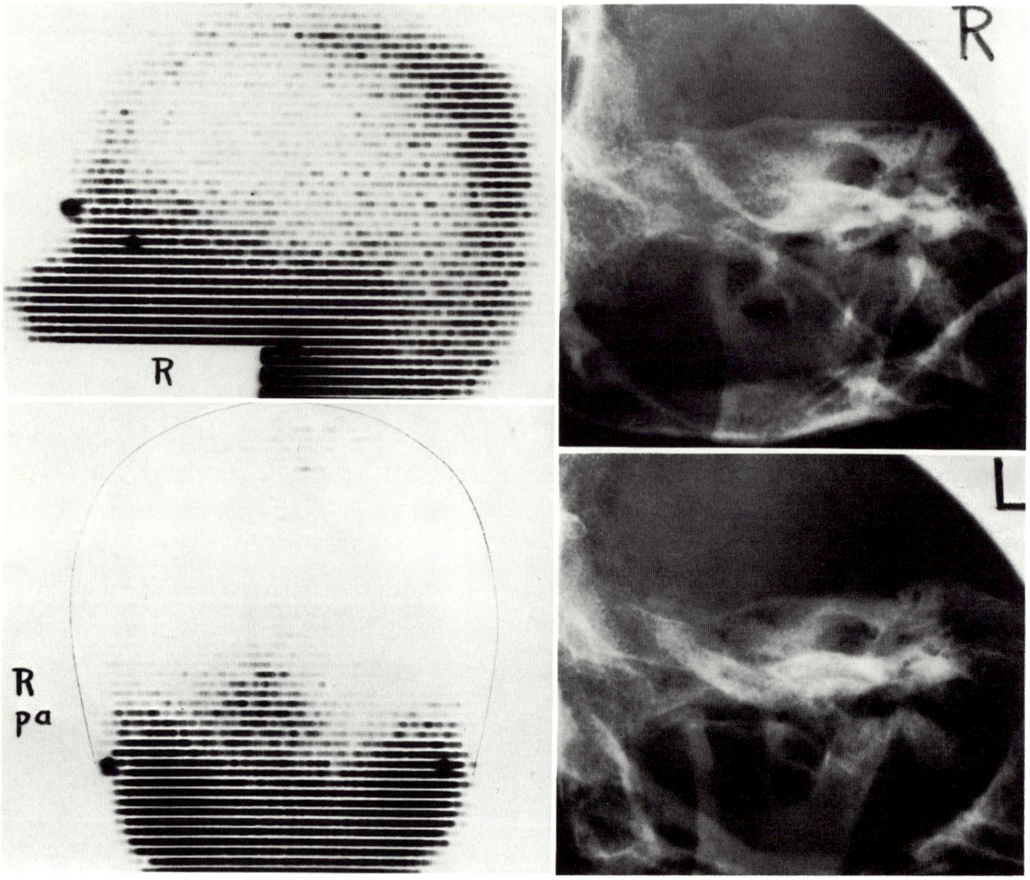

Fig. 3. Right acoustic neurinoma of more than 3 cm in diameter. No significant pathological findings in STENVERS' view (diameter of the right IAC 5.5 mm, left IAC 5.0 mm, no erosions). The scan shows the large tumor in the right cerebellopontine angle region

The Diagnostic Value of Brain Scan in Cerebello-Pontine Angle Tumors

H. ALTENBURG and W. WALTER

Until a few years ago, the value of diagnostic isotope investigations for the detection of tumors and other lesions of the cerebellum and the posterior fossa was controversial because of technical difficulties and the anatomical peculiarities of this area. Due to technical progress, the use of newer diagnostic isotopes, and greater experience in interpretation in recent years, it has become increasingly easier to allay the basic doubts expressed by many authors about the value of brain scans in the diagnosis of infratentorial lesions. In the meantime thoroughly satisfactory results have been achieved.

Our experience is based on 25 cases of tumors in the cerebello-pontine angle, operated on during the last 3 years and confirmed by surgery and histology. 20 of these were neurinomas and 5 meningiomas. The other rare types of tumor in this localisation will not be considered here.

In all 25 tumors of the cerebello-pontine angle where the diagnosis was suspected on the basis of the clinical, radiological and echoencephalographic findings, an unequivocally pathological concentration of 99m Tc pertechnetate confirmed the localisation and size of the tumor before further, more involved diagnostic procedures were performed. Conclusions about the type of tumor could not be drawn.

We are aware of the fact that smaller tumors, located primarily in the porus acusticus can escape detection by scintigraphy. However, the tumors we diagnosed could be clearly verified on the p.a.-scan as well as on the corresponding lateral scan. Beyond this, large tumors could be recognized even on the p.a.-scans.

In every case vertebral angiography via the brachial artery was performed, and in most cases central ventriculography with Dimer-X was also carried out in order to confirm the diagnosis further.

Although vertebral angiography revealed indirect signs of an infratentorial lesion in most cases, only 20% of tumors detected with the brain scan showed a corresponding pathological vascular tumor blush. These were exclusively meningiomas and unusually vascular neurinomas.

At ventriculography, the signs of tumor growth in the cerebello-pontine angle were also only indirect and included lateral and upward displacement of the aqueduct, as well as stenosis of the aqueduct.

Finally, it should be emphasized that brain scintigraphy is a genuinely valuable addition to the diagnostic methods for detecting cerebello-pontine angle tumors. Since it is harmless, it can be applied even before the use of contrast medium methods, in many cases on an ambulant basis, in order to confirm the typical clinical syndrome, so that further, more stressful diagnostic procedures can even be avoided in some high-risk patients. It is not suited for the early diagnosis of such lesions.

Radio-Isotope Cisternography for the Diagnosis of Cerebello-Pontine Angle Tumors

M. SUNDER-PLASSMANN+)

In 1972, MAMO and HOUDART described radio-isotopic cisternography as being superior to conventional neuroradiological techniques in diagnosing cerebello-pontine angle tumors down to a diameter of 1 cm. But the authors left aside the results obtained with the STENVERS' technique and with cisternography using positive radiopaque substances, when assessing the merits of the isotope procedure.

To verify the diagnostic value of radio-isotopic cisternography we decided to employ this technique on our material, that has, however, not included any tumor with a diameter below 3 cm in the past 6 months on which radio-isotopic cisternography could have been tried.

Method

100 μC ^{131}I-human serum albumin (RIHSA) were diluted to 2 ml in physiologic saline solution and injected into the cisterna magna by sub occipital puncture. Patterns were recorded with the Anger-Camera (Ph. Gamma III) in the exact lateral and postero-anterior views with the head in maximum extension. Recording was started immediately after application of the isotope and continued for 2 hours at intervals of 15 to 20 minutes.

Material

Since December 1972, radio-isotopic cisternography was performed in 12 patients showing symptoms referable to the cerebello-pontine angle. In all of them vestibular and cochlear function was either reduced or completely lost. The STENVERS' technique and Pantopaque cisternography were added to the radio-isotope method in all cases. The table shows the results obtained (Table I). Surgical findings were added for comparison. In cases 1 through 4 the data of the diagnostic procedures were found to correlate well with the surgical findings. In case 5, a patient with a tumor, measuring more than 5 cm in diameter which had pushed the brainstem far towards contralateral, Pantopaque cisternography failed. Attempts at visualizing the tumor contour on the side affected and at introducing the radiopaque substance into the contralateral porus acusticus were unsuccessful. In case 6, an arched contour typically seen in the tumors was visualized in the caudal section of the right cerebello-pontine angle on Pantopaque cisternography. Radio-isotopic cisternography, by contrast, showed an obstacle to isotope passage in the cisterna magna area which was demonstrable for 24 hours. On surgery the cisterna magna was found to be occupied by an arachnoidal cyst. Additionally, arachnoidal adhesions

+) With technical assistance of Miss W.U. SCHUSTER

Table I. Diagnostic and surgical findings in 12 patients with cerebello-pontine angle symptoms

Case	STENVERS' technique	Radioisotopic cisternography	Pantopaque cisternography	Surgical findings
1	pos. l	Lesion l: CP, CM and CCP	pos. l	Acoustic neurinoma
2	pos. r	Lesion r: CP and CCP	pos. r	Acoustic neurinoma
3	pos. l	Lesion l: CP	pos. l	Acoustic neurinoma
4	pos. r	Lesion r: CP and CCP	pos. r	Acoustic neurinoma
5	pos. r	Lesion r: CP and CM	unclear bilateral	Acoustic neurinoma
6	neg.	Block in CM	pos. r	Arachnoidal cyst in CM
7	neg.	neg.	pos. r	Lipoma
8	neg.	Lesion r: CP and CM	neg.	Scheduled for surgery
9	neg.	neg.	neg.	neg.
10-12	neg.	neg.	neg.	-

CP = Cisterna pontis, CM = Cisterna magna, CCP = Cisterna cereb. pontis

were present in the area of the right cerebello-pontine angle. In case 7, Pantopaque cisternography was the only technique to successfully visualize the tumor, a patchy lipoma of the right cerebello-pontine angle extending a cylindrical tongue into the porus acusticus internus. In case 9, a patient with atypical trigeminal neuralgia, both neuroradiologic techniques and scanning failed to visualize any tumor. The absence of a neoplasm was confirmed on surgery using the Dandy neurotomy technique. In cases 10 through 12 none of the diagnostic procedures mentioned revealed a tumor of the cerebello-pontine angle. Surgery was not attempted in these cases.

In conclusion radio-isotopic cisternography is superior to the Pantopaque technique in visualizing extensive tumors associated with lateral displacement of the brain-stem. On account of arachnoidal adhesions Pantopaque cisternography often fails to visualize the tumor contour, and the radiopaque substance can, at times, not be introduced into the porus acusticus internus on the contralateral, intact side. Minor tumors which do not reach far beyond the porus acusticus internus are likely to escape radio-isotopic visualization. In these cases the Pantopaque technique combined with tomography is superior to the isotope procedure.

Where the clinical signs and symptoms are beyond doubt and distension of the porus acusticus internus is verified radiologically, further diagnostic evidence is surely unneccessary. But valuable information can be obtained both from the radio-isotopic and the Pantopaque techniques on the extension of the tumor.

As radio-isotopic cisternography exposes patients to fewer stresses, it should invariably be preferred to the Pantopaque technique.

REFERENCES

1. MAMO, L. and R. HOUDART: Radioisotopic cisternography - contribution to the diagnosis of cerebellopontine angle tumors. J. Neurosurg. 37, 325-331 (1972)

Duroliopaque Cisternography in Cerebello-Pontine Angle Tumors (Abstract)

P. R. Dorland, J. M. Sterkers, R. Billet, and J. P. Chodkiewicz

During the past four years we have been using Pantopaque-Cisternography as a routine procedure to identify cerebello-pontine angle tumors, mostly acoustic neurinomas. Pantopaque Cisternograms are used for every patient with clinical symptoms or signs of acoustic tumor, except in the presence of increased intracranial pressure.

The technique is very simple: 1 or 2 cc. of contrast material are introduced by lumbar puncture; the head is then rotated and positioned to have the pantopaque flowing into the posterior fossa under fluoroscopic control.

In normal patients, the auditory canal can be filled completely, while in case of acoustic neurinoma, the canal cannot be filled and the contrast material outlines the tumor in and outside the canal, depending upon its size.

We have performed more than 100 Pantopaque cisternographies with no incident; the procedure which always lasts less than one hour, is well tolerated.

The results, as fas as the last 70 patients are concerned, are very encouraging:

In 25 cases in which the auditory canal could not be filled correctly there were 18 verified tumors in the angle (15 neurinomas and 3 meningiomas).

In six other cases the tumor was strictly within the auditory canal and almost impossible to demonstrate by the usual radiological procedures.

In the last case of unfilled canal, the operation failed to identify a tumor.

In our hands, when properly performed, pantopaque cisternography has proved to be a benign and faithful test to identify small tumors in the cerebello-pontine angle; the procedure is of great help to the neurosurgeon in selecting the adequate approach based on tumor size and extension.

The Use of Vertebral Angiography in the Differential Diagnosis of Cerebello-Pontine Angle Lesions

L. SYMON and B. KENDALL

In recent years, vertebral angiography has been increasingly used to provide details of the exact site and probable nature of posterior fossa tumors, in a fashion similar to carotid angiography which has largely replaced air study as the definitive neuro-radiological investigation in cases of supratentorial tumor. Angiography has additional advantages in showing the relationship of the tumor to the major blood vessels, which is helpful in planning surgery and, particularly if performed under basal sedation, of carrying little risk of disturbance of intracranial dynamics. In large posterior fossa tumors, it is less liable, therefore, to cause deterioration in the patient's state than encephalography or ventriculography. Vertebro-basilar angiography in combination with plain film findings will usually give enough information to make further neuro-radiological investigations unnecessary. This view is illustrated by review of 30 recent cerebello-pontine angle masses in which vertebral angiography was used to elucidate the clinical picture. The tumors, which presented over the past two years in The National Hospital, Queen Square, and Maida Vale Hospital, all had signs which made the diagnosis of a C. P. angle lesion certain on clinical grounds. There were no cases in which the potential diagnosis of a small acoustic neuroma was being considered and we do not necessarily use angiography as the primary contrast study in such cases.

The 30 cases were 15 acoustic neuromas, 4 angle meningiomas, 2 trigeminal neuromas, 2 brain stem gliomas, 1 epidermoid tumor, 1 chordoma, 1 arachnoid cyst, 2 giant aneurysms of the basilar artery and 2 ectatic atheromatous vertebro-basilar arteries presenting in the angle. Specific changes, erosion of the internal auditory canals, was shown in the plain skull films of 13 of the 15 cases of acoustic neuroma, but in only one of the four posterior fossa meningiomas, which had sclerosis of the petrous bone. Both trigeminal neuromas showed apical petrous erosion with a smooth edge highly suggestive of the condition; the chordoma, however, also showed similar apical petrous erosion and such erosion is not of itself specific. Curvilinear calcification was seen in one of the giant vertebro-basilar aneurysms and a slight expansion of the posterior fossa, indicative of the presence of a large mass, was seen in the case of the arachnoid cyst. In two of the acoustic neuromas, three of the meningiomas and in the cases of brain stem glioma, ectatic arteries, epidermoids and one of the aneurysms, the straight films of the skull were normal.

Any mass within the cerebello-pontine angle will displace vessels away from the petrous bone. Small masses usually displace first the complex of veins running towards the petrosal vein which passes from the lateral aspect of the pons to the superior petrosal sinus. These are the descending brachial vein which frequently receives the lateral mesencephalic vein, the ascending vein of the lateral recess of the 4th ventricle, transverse pontine veins and hemispheric veins from the cerebellum. transverse pontine veins and hemispheric veins from the cerebellum. Fig. 1 shows the normal disposition of these veins on the right side and the complex of veins (arrow heads) displaced away from the petrous bone on the left side by a moderate-sized acoustic neuroma. It should be noted that the displacement of the veins, although curvilinear, does not of itself necessarily outline the maximum circumference of the lesion and that the tumor may be considerably larger than the displacement of the veins suggests. If the mass is large, it will displace the vessels adjacent to the anterior or lateral aspects of the brain stem posteriorly and/or medially. It may cause an increase in the distance between vessels on the anterior and posterior surfaces of the brain stem by flattening it due to compression from one side. An intrinsic brain stem mass may cause similar findings in the lateral projection, but usually expands the transverse diameter also and separates the brain stem vessels in the antero-posterior plane also. The use of vertebro-basilar angiography in differential diagnosis depends upon assessment of all the vascular displacements. In an endeavour to suggest the direction in which growth has occurred. The presence or absence of a pathological circulation and its source of filling will also provide an indication of the character of the lesion.

The acoustic neuromas: This group of tumors forms the largest proportion of any series of angle lesion, and presents fairly typical features on vertebro-basilar angiography. In our own series, 10 of the 15 cases showed pathological circulation of a consistent type. An example is shown in figure 2. The pathological circulation of an acoustic neuroma is typically patchy, is usually filled from small branches of the anterior inferior cerebellar artery, and in the capsule there are often early draining veins. These will usually outline with accuracy the surface of the tumor and when present are the best guide to its size and extent. The anterior inferior cerebellar artery is typically displaced posteriorly and superiorly, the former being evident in the Townes and the latter in the antero-posterior view. Not infrequently, the AICA may be displaced only superiorly and more rarely inferiorly, the patterns of its distribution depending very much on the height of origin of the vessels from the vessel from the basilar artery. Fig. 3, for example, is an antero-posterior projection in which the antero-inferior cerebellar arteries (large arrowheads) show different displacements by bilateral acoustic neuromas. The tumour on the left side displaced a small branch of the AICA running on the lateral aspect of the brain stem (small arrow) medially, but did not affect the normal course of the main artery or its hemispheric branches. The larger tumour on the right side elevated the AICA and sisplaced a hemispheric branch around it. The superior cerebellar artery is also elevated (arrowhead). This was a young lady with neuro-fibromatosis in whom both tumours were successfully removed with preservation of the facial nerves. If very large, the mass may so indent the brain stem as to pass behind the basilar artery, carrying the anterior inferior cerebellar artery of the affected side across the midline before running back on the posterior aspect of the tumour. The vertebro-basilar appearances of a moderate or large acoustic neuroma are virtually diagnostic.

Trigeminal neuroma: The two trigeminal neuromas in this series were both large lesions and the displacement of the vessels seen in these circumstances is again characteristic. Pathological ciruclation was not a feature of either of these lesions. Although, if present, it is usually from the meningo-hypophyseal trunk of the carotid artery. Classically, the trigeminal neuroma displaces the veins of the angle from the upper part of the petrous bone, and laterally indents the upper brain stem, separating the anterior inferior cerebellar artery which is bowed inferiorly or if the tumor is very large, even directly medially from the superior cerebellar artery which is commonly stretched upwards and medially. The posterior cerebral artery itself may also be similarly displaced. The tumor pushes the lateral mesencephalic vein posteriorly and increases the space between it and the anterior pontomesencephalic vein. The posterior and lateral mesencephalic veins are also displaced medially. A typical trigeminal neuroma is shown in fig. 4, in which the small arrowhead indicates the superior cerebellar artery, the medium arrowhead points to the AICA and the large one to the superior cerebellar artery.

Meningiomas of the angle: These may present a pathological circulation which aids appreciably in diagnosis. It is usually derived from the meningeal branches of the carotid arteries and is homogeneous and tends to persist in the venous phase, in contrast to the patchy, more rapid circulation of an acoustic neuroma. The meningioma also tends to encircle vessels in the upper part of the angle, and in this respect resembles basal meningiomas elsewhere, where suspiciously straight or suddenly narrowed portions of major arteries suggest the presence of an encircling meningioma. Such findings were evident in two of the four angle lesions in the present series, where the posterior cerebral and internal carotid arteries were shown to be involved in the tumor on preliminary angiography.

Tumors of the brain stem: Intrinsic brain stem tumors presenting with masses in the angle may occasionally cause difficulties in pre-operative diagnosis. The vertebrobasilar angiogram shows splaying of some vessels around the brain stem, due to expansion of both the sagittal and transverse diameters, in addition to the displacement of the vessels in the cerebello-pontine angle.

Chordoma: The chordoma in the present series displayed an apical petrous erosion on the straight films and displacement of the AIC and superior cerebellar arteries suggestive of an apical petrous mass, such as a trigeminal neuroma. In this instance, the irregular pathological circulation sometimes seen in chordomas was not in evidence, and the angiogram could not be regarded as having given specific information as to pathology.

Cholesteatoma: This avascular lesion is often a flat plaque in the angle causing only a slight displacement of the vessels away from the petrous bone over a wide extent. The shape of the lesion and absence of circulation should suggest the diagnosis.

Arachnoid Cyst: These avascular lesions in the cerebello-pontine angle are often extensive and multilocular and may pass through the tentorium into the interpeduncular and parasellar regions. They frequently expand the adjacent part of the skull. The extent of displacement of the vessels with the posterior cerebral and superior cerebellar carried upwards and medially, anterior inferior cerebellar medial and the posterior inferior cerebellar depressed, together with complete avascularity in the capillary phase of the angiogram, lead to consideration of an arachnoid cyst in our case. This patient had originally been regarded as a case of communicating hydrocephalus and had had a ventriculo-caval shunt inserted in childhood without detailed neuro-radiological studies. The presentation of a cerebello-pontine angle lesion syndrome in the fifth year of life, despite revision of the shunt, led to detailed investigation and the removal of the benign arachnoidal cyst with complete cure.

Vascular lesions: These are directly elucidated by vertebro-basilar angiography. In the present group of cases, two ectatic vessels in the angle were present, both of which had presented with tinnitus, a partial deafness and cranial nerve palsies, in one instance involving the 7th nerve alone, in the other instance involving the 5th, 7th and 9th as well as the 8th. Exploration of these lesions is not as a rule indicated, unless for trigeminal pain, and the use of vertebro-basilar angiography will, therefore, avoid purposeless operation. Giant aneurysms of the basilar artery or giant ectatic basilar arteries are also not amenable to surgery. One of the present cases presented with 9th cranial nerve palsy, together with a cerebellar syndrome. Air encephalography elsewhere had shown a very large mass in front of the brain stem and in the angle. Vertebral angiography confirmed this mass to be the largely thrombosed giant sac of a basilar aneurysm which involved the whole length of the basilar artery from the vertebral junction to the origin of the posterior cerebral arteries. Exploration in this case, which would have been of no value and might possibly have been dangerous, was avoided by the use of angiography.

Summary

It appears to be a characteristic of European neurosurgery that cerebello-pontine lesions have reached a fairly large size by the time of presentation to the neurosurgeon. We do not claim that in the case of small lesions of the angle vertebral angiography will give unequivocal diagnostic results, but in moderate or large-sized angle lesions the site of the tumor has been localised correctly in every case, its size accurately outlined in over 80 % of cases, and its pathological nature suggested from pathological circulation or other findings in the majority of these cases. Subtraction studies were routinely performed, but magnification which further enhances the value of vertebral angiography was not used in the small series.

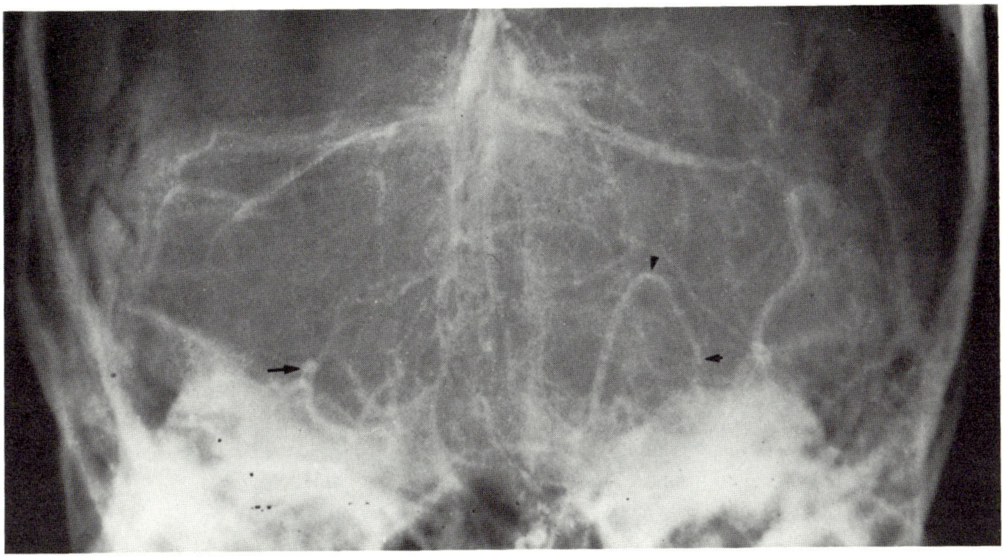

Fig. 1. (see text)

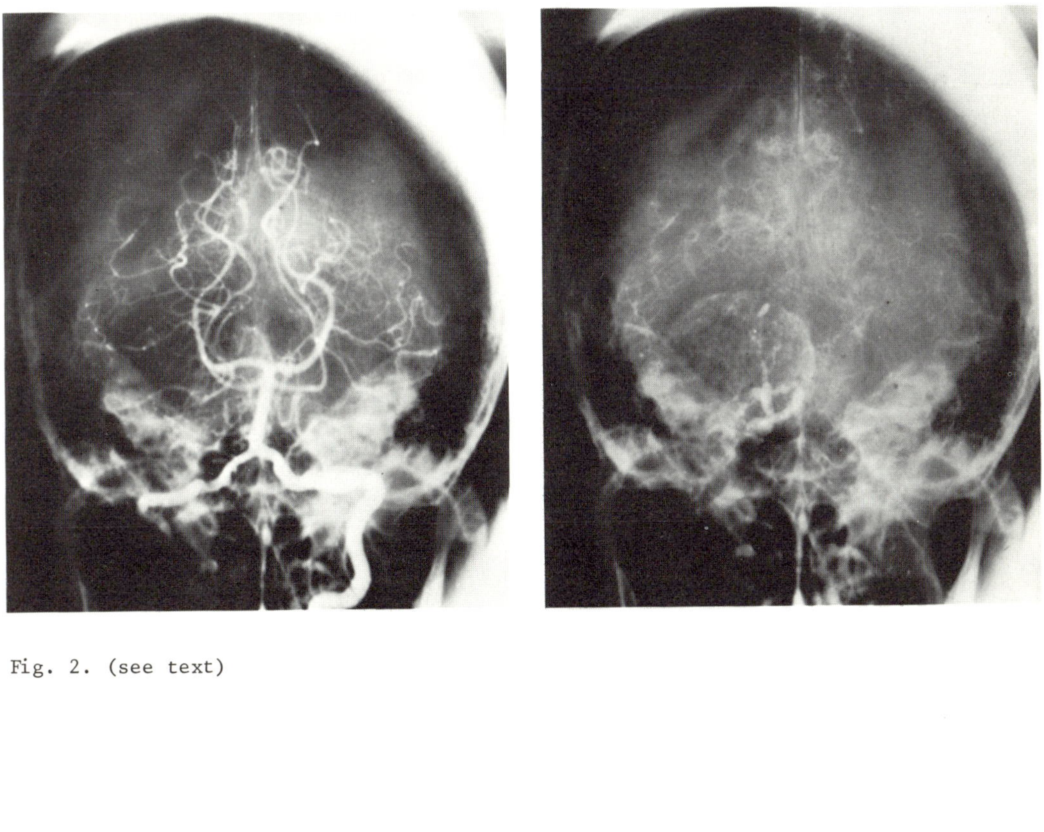

Fig. 2. (see text)

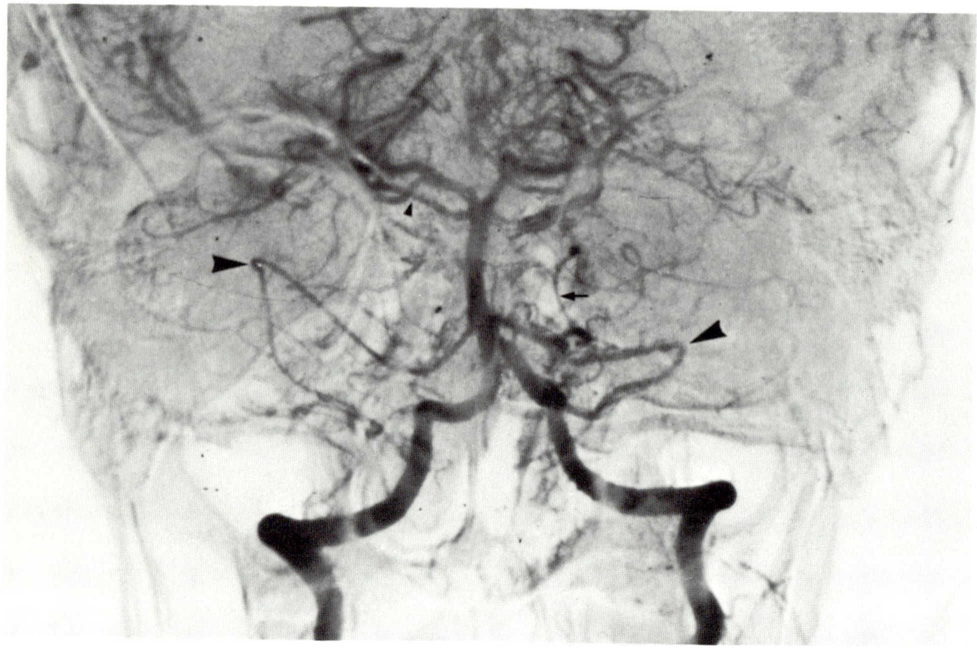

Fig. 3. (see text)

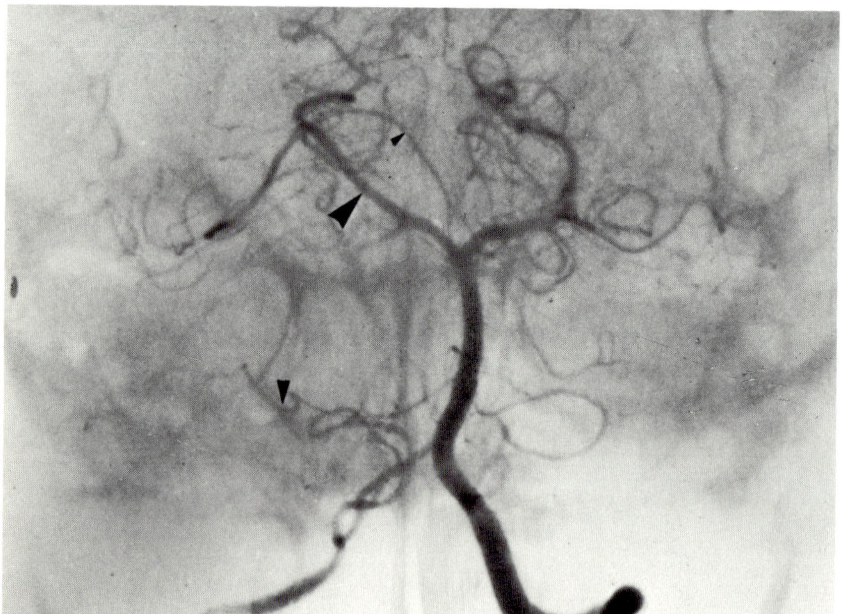

Fig. 4. (see text)

Chapter V.

Surgery of Cerebello-Pontine Angle Tumors

Experiences and Results with the Translabyrinthine Approach and Related Techniques (Abstract)

W. E. HITSELBERGER and W. F. HOUSE

Since 1963, the authors have collaborated in carrying out over 600 explorations of the cerebellopontine angle for various types of tumors. During this period of time, there has been a gradual evolution in the surgical approaches to this area. Initially there were considerable limitations placed on the translabyrinthine approach, i.e., it was felt only suitable for use in small tumors. However, with an increase in our understanding of this tumor we have been able to apply this operation for even large tumors. This has resulted from primarily an improvement in instrumentation, the use of the operating microscope and high speed drills and certainly the increasing experience of the surgeons. However, we have felt that these techniques are of no value if they cannot be taught to other physicians; instead of being the type of operation that will be perpetuated and will be used, they become more of a stunt or even an experiment if the physicians who originated them, cannot teach them to other doctors. It is our hope that the techniques that have been developed in this area, will continue to be used and even improved upon by others who have taken up this type of work.

These authors will discuss the results of their surgery as regards mortality and morbidity, especially preservation of facial nerve function. Appropriate movies will be used to demonstrate the different surgical problems that one encounters in this region.

Experiences and Results with Posterior Approaches (Abstract)

C. G. Drake

The surgical treatment of acoustic neuroma has reached the stage when it is not a question whether the facial nerve can be saved, but rather that it should be saved or reconstituted in the posterior fossa during total removal of large (and small) tumors except in unusual circumstances.

In a series of 51 large tumors, 14 were completely removed and the facial nerve could be saved or reconstituted in all but nine cases which were chiefly early in the series (Table I).

Table I. Acoustic Neuroma - 55 Cases - Fate of Facial Nerve and its Function

Tumor Size	Procedure		No. Cases	Excellent	Good	Poor
Large	Intracapsular Removal		7	7		
		C7 sacrificed	9			9
		C7 saved	27+)	5	10	8++)
	Total removal	Extrapetrous graft	4		3	1
		Intracranial anastomosis of C7	8		5	3
Small	Total removal		4	3		1

+) 4 deaths with post-operative clots early in series

++) 2 too recent to assess

Excellent = No mass movement

Good = with mass movement

The four deaths occurred early in the series, all from postoperative clots after the patient had come around from the procedure initially.

The extrapetrous grafts were done early in the series. There will be little need for this method in the future as it is possible now either to save the whole nerve or, where it is frayed or incorporated in the capsule, to anastomose the elongated pontine and meatal segments in the posterior fossa.

Only four small tumors have been seen and there was no problem with preservation of the facial nerve and its function, except in one case where the tumor was peculiarly en plaque and invading the petrous bone. The future lies in the early recognition of these tumors when the problem will be to preserve useful hearing.

A reassessment of the posterior fossa technique will be given emphasizing the features for preserving or reconstituting the facial nerve in the total removal of large tumors.

Surgical Reconstruction of Intracranial Lesions of Cranial Nerves

F. LOEW and R. KIVELITZ

In only a few cranial nerves is direct intervention possible on the nerve itself to alleviate intracranial lesions. This is totally impossible for those cranial nerves which actually are brain appendices such as the olfactory and optic nerves. To the best of our knowledge, attempts at nerve suture or anastomosis of the oculomotor nerves have never been made[+]; perhaps because their path, in the sinus cavernosus, is not accessible to operative approach and their other intracranial paths are reached only with difficulty. Perhaps also owing to the extremely differentiated interplay on the reacting organ, the eye muscle coordination, makes a satisfactory result after nerve suture, unlikely. Yet the possibility exists that merely no one has been interested in this problem. Whatever the case may be, up to now, one had to be satisfied in cases of functional loss of the third, fourth and sixth cranial nerves with a positional correction of the eyeball using surgical manipulation of the eye muscles, primarily an ophthalmological domain with which neurosurgeons are usually not confronted and therefore excluded from this report.

Furthermore, we know of no attempts at reconstruction after lesions of the statoacoustic nerves as well as following intracranial lesions of the caudal cranial nerve group. As the extracranial lesions of cranial nerves are not directly related to our topic, we have not taken into consideration individual successes of extracranial nerve sutures, transplantations and neurolysis following lesions of the last three cranial nerves, as well as of trigeminal defect-bridging in connection with oral surgical procedures and the reconstruction of the extracranial portion of the facial nerve following injuries and operation in the facial region.

Thus, our report restricts itself to reconstructive measures in cases of intracranial lesions of the trigeminal and facial nerves.

It is certainly easier to eliminate a trigeminal neuralgia by cutting off the nervus trigeminus than to attempt a reconstruction, although it may be indicated. To the best of our knowledge, SAMII has been the only neurosurgeon to date reporting on a successful trigeminal reconstruction through nerve transplantations.

A boy with post-traumatic optical nerve functional loss on the one side and trigeminal functional loss on the other was reported on. Because of the trigeminal lesion and resultant trophic disturbances, a cloudiness of the cornea of the healthy eye was observed. On account of this, the first corneal transplant was

[+] Meanwhile Prof. Yasargil told us that he sutured in one case the oculomotor nerve which had been damaged during the operation of an aneurysm. The nerve function partially recovered.

unsuccessful. Here the restoration of corneal sensibility was prerequisite to a repeated attempt at corneal plastic. MILLESI and SAMII, using an autologous nerve transplant, connected the major occipital nerve to the ophthalmic nerve, reporting that five months thereafter, the trophic disturbances regressed.

We are convinced that after treatment of trigeminal neuralgia, a similar indication for this operative procedure is occasionally present, then namely, when accidently the first trigeminal branch is damaged causing desensibilisation of the cornea of the only eye, or when the patient is employed such that the eyes are particularly susceptible to foreign bodies. Similar situations are seen after operation of cerebellopontine angle tumors, when the trigeminal root cannot be preserved. In any event, future cases of this nature will be treated by us in the manner described by SAMII.

As opposed to the trigeminal nerve, where the possibility of connective restoration has just recently been discovered and the indications for which must first be adopted, the reconstructive problems of facial nerve function have concerned neurosurgeons since 1898. At that time, FAURE first reported a nerve anastomosis, the accessory-facial nerve anastomosis frequently employed even nowadays. Depending on the school, neurosurgeons today prefer the one or other type of nerve reconstructive plastic, as a rule either the accessory-facial nerve or hypoglossal-facial nerve anastomosis. There appears to be, at least among German neurosurgeons, agreement on the fact, that if no possibility for reconstruction of the facial nerve continuity through direct suture or nerve transplant exists, the anastomosis with other nerves has the prerogative for a plastic surgical reconstruction of facial symmetry. We are convinced that the anastomosis usually gives good results; the patient is thereby satisfied, and naturally, the neurosurgeon too. Depending on the intensity of training adequate involuntary symmetric mimic can be learned additionally to the restoration of a symmetric resting muscle tone and to voluntary nervous control over the mimetic musculature. In this manner, Mr. KIVELITZ and I prepared this discussion with the somewhat pessimistic feeling that nothing new would be presented. Let me make clear in advance that we underestimated this topic and surprisingly found ourselves in a position to revise a number of otherwise unreflected assumed opinions. We, in any event, have learned from preparation of this paper.

We, neurosurgeons, are mostly confronted with the question of facial nerve reconstruction in conjunction with cerebellopontine angle tumors. We, therefore, wish to handle the problem from this viewpoint. Regarding Mr. MIEHLKE's report, we consciously excluded traumatic facial nerve paralysis in connection with skull-base fractures.

That even the best nerve suture, transplant or substitution plastic is not nearly as good as the primary maintenance of facial nerve continuity, does not need further mentioning. As Mr. DRAKE clearly demonstrated in his report, we must strive to attain results approximating his own excellent ones.

If maintenance of nerve continuity is not possible, the best results can be obtained by direct facial nerve suture in the cerebellopontine angle as DRAKE demonstrated as a possibility, or facial nerve plastic after DOTT. In DOTT's procedure, an autologous transplant is sewn onto the central stump of the facial nerve root and positioned near the mastoid process, where it is connected again to the facial nerve. The intra-temporal course of the facial nerve is thus bypassed. The results are positive as, among others, DOTT, DRAKE and myself have shown and also yield a satisfactory involuntary mimic. Our experience has shown that through this plastic-surgical technique, the operation time is lengthened by approximately one hour. This is by no means detrimental with good anesthesia, from the patient's viewpoint. In our last operation of this type, the surgical team was exchanged after the removal of the tumor, for the sake of operative efficiency. This tactic is for me recommendable. Unfortunately, the prerequisite maintenance of a central stump of the facial nerve root on the pons for DOTT's plastic technique is only seldomly present so that in most instances other methods of facial nerve plastic must be sought.

Other possibilities include, on the one hand, the anastomosis of the facial nerve to another nerve, and on the other hand, a plastic-surgical procedure for reconstruction of the facial symmetry, non-dependent on the reinnervation of the mimetic musculature.

Reviewing the literature regarding nerve anastomosis, besides the well-known accessory-hypoglossal anastomosis, three other reinnervation processes can be found: use of the glossopharyngeal nerve, anastomosis with the platysmal facial nerve branch of the healthy side using an intermediate autologous nerve transplant, and anastomosis with the phrenic nerve.

Only one report by WATSON-WILLIAMS in 1927 concerning the glossopharyngeal-facial nerve anastomosis could be found. By right, this technique has found no imitation, although at that time, the reinnervation of the mimetic musculature was successful. Swallowing difficulties are occasionally observed after cerebello-pontine angle tumors, if the glossopharyngeal nerve is unintentionally injured, such complications being avoided if other possibilities exist.

Unfortunately, I cannot say much concerning the reinnervation by means of the opposite facial nerve. We were only able to locate a brief report in the popular medical journal "Medical Tribune", and it has not been possible to date, to obtain the original work. Principally, it is conceivable to conduct symmetric mimetic impulses from a platysmal branch of the healthy side to the paretic facial nerve via nerve transplant, however, a quantitative problem is present in this case. The number of neuraxons and corresponding innervation impulses from the small donator facial nerve branch is inadequate for a truly symmetric innervation.

As opposed to this, it seems to us that the phrenic-facial nerve anastomosis is unfortunately too little known. It was discussed in 1957 by HARDY, PERRET and MEYERS. Besides that, we were able to locate a Russian report in 1962 over a series of 110 cases. The results of this procedure seem to compare favorably with the later discussed accessory-facial nerve and hypoglossus-facial nerve anastomosis. However, the disadvantages inherent in these procedures, the hemi-atrophy of the tongue and/or a reduction in strength of the muscles supplied by the accessory nerve are avoided. In spite of this, a hemilateral diaphragmatic paralysis must be acceptable. This is, however, as extensive experience connected with pulmonary tuberculosis has shown, functionally insignificant. In 20 - 30% of the cases of phrenic nerve disconnection, continuing kinesthetic disturbances of the diaphragm are not even to be observed. With a degree of reservation, as my own experience is limited in this method, I must state that based on the literature, if an operative reinnervation of the mimetic musculature using another nerve is decided upon, the phrenic-facial nerve anastomosis is preferable to the accessory or hypoglossal anastomosis.

According to the literature, facial nerve anastomosis with the accessory or hypoglossal nerve are comparable with respect to the restoration of the facial nerve function. In 2/3 to 3/4 of the cases good to satisfactory facial innervation is attained. These figures correspond to our own follow-up study of 14 cases with facial-accessory nerve anastomosis, which, without exception, lead to reinnervation of this region.

In both methods, the donator nerve function must be sacrificed; that is to say, one must accept a disturbance of the tongue mobility with hemi-lateral atrophy, or at least the loss of one sternocleidomastoid muscle.

Trapezius loss can be prevented, if, after the technique described by COLEMAN and WALKER in 1950, only that portion of the accessory nerve is used for anastomosis which supplies the sternocleidomastoid muscle and preserves the nerve portion supplying the trapezius.

However, what does the classification "good to satisfactory" function of the nerve anastomosis mean for the patient?

To answer this question, we not only undertook critical analysis of the literature, but also carried out detailed follow-up examinations of our own cases. To prevent misunderstandings, I repeat that all anastomoses in our series are functioning, yet the objective results remain in sharp contrast to the level of patient satisfaction and our thereby subjectively induced and recollected impressions to date.

It must clearly be stated that even the best results are objectively unsatisfactory. Although nerve anastomosis restores the resting facial symmetry in many cases, no one, no matter how differentiated and vain the personality, can learn a truly symmetric, comparable to the norm, involuntary mimic.

Symmetric innervation of the mimetic musculature is more or less possible for brief periods of time with concentrated attentiveness and great momentary effort. As soon as the attention is concentrated elsewhere, the symmetry is lost and the mimic, mirror of the soul, is distorted.

This is, in advantageous cases somewhat more, in many cases unfortunately less, than is attainable by plastic-surgical procedures. These have the distinct advantage, as opposed to nerve anastomosis, that no other nerve with its function must be sacrificed for questionable results.

From all these results, it could be concluded:

1. In cases of simultaneous homolateral trigeminal lesions, the patient is not in the position to relearn usage of the mimetic musculature after a reinnervation through nerve anastomosis. In such cases, plastic-surgical correction is indicated over every other form of nerve anastomosis.

2. The facial-accessory nerve anastomosis is contra-indicated when
   a) the homolateral upper extremity is affected,
   b) the affected patient requires the full strength of his shoulder girdle in his job
   c) during the operation, lesions of the caudal cranial nerve group occurred,
   d) a homolateral trigeminal loss is present.

3. The facial, hypoglossus anastomosis is contra-indicated when

a) operation produced lesions of the caudal cranial nerve group,
b) in patients with homolateral trigeminal loss and
c) patients requiring speech in their employment.

4. The facial-phrenic anastomosis is contra-indicated
   a) in the infrequent cases of reduced pulmonary function
   b) in patients with homolateral trigeminal loss.

   The phrenic facial nerve anastomosis should be preferred to the aforementioned procedures.

5. The results of skilled plastic-surgical treatment are frequently better than poorly functioning nerve anastomosis.

REFERENCES

1. BRAGDON, F.H. and G.H. GRAY, Jr.: Differential spinal accessory-facial anastomosis with preservation of function of trapezius. J. Neurosurg 19, 981-985 (1962)
2. COLEMAN, C.C. and J.C. WALKER: Technic of anastomosis of the branches of the facial nerve with the spinal accessory for facial nerve paralysis. Ann. Surg. 131, 960-966 (1950)
3. CUSHING, H.: The surgical treatment of facial paralysis by nerve anastomosis. With the report of a successful case. Ann. Surg. 37, 641-659 (1903)
4. DOTT, N.M.: Facial paralysis restitution by extrapetrous nerve graft. Proc. Roy. Soc. Med. 51, 900-902 (1958)
5. DRAKE, C.G.: Acoustic neurinoma. Repair of facial with autogenous graft. J. Neurosurg. 17, 836-842 (1960)
6. FAURE, J.L.: Traitement chirurgical de la paralysie faciale par l'anastomose spino-faciale. Rev. Chir. (Paris) 1098-1099 (1898)
7. HARDY, R.C., G. PERRET and R. MEYERS: Phrenico-facial nerve anastomosis for facial paralysis. J. Neurosurg. 14, 400-405 (1957)
8. KÖRTE, W. and M. BERNHARDT: Ein Fall von Nervenpropfung des Nervus facialis auf den Nervus hypoglossus. Dtsch. Med. WSchr. 29, 293-295 (1903)
9. LOEW, F.: Die kombinierte intrakranielle-extratemporale Fazialisplastik nach DOTT. Langenbecks Arch. Klin. Chir. 298, 934-935 (1962) und Saarl. Ärzteblatt 9 (1962)
10. LOVE, J.G. and B.W. CANNON: Nerve anastomosis in the treatment of facial paralysis. Special consideration of the etiologic role of total removal of tumors of the acoustic nerve. Arch. Surg. (Chicago) 62, 379-390 (1951)
11. McKENZIE, K.G. and E. ALEXANDER Jr.: Restoration of facial function by nerve anastomosis. Ann Surg. 132, 411-415 (1950)
12. MIGLIAVACCA, F.: Facial nerve anastomosis for facial paralysis following acoustic neurinoma surgery. Acta Neurochir. 17, 274-279 (1968)
13. SAMII, M.: Diskussion zum Vortrag von H. MILLESI: Indikation und Technik der autologen und interfaszikulären Nerventransplantation. Mels. Med. Mitteilungen 46, 189-194 (1972)

14. SUNDER-PLASSMANN, M., V. GRUNERT und J. A. GANGLBERGER: Über die Ergebnisse der Akzessorius- und Hypoglossusanastomosen zur chirurgischen Therapie der Fazialisparese. Wien. Med. WSchr. 47, 880-882 (1970)

15. WATSON-WILLIAMS, E.: Glossopharyngeal-facial nerve anastomosis. Proc. Roy. Soc. Med. 20, 1439-1442 (1927)

Advances in Surgery for Acoustic Neurinoma (A Synopsis)

H. KRAUS, F. BÖCK, V. GRUNERT, and W. KOOS

Radical surgery has always been the ultimate objective of any operative treatment in cases of acoustic neurinomas. The degree of radicality obtainable depends on various factors, including the size and localization of the tumor and, more prominently, its orientation and relationship to adjoining structures, particularly the brainstem. But the obtainable radicality is decided by the surgical technique, the choice of a suitable anesthesia, an optimal view of the surgical field and an optimal access to the tumor by appropriate positioning of the patient. We should like to report on some modalities developed in the Vienna clinic for the purpose of advancing the radicality of acoustic neurinoma surgery.

Since 1958, 147 operations for acoustic neurinoma have been performed on 128 patients. In 23 cases surgery was done for relapses or as a secondary procedure in bilateral tumors. The patients' age ranged from 13 to 73 years, the average being just below 5O.

From 1958 to 1964, 55 patients were operated on in a prone position. A sitting posture was adopted in 1964 and applied in 32 cases until 1969. From 1969 onwards we have opted for a lateral position, which was applied in 34 cases. The surgical microscope was first used in 1971 and has since been employed in 26 patients, some undergoing surgery in a sitting and some in a lateral position.

The table clearly documents that results were poorest with the patients in the prone position, while they improved considerably when we opted for a sitting posture. With the patients sitting there is, however, the danger of major variations in blood pressure in terms of a BP drop. In addition, air embolism may necessitate overpressure anesthesia. Both these untoward effects are excluded in the lateral position. Beyond that, the lateral position offers the best access to the tumor, as the cerebellum automatically drops backwards and is thus not exposed to pressure by the surgical instruments. As in the other positions, the surgical microscope can be used without obstacles.

The introduction of the surgical microscope and the use of bipolar coagulation marked the most recent advances in surgery for acoustic neurinomas.

Prior to employing these techniques we had felt that postoperative mortality was mainly due to the size and localization of the tumor. However, this is not consistently so. As seen from the reports by various co-workers of our clinic, the postoperative course is decided by the functional blood supply of the brain stem, while the tumor size will only be of influence in terms of mechanical interference with brain stem function. With the aid of the surgical microscope important vessels, including minor arteries, can almost invariably be identified. The significance of preserving the brain stem circulation is documented by the fact that of our 23 cases we did not loose a single patient.

The surgical microscope helped in preserving the facial nerve in 19 cases. Attempts at preservation failed in 7 patients, because the fasicles were split up by the tumor mass.

Temporary facial palsy persisted for weeks to months in 14 cases with preserved facial nerve. In 4 patients motor function was fully retained, while complete facial palsy persisted in one case in spite of a macroscopically intact nerve.

This brief synopsis was meant to illustrate the progress made in recent years with modified techniques and advanced instrumentation, such as the surgical microscope. Acoustic neurinomas initially dreaded as most dangerous, have thus lost much of their horrors. With painstaking, technically adequate surgery they range, in fact, among the tumors that offer the best prospects for operative treatment.

THE POSITION OF THE PATIENT AND THE RADICALITY OF THE OPERATION

(quotations between brackets: postoperative mortality)

Position		Number of all operations	Total removal	Subtotal removal
Prone	1958-1964	55 (13)	4 (1)	51 (12)
Sitting up	1964-1969	32 (4)	14 (2)	18 (2)
Recumbent lateral	1967-1969	34 (3)	28 (2)	6 (1)
Microsurgery	1971-1973	26 (O)	23 (O)	3 (O)
Total		147 (2O)	69 (5)	78 (15)

Microsurgical Experience in Surgery of Acoustic Neurinomas (Abstract)

M. G. YASARGIL

During the last 6 years (1967-1973) 120 patients have been operated on at the Kantonsspital Zurich; 40 small tumors (1,0 - 2,5 mm diameter) were operated on in the ENT-Department by Prof. U. Fisch. In 25 cases, during the translabyrinthine exploration, the tumor was found to be larger than anticipated by the preoperative neurological and radiological investigations; in these cases the tumor was partially removed and the facial nerve was dissected in the meatus; 4 - 7 days later a suboccipital exploration was performed at the neurosurgical department and the tumor radically extirpated.

In 55 cases the primary suboccipital-transmeatal approach allowed radical excision of larger tumors, which was carried out at the neurosurgical department. After having some unfavourable experience with patients in the prone position in 1967, the author prefers the sitting position of the patients during surgery; the head is tilted forward and slightly turned to ipsilateral side and fixed with the Mayfield-Kees headholder. This position provides ideal visualization and facilitates the surgical manipulations of the procedure with only slight retraction of the uncongested cerebellar hemisphere.

The applied microtechnique allowed a remarkable decrease of the mortality and morbidity rates.

Experiences in Microsurgery of Acoustic Neurinomas (Abstract)

W. T. Koos, F. W. Böck, and S. Salah

The use of the operating microscope for modification of the classical suboccipital removal of cerebellopontine angle tumors has now advanced to the point where acoustic neurinomas, from the small intracanalicular lesions to the more common giant tumors may be most reasonably resected by this technique. At the Neurosurgical Department in Vienna, 24 cases of acoustic neurinomas have been subjected to microsurgery since 1971. In 20 cases we were dealing with unilateral neurinomas, while multiple tumors consistent with von Recklinghausen's disease were found in the cerebellopontine angle bilaterally in 4 patients. In 20 cases the angle tumor measured more than 4 cm in diameter, only in 4 patients were we dealing with 2 to 3 cm tumors.

A two-stage procedure was used only once to remove an extremely large unilateral tumor. In bilateral cerebellopontine angle tumors, the larger tumor was extirpated first, while the contralateral process was attacked about 2 to 3 weeks following the initial intervention.

In 73% of the patients the facial nerve was fully preserved. Postoperative facial weakness due to manipulation on the stretched and greatly thinned nerve was invariably found to disappear provided nerve continuity was preserved. Where anatomical preservation of the facial nerve failed, hypoglossal-facial anastomosis was performed 4 to 8 weeks following primary surgery. Complete deafness of the involved side was present after these large lesions were removed totally, but deafness was total already preoperatively in 82 of our cases.

For all procedures performed during the past 18 months a special method of controlled arterial hypotension has been used which permits to work in a surgical field virtually free from bleedings.

Critical Observations Concerning the Diagnosis and Clinical Features in 100 Cases of Tumors in the Cerebellopontine Region

G. THOMALSKE, I. KIENOW-RIEG, and G. MOHR

The 100 non-selected cases studied comprised:

- 69 acoustic neurinomas
- 13 meningiomas
- 6 epidermoids
- 5 gliomas
- 7 different tumors

(1 chordoma, 1 chondroma, 1 fibrosarcoma, 1 LINDAU-tumor, 2 carcinomas, 1 case without histological examinations)

The average duration of the case histories as shown in Fig. 1 was shortest in gliomas (average 4.8 months), increasing further in the following sequence: meningiomas (3.3 years), acoustic neurinomas (4.5 years) up to the epidermoids (10.4 years).

In analysing the symptomatology we differentiated between the initial symptom (i.e. the very first symptom noticed by the patient), the other early symptoms (i.e. further symptoms occurring early during the course of the disease) as well as the late symptoms of the fully developed clinical syndrome just before or at the time of hospital admission.

Fig. 2 shows the four initial symptoms most commonly noticed in the patients in their relative distribution among the various space occupying lesions. Impairment of hearing, which occurs relatively often as initial symptom, was most commonly noticed as such by patients with neurinomas, epidermoids and meningiomas. Incoordination , on the other hand, manifested itself as the first symptom only in the patients with epidermoids, and tinnitus only in patients with acoustic neurinomas.

The most diversified spectrum of the initial symptoms occurs in the cases of acoustic neurinoma, whereas the number of the various symptoms manifesting themselves initially was less in the other tumor cases (Fig. 3). There were considerable fluctuations in the relative distribution of the various symptoms depending on the stage of the illness, as seen in Figs. 4 and 5 in neurinomas and meningiomas. When comparing the percentage distribution of the cochlear and vestibular signs in the fully developed clinical syndrome we found it equal for both in each tumor group (acoustic neurinomas, meningiomas, epidermoids and the 7 different tumors, except in gliomas where there was a predominance of vestibular symptoms over hearing disturbances. See Fig. 6 for the distribution of symptoms in acoustic neurinomas and meningiomas. Symptoms of the trigeminal nerve were more often found in acoustic neurinomas than in the other tumor types. Caudal nerve signs were most frequent in meningiomas. Brain stem symptoms involving the long tracts (disturbances of sensibility, reflex activity and motility, spastic signs, urinary bladder symptoms) as well as bulbar speech were relatively frequent in acoustic neurinomas, but even less than in the other tumors.

In space occupying lesions of a certain size neuroradiology is the most important diagnostic method, whereas in cases of small and smallest tumors the results of the ENT examinations, especially the negative recruitment, can often be of conclusive value even in cases where the other symptoms and investigation findings are not yet definitely helpful. Nevertheless, with the necessary experience, especially the positive contrast cisternography can be of immense help in the diagnosis of even the smallest tumors.

Unfortunately the otologic diagnosis was often impracticable because of the presence of marked intracranial hypertension or vertigo. 80-100% of our patients already had signs of raised intracranial pressure by the time of hospital admission. Especially early otological examinations could of course enable an optimal diagnosis and lead to earlier operations.

So it is not surprising that only 39 audiograms with 14 recruitment-diagnosis were of any value, since for example 12 patients who were already unilaterally deaf could not be examined by this method. In 10 of the above-mentioned 14 cases the recruitment was negative, thus proving a retrocochlear lesion. In a larger statistical study PERTUISET (3) stated that recruitment was negative in 80% of acoustic neurinomas whereas it was positive in 90% of MENIERE' s disease.

We have also had cases in whom the most important early diagnostic criterium was a negative recruitment, thus enabling the definite early diagnosis and early operation of tumors of smallest size. In a former publication by our clinic the reduction of the warm water irrigation reaction during vestibularis investigation was shown also to be an early sign of vestibular impairment.

Nevertheless it must be emphasized that negative recruitment does not occur only in acoustic neurinomas, and that on the other hand in rare cases even positive recruitment can occur in acoustic neurinomas. Even acoustic impairment may be absent, as reported by ALVING (1) in a case of acoustic neurinoma of 4 x 5 x 6 cm size. Table I shows the frequency of relevant neuroradiological findings in the different tumor groups (in plain films, vertebral angiograms and PEG). The value of plain film diagnosis cannot be overemphasized. Because of the small number of gliomas we cannot, of course, claim statistical significance for this group.

In neurinomas the EEGs with unilateral focal signs showed ipsilateral manifestations twice more frequently than contralateral ones. However, the unilateral ipsilateral focal signs comprised only one seventh (1/7) of all the pathological EEG findings in all the tumor cases (Table II).

It is worth mentioning that we found an increased albumin content in the CSF in about 82% of our neurinoma cases whilst this occurred only in somewhat more than 1/4 (= 27.65%) in the other tumor cases, i.e. in some of the meningiomas, the fibrosarcoma and a carcinoma. All the epidermoids and gliomas were not accompanied by an increased albumin content in the CSF.

In conclusion, we must admit that in our patients, unfortunately, for the above-mentioned reasons, the modern cochleo-vestibular examination techniques and finer neuroradiological contrast methods had not been exhaustively employed for the early diagnosis of small and smallest cerebellopontine tumors. It appears necessary to continue emphasizing the importance of such methods for finding

Table I. Relevant neuroradiologic findings

	plain films	vertebral angiogram	PEG
Neurinomas	76, 9 %	33, 3 %	63, 6 %
Meningiomas	61, 5 %	28, 6 %	44, 4 %
Epidermoids	60, 0 %	20, 0 %	25, 0 %
Gliomas	66, 7 %	0 %	50, 0 %
Various tumors	83, 3 %	50, 0 %	50, 0 %

Table II. E E G

	Neurinomas	Meningiomas	Epidermoids	Gliomas	various tumors
N = 69	46	9	5	4	5
ipsilat. focus	6 (13, 0%)	1 (11, 1%)	1 (20, 0%)		2 40, 0%)
bilat. pathol. waves ipsilat. predominant	6 (13, 0%)			1 (25, 0%)	
contralat. focus	3 (6, 5%)			1 (25, 0%)	
bilat. pathol. waves contralat. predominant	3 (6, 5%)	1 (11, 1%)			
bilat. pathol. waves	6 (13, %)	2 (22, 2%)	1 (20, 0%)	2 (50, 0%)	1 (20, 0%)
pathol. EEG without focus	9 (19, 7%)	1 (11, 1%)	2 (40, 0%)		
normal	13 (28, 3%)	4 (44, 4%)	1 (20, 0%)		2 (40, 0%)

these small tumors, in order to improve the operative prognosis. The collaboration between the general practitioners, otologists, neurologists and neurosurgeons must be intensified. Only then can it be expected that enough patients will come to the surgeon long before intracranial hypertension has become a life-endangering complication with an unfavorable influence on the prognosis.

REFERENCES

1. ALVING, J.: Akustikusneurinom mit während des ganzen Verlaufs normal bleibendem Hörvermögen. Ugeskr. Laeg. 134, 2593 (1972)
2. KAEMMERER, E. and G. ROSSBERG: Zur Frühdiagnose des Akustikus-Neurinoms. Münch. Med. Wschr. 103, 212) (1961)
3. PERTUISET, B.: Les neurinomes de l'acoustique. Neurochirurgie, Paris, 16, Suppl. 1 (1970)

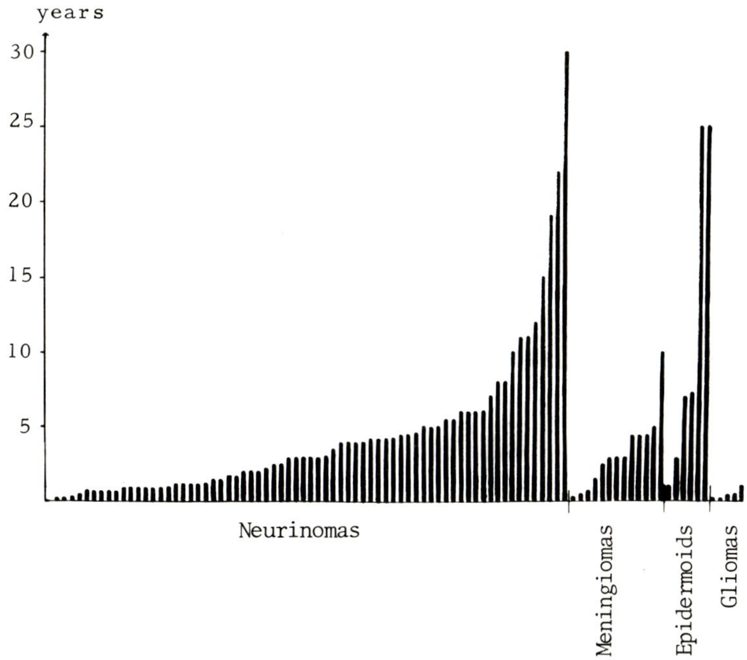

Fig. 1. Length of case history

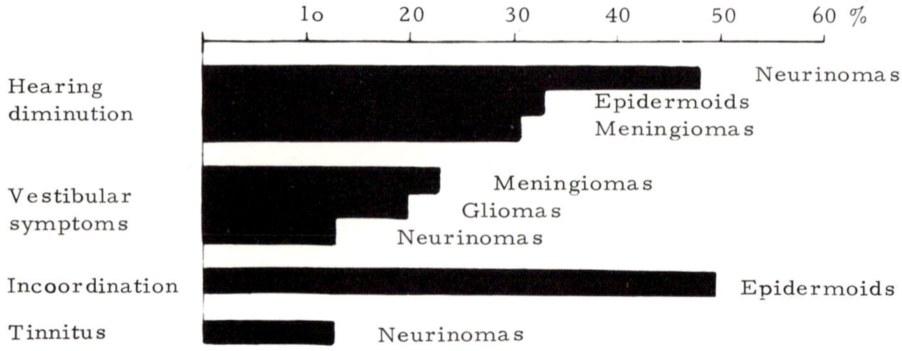

Fig. 2. Most frequent initial symptoms

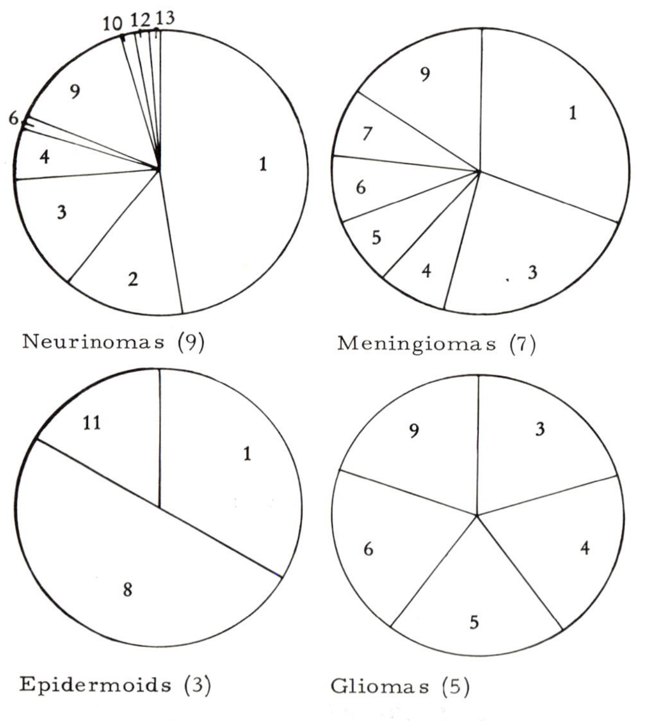

Fig. 3. Initial symptoms

1 Hearing diminution
2 Tinnitus
3 Vestibular symptoms
4 Trigeminal symptoms
5 Abducens symptoms
6 Facial-nerve symptoms
7 Symptoms of caudal group
8 Incoordination
9 Cephalea
10 Vomiting
11 Trouble of vision
12 Fits
13 Weakness of extremities

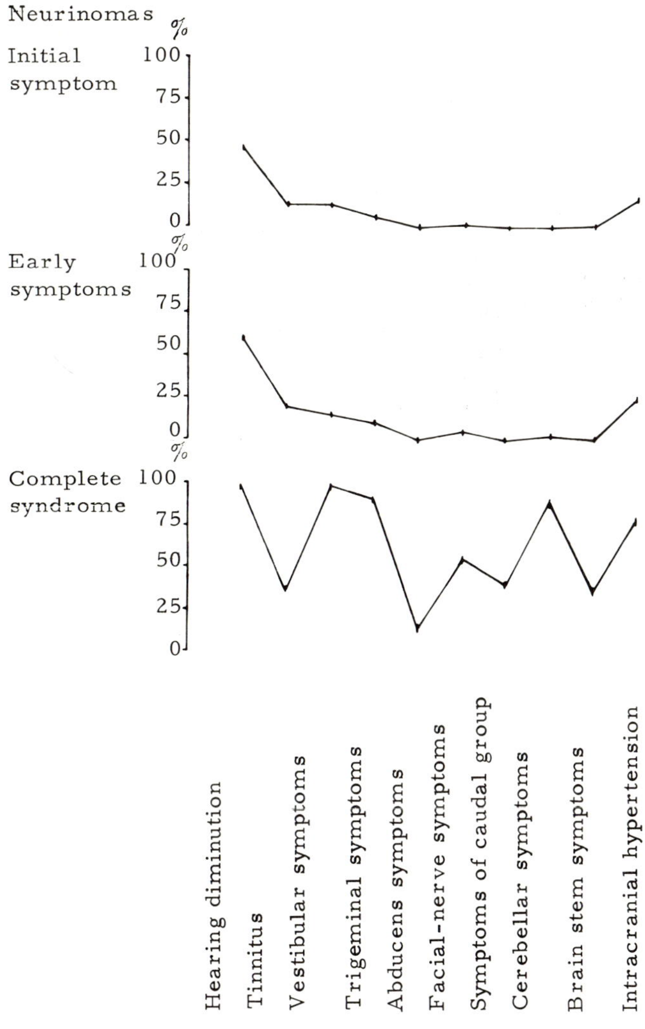
Neurinomas
%
Initial symptom
100
75
50
25
0
%
Early symptoms
100
75
50
25
0
%
Complete syndrome
100
75
50
25
0
Hearing diminution
Tinnitus
Vestibular symptoms
Trigeminal symptoms
Abducens symptoms
Facial-nerve symptoms
Symptoms of caudal group
Cerebellar symptoms
Brain stem symptoms
Intracranial hypertension

Fig. 4.

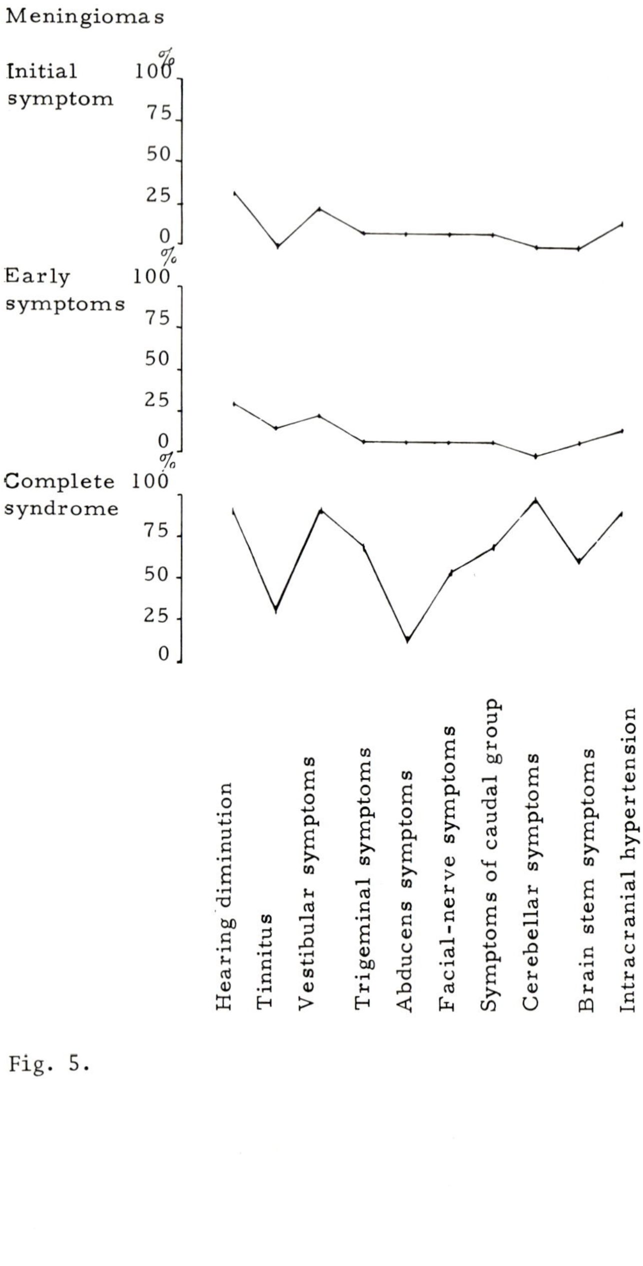
Meningiomas
Initial symptom
%
100
75
50
25
0
Early symptoms
%
100
75
50
25
0
Complete syndrome
%
100
75
50
25
0
Hearing diminution
Tinnitus
Vestibular symptoms
Trigeminal symptoms
Abducens symptoms
Facial-nerve symptoms
Symptoms of caudal group
Cerebellar symptoms
Brain stem symptoms
Intracranial hypertension

Fig. 5.

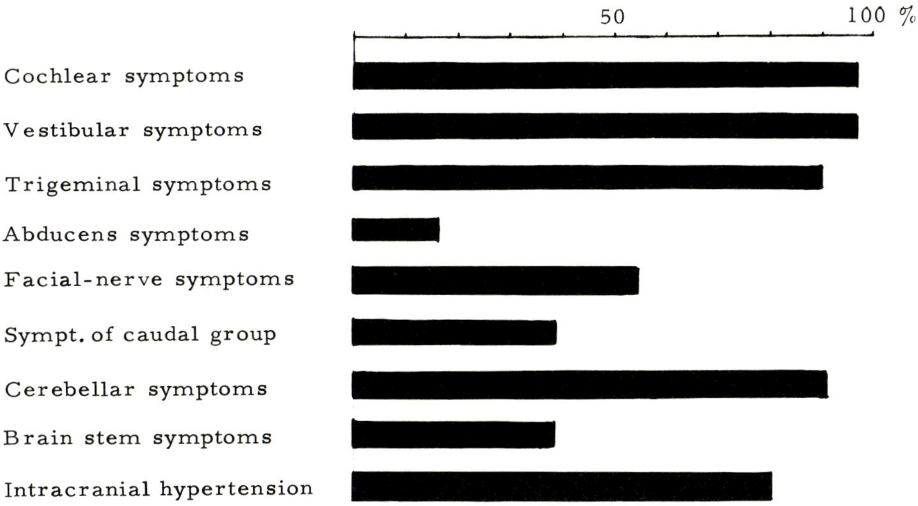

Complete syndrome in neurinomas

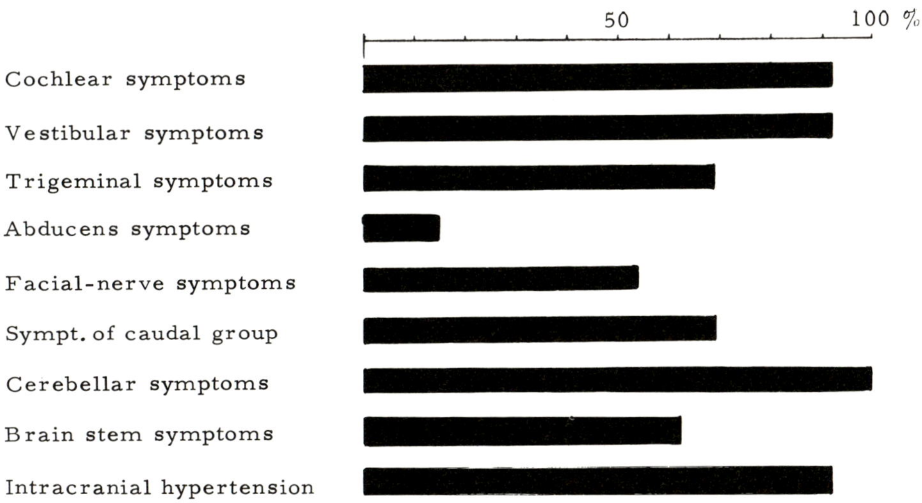

Complete syndrome in meningiomas

Fig. 6.

Operations and Results in 102 Tumors of the Cerebellopontine Angle

H. FROMM, H. HUF, and M. SCHÄFER

A non-selected series of 102 tumors of the cerebellopontine angle region is presented. These tumors were operated on by several surgeons of the Neurosurgical Clinic of the University Hospital at Frankfurt/Main. In all cases the diagnosis was verified histologically:

74 Acoustic Neurinomas
18 Meningiomas
7 Cholesteatomas
2 Chordomas
1 Fibrosarcoma

As shown above, about three quarters of all cases were acoustic neurinomas. We feel it essential to point out that the majority of these patients operated on was admitted in a rather advanced state, frequently with symptoms of a markedly increased intracranial pressure. Most of the tumors had a diameter of at least 3 to 4 cm.

In such cases intracranial pressure was lowered by ventricular tapping before opening the dura. All patients were operated on in a lateral position. As usual, for smaller tumors, a direct approach was obtained by a suboccipital trepanation measuring 3 x 3 cm. As the postoperative recovery may be seriously influenced by a reactive edema of the brainstem and the pons, in large tumors a prophylactic decompression of sufficient size was performed in the atlanto-occipital region, including a dura graft.

It is well known that in large tumors, even when microsurgical technique and electrical stimulation are combined, it is not always possible to identify and to preserve the facial nerve. In some cases where the structure of the facial nerve seemed to be intact, its function gradually diminished within a few days postoperatively. Full function of facial nerve could be preserved in 40% of our acoustic neuromas. In cases of lost facial function an anastomosis between facial nerve and accessory nerve performed after a latency of about 3 months led to fair or satisfactory results.

The usual postoperative treatment including fluid, electrolyte and blood gas balance needs no special mention. The use of a gastric tube in preventing aspiration and in early detection of stress-ulcer-bleeding is important. Hyperthermia should as far as possible be avoided, since it favours the development of brain swelling. If necessary, the normalisation of temperature is accomplished immediately by simple cooling methods such as ice-packs and ventilators. If there is prolonged insufficient vigilance during postoperative period, we prefer to shorten this state by giving such patients Pervitin. No unfavourable side effects have been noted. If necessary, tracheostomy is promptly performed.

The operative results in acoustic neurinoma are as shown in the Table below:

Neurinomas	operated	74 = 100%
	dead	15 = 20%

1.-10 postop. day	11.-20. postop. day	up to 130 postop. days
12	2	1
cause of death		
central 7		
pulmonary embol. 4	pulmonary embol. 2	
myocardial infarct. 1		marasm 1

It is remarkable that the cause of death in more than one half of the lethal cases was not central. Even during the first 10 postoperative days autopsy showed massive pulmonary embolism in 4 cases and acute myocardial infarction in one. The occurrence of pulmonary embolisation was apparently favored by long periods of preoperative bedrest at home or other hospitals. In other words, only 10% died as the result of the operation. It should be emphasized however, that 80% of the patients who died were older than 50 years.

In 6 cases there was a recurrence of the tumor after an average interval of 5 years. These reinterventions took place under rather unfavorable circumstances (usually as an emergency). This is the reason for the high rate of mortality (4 patients).

In cases of meningioma and cholesteatoma we almost always found extremely large tumors with corresponding surgical risk, leading to the rather high mortality of 25%.

Preservation of the Facial Nerve in Acoustic Neurinoma Surgery (Abstract)

I. M. VAN DER WERF

Preservation of the facial nerve in acoustic neurinoma surgery has become a challenge to both the otologist and the neurosurgeon. Since these tumors can now be detected at an early stage, when they are relatively small, on the one hand, and since microscopic techniques became available, on the other hand, the facial nerve can be saved in an increasing number of cases. In a consecutive series of 19 patients and 21 neurinomas - two patients had bilateral tumors - the facial nerve could be preserved anatomically 11 times and functionally 7 times. Technical details concerning the possibilities as well as the limits of surgery are discussed and illustrated by a movie.

Crossed Cranial Nerve Anastomosis for Re-Innervation of Muscles Supplied by the Facial Nerve

V. GRUNERT and M. SUNDER-PLASSMANN

In lesions of the facial nerve following extirpation of cerebello-pontine angle tumors the best results are undoubtedly obtained by direct anastomosis of the facial nerve ends, if preserved, or by Dott's operation, if only the cranial nerve end is available. We have never had an opportunity of performing any of these two techniques, as the remaining nerve ends in all of our cases proved to be unsuitable for direct anastomosis. Consequently we were compelled to resort to cross anastomosis for re-innervation of the facial muscles in those cases where the facial nerve was injured intraoperatively.

Between 1967 and 1973 we attempted re-innervation of the facial muscles by cross anastomosis following removal of a cerebello-pontine angle tumor in a total of 32 patients. In 14 cases the accessory nerve was used, in the remaining 18 the facial nerve was conneeted to the hypoglossal nerve. Almost all patients presented satisfactory results within 6 to 9 months postoperatively. These were already reported in September 1972 in Vienna.

Time does not permit a detailed account of our material. Instead, we will try to highlight some specific problems involved. In the literature, hypoglossal anastomosis is claimed to produce better results than accessory anastomosis. These findings were confirmed by our experience in as far as we found re-innervation potentials in the cheek muscles to recur considerably earlier when the hypoglossal technique was employed. But we have now come to opt for routine anastomosis with the accessory nerve, since the long-term results are apparently the same as for the hypoglossal technique and functional loss of the muscles supplied by the accessory nerve is apparently better tolerated by the patients than paresis of the tongue muscles.

Hypoglossal-facial anastomosis is performed in sporadic cases if pareses of the muscles supplied by the accessory nerve can be expected to constitute a vocational handicap for the patient. The case of a contrabass player whom one would probably enjoy listening to, though not watching, is an appropriate example.

Another problem is encountered in cases where the tumor can be removed under the surgical microscope with preservation of facial nerve continuity, but the postoperative electromyogram shows loss of nerve function. We have come across one such case. After attempting conservative treatment for one year, we ultimately performed cross anastomosis. Intracranial reconstruction of the nerve was not considered in this case due to the high risk involved in re-craniotomy and since identification of the functional facial nerve segments in the cerebello-pontine angle appeared to be impossible.

Facial Paralysis Secondary to Skull Fractures New Approaches in Management (Abstract)

A. MIEHLKE

Facial paralysis following skull fracture or penetrating lacerations is occurring more frequently in clinical practice. Accordingly, the surgeon has had to adapt his diagnostic skills in order to allow immediate facial nerve repair when indicated as well as elaboration of regional plastic or reconstructive surgery, when required.

Both longitudinal and transverse fractures of the base of the skull may cause facial nerve injury. Nerve lesion occurs in 10-25% of patients with longitudinal fractures, but increases to 30-50% of patients with transverse fractures. Of the total number of nerve lesions, 75% of early lesions and 90% of late onset lesions will resolve without medical intervention. However, it remains to be defined which group will require operative care.

Indications for decompression of the facial nerve in early phases of injury at the Göttingen E.N.T. Department are based on the transcutaneous nerve excitability test. This test becomes significant four days following injury, thus allowing clinical stabilization of the injured patient. A greater than 3,5 milliamp side differential in nerve stimulation or progressive limitation of nerve function indicates irreversible nerve injury, and the need for operative intervention.

Discussion will elaborate upon the pathology of facial nerve lesion, as well as early and late management of the involved lesions. Stress will be placed on the various surgical means available for repair of intra-temporal nerve injuries, particularly as related to injuries of the nerve within the internal auditory canal and its intralabyrinthine segment. Examples will include injuries subsequent to bone splinters, lacerations as well as traction-lesions of the nerve. Note will be given to the role of regeneration fibers passing through the greater superficial petrosal nerve inhibiting normal regeneration of facial motor-fibres, and appropriate management of this problem by rerouting of the VIIth nerve.

Cerebello-Pontine Angle Arterio-Venous Malformations (Abstract)

C. G. DRAKE

Large AVMs of the brain stem have been considered to be inoperable because of the conception that they are embedded in the brain stem. Surgical experience with three cases suggests that may not always be the case.

The AVMs appeared to lie in the pons and cerebello-pontine angle in two cases and in the other to occupy one-half of the midbrain. Each patient had a severe neurological deficit as the result of multiple hemorrhages. As a result of an operation designed to clip feeding vessels in a critically ill boy of 14, it was found that the AVM could be completely removed from the surface of the pons, midbrain, cranial nerves and cerebello-pontine angle. His recovery has been virtually complete except for unilateral deafness.

Similarly, a larger AVM including a peripheral AICA aneurysm sould be totally removed from the surface of the pons, cerebellar peduncle and angle in a 21 year old woman. In the last case, the AVM which appeared on angiography to be in the midbrain actually lay on the lateral surface, the crus and the interpeduncular fossa. In these two cases, there has been to date only mild improvement of their severe pre-existing neurological deficits.

This experience suggests that in some cases AVMs seeming to lie within the brain stem are actually on the surface alike to most spinal AVMs and may be totally removed without great jeopardy to the integrity of the brain stem.

Cerebellopontine Angle Meningiomas

O. WILCKE

The most common cerebellopontine angle tumors are acoustic neurinomas and the second most common are meningiomas. Acoustic neurinomas are about 7 to 10 times more common than meningiomas; then follow gliomas which extend into the cerebellopontine angle, and cerebellopontine angle epidermoids are about half as common as meningiomas.

From our data of 55 infratentorial meningiomas (Table I) observed during the last ten years in our hospital under comparable diagnostic conditions, cerebellopontine angle meningiomas were, after tentorial meningiomas which extended into the supra-tentorial or infratentorial region, the second most common amounting to 31%. Most of the patients were female (71%). It can be seen from the larger surveys in the literature that cerebellopontine angle meningiomas (Table II) are the most common among meningiomas in the posterior fossa, and 42% of the meningiomas are petrosal. Unlike acoustic neurinomas, meningiomas are not always found in the same place and therefore their effects on neighbouring formations differ.

Table I. Incidence and sex distribution of 55 infratentorial meningiomas

Localisation	Σ	%	♂	♀
Tentorium	25	45	8	17
Cerebellar convexity	7	13	2	5
Cerebellopontine angle	17	31	5	12
Clivus	3	5	1	2
IV. Ventricle	1	2		1
Multiple Meningiomas	2	4		2
	55		16	39
			29%	71%

Table II. Survey of the literature concerning the incidence of tentorial and infratentorial meningiomas

Author	Clinic	Number of cases	Tentorium	Ridge of the tentorium	Cerebellar convexity	Petrous pyramid	Clivus	fourth ventricle and multiple meningiomas
Castellano and Ruggiero (1953)	Stock-holm	71	16	5	7	30	8	5
Tristan and Hodes (1958)	Philadel-phia	59	8	-	14	28	2	7
Markham and coll. (1955)	Boston	29	3	3	6	13	2	2
Russel and Bucy (1953)	Chicago	15	2	-	4	8	-	1
Petit - Dutaillis and coll. (1949)	Paris	41	5	2	5	21	2	6
Lecuire and Dechaume (1971)	Lyon	244	46	10	26	99	17	46
Own cases (1961-1971)	Köln	55	25	-	7	17	3	3
		514	105 20,4%	20 3,1%	69 13,4%	216 42%	34 6,6%	70 13,6%

Table III. First symptoms of cerebellopontine angle neurinomas and meningiomas

	Cerebellopontine angle	
	Neurinomas	Meningiomas
Number of cases	234	45
Impairment of hearing	45%	17%
Tinnitus	6%	
Disturbance of equilibrium	15%	11%
N. V disorder	6%	7%
N. VIII disorder	2%	
Headache	11%	40%
Intracranial pressure	3%	13%

Table IV. Clinical symptoms of cerebellopontine angle neurinomas and meningiomas

		Acousticus-Neurinomas	Cerebellopontine angle Meningiomas
Number of cases		234	45
Cochlear disorder		96%	71%
Vestibular disorder		80%	64%
Disorder of	N. IV	33%	25%
	N. V	74%	54%
	N. VII	61%	25%
	N. IX	16%	25% (N. IX, N. X, N. XII together)
	N. X	6%	
	N. XII	10%	
Intracranial pressure		66%	75%
Motor and sense disorders		25%	22%
Psychic disorders		19%	10%

Although clinically cerebellopontine angle tumors are all similar, there are specific criteria which enable a diagnostic prediction about the type of tumor. There is, first of all, a significant observation to be made here with regard to the first symptoms and their frequency (Table III). I am basing my observation here in part on a survey of 234 acoustic neurinomas by REMBOLD and TÖNNIS (7). Whereas impairment of hearing is the most frequent initial symptom (42%) of acoustic neurinomas, it is the first symptom of cerebellopontine angle meningiomas in only 17% and the most frequent first symptom (40%) is a continuing headache - usually at the back of the head. A continuing headache is the first symptom in only 11% of neurinomas. Signs of intracranial pressure were four times more frequent in cases of meningioma than in cases of neurinoma.

The average time of evolution for cerebellopontine angle meningiomas is 3, 6 years, but short evolutions of about 6 months are more frequent than in cases of other meningiomas of the posterior fossa. The average evolution time for acoustic neurinomas is 4, 6 years according to REMBOLD and TÖNNIS (7).

The most frequent clinical symptom (Table IV) of cerebellopontine angle meningiomas is papilledema and increased intracranial pressure, which is found in 75% of the cases, more often than with acoustic meningiomas. Then follow symptoms of the eighth brain nerve; these are the most significant symptoms for acoustic neurinomas, where cochlear disorder is almost always observed. The other brain nerves, especially the trigeminus and facialis are more often affected by neurinomas than by meningiomas. Altogether it is more usual to find several brain nerves affected with acoustic neurinomas than with cerebelloponine angle meningiomas, although according to the findings of LECUIRE and DECHAUME (2) and also to a certain degree our own observations, damage to the contralteral trigeminus is, to a certain extent, indicative of cerebellopontine angle meningiomas, and this can lead to a false localisation.

The protein content of the CSF is of considerable diagnostic value. The protein content was over 50 mg% in only 15% of the cerebellopontine angle meningiomas but in 97% of the neurinomas. The average protein content was 46 mg% for meningiomas and 146% for neurinomas. For cerebellopontine angle epidermoids, arachnoiditis and metastases protein values of higher than 50 mg% are almost never encountered.

Isotope investigations can be of geat diagnostic help in recognizing cerebellopontine angle meningiomas. Meningiomas increase the activity more than neurinomas but to different extents (Fig. 1) and a correct diagnosis of the type of tumor was possible in 60% of the cases investigated and a correct localisation was possible in all cases.

X-ray evidence of intracranial pressure - secondary elargement of the sella or decalcification - is found in about 45% of cerebellopontine angle meningiomas and thus more commonly than in other cerebellopontine tumors. An expansion of the porus acusticus internus, however, is found in about 60-80% of acoustic neurinomas but in only 20% of the cerebellopontine angle meningiomas.

Clear destruction of the petrous pyramid or changes in the calcium structure was radiographically verifiable in 35% of cerebellopontine angle meningiomas. Calcification of the tumor is very rare.

Encephalography or ventriculography need only rarely be used to substantiate a clinical diagnosis. A view of the cerebellopontine angle cisterns (Fig. 2) or the arachnoidal regions (Fig. 3) can give more conclusive evidence of a cerebellopontine angle tumor than the inconclusive evidence from a view of the displaced fourth ventricle (Fig. 4).

Angiographic evidence of cerebellopontine angle meningiomas is less characteristic than with meningiomas in other locations. Usually there is no tumor flush typical of meningiomas and from a vertebral angiogram (Fig. 5) one can only conclude that there is a tumor from the vascular displacement (Fig. 6). The raising of the superior cerebellar artery and the fact that the basilar artery runs close to the clivus are the most obvious pieces of evidence. Sagittal views (Fig. 7) also often show a clear raising of the posterior in the arterial phase and a pathological course of the superior cerebellar artery. It is often the case that a carotid angiogram (Fig. 8) shows small vessels leading from the internal carotid to the cerebellopontine angle and this is evidence of a meningioma, especially when a vascular hilus is to be seen.

Without wishing to go into details of surgical technique, the literature and our own experience show a surgical mortality of 30-40%. ZOLTAN and collaborators (8) were able to demonstrate what CUSHING had already observed with a small number of patients, namely that partial removal of cerebellopontine angle meningiomas is associated with a considerably higher mortality than total extirpation. Thus a clarification of the type of tumor involved seems desirable before an operation is planned. Contrast medium methods are not suitable for this. A combination of clinical features - sex, typical first syndrome, investigation of the CSF, displacement, damage to the brain nerves and radiographic and scintigraphic evidence enable us to clarify, to a large extent, as I have tried to show, what kind of tumor is involved.

REFERENCES

1. CASTELLANO, F. and G.RUGGIERO: Meningiomas of the posterior fossa. Act. Radiol. (Stockholm) Suppl. 104 (1953)

2. LECUIRE, and J.P. DECHAUME: Les Méningiomes de la fosse cérébrale postérieur. Bd.d.Neurochirurgie, Supplement II (1971)

3. MARKHAM, J.W.: Meningiomas of the posterior fossa. Arch.Neurol.Psychiat. (Chicago) 74, 1963-1970 (1955)

4. PETIT-DUTAILLIS, D.: Les Meningiomes da la fosse postérieur. Rev.neurol. Par. 81, 557-572 (1949)

5. RUSSEL, J.R. and P.C.BUCY: Meningiomas of the posterior fossa. Surg. Gynec.Obstet. 96, 183-192 (1953)

6. TRISTAN, T.A. and Ph.J.HODES: Meningiomas of the posterior cranial fossa. Radiology 70, 1-14 (1958)

7. REMBOLD and W.TÖNNIS: Die Differentialdiagnose der Erkrankungen des Kleinhirnbrückenwinkels. Dtsch. Zeitschrift f.Nervenheilkunde 175, 329-353 (1956)

8. ZOLTAN, L.: Aus dem Problemkreis der Meningiome der hinteren Schädelgrube. Act.Neurochir. (Wien) 15, 249 (1966)

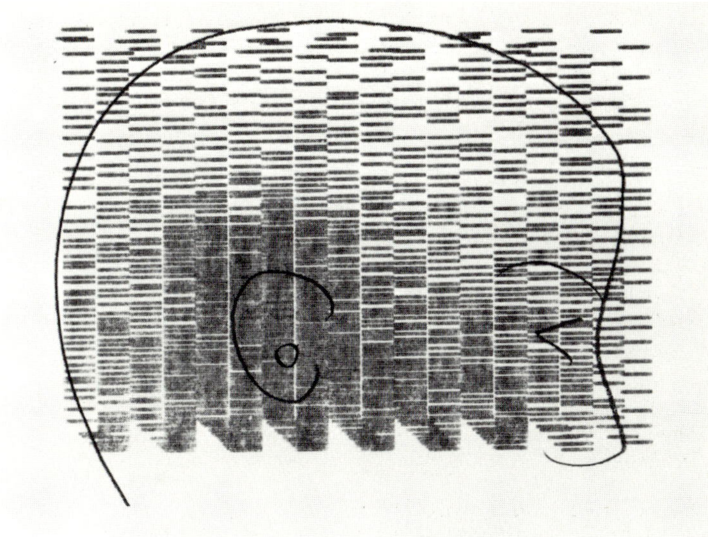

Fig. 1. Positron-scan of a left sided cerebellopontine angle meningioma

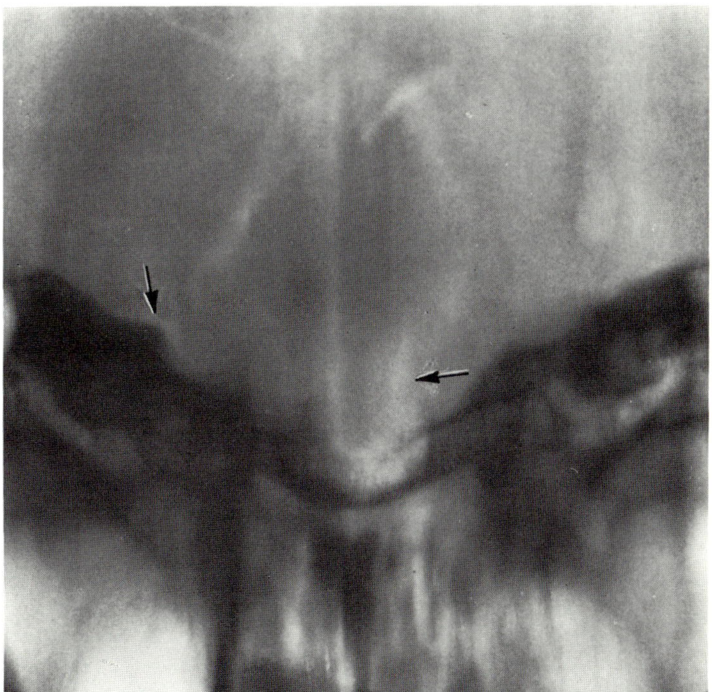

Fig. 2. Displacement of the cerebellopontine cistern in a case of a left sided cerebellopontine angle tumor

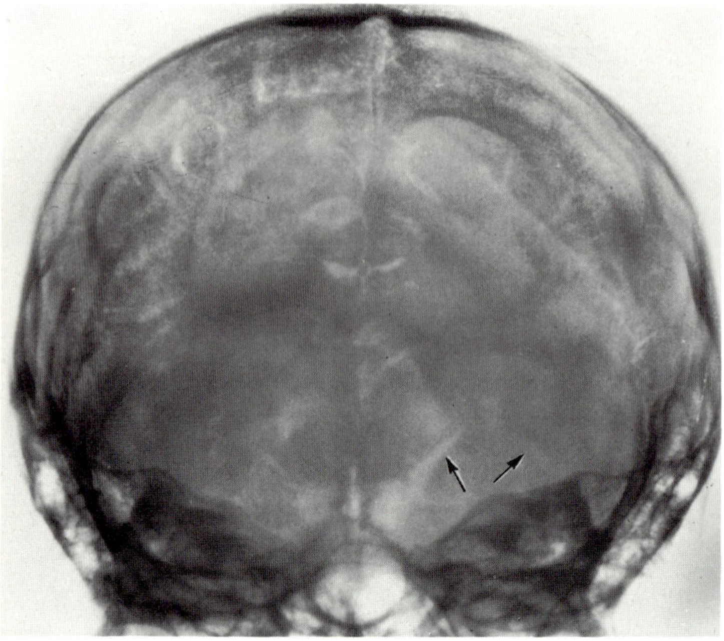

Fig. 3. Meningioma in the cerebellopontine covered by an arachnoidal air cap

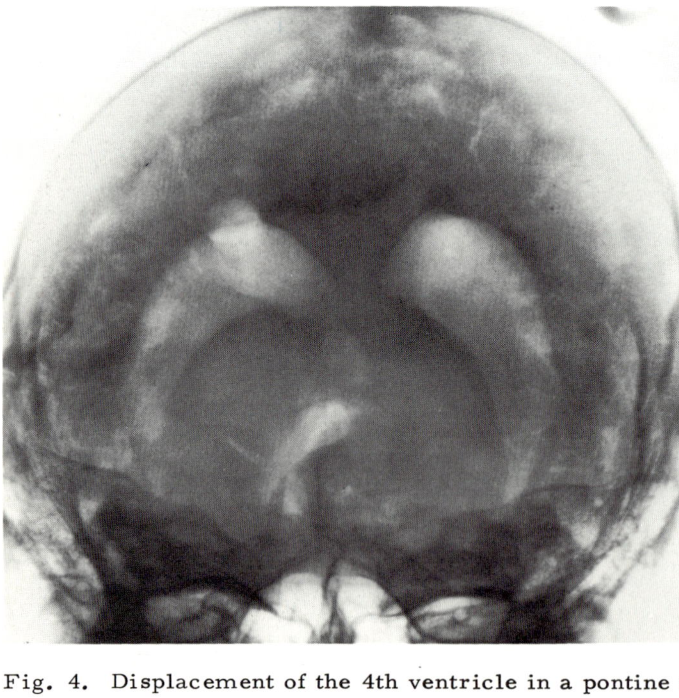

Fig. 4. Displacement of the 4th ventricle in a pontine angle meningioma

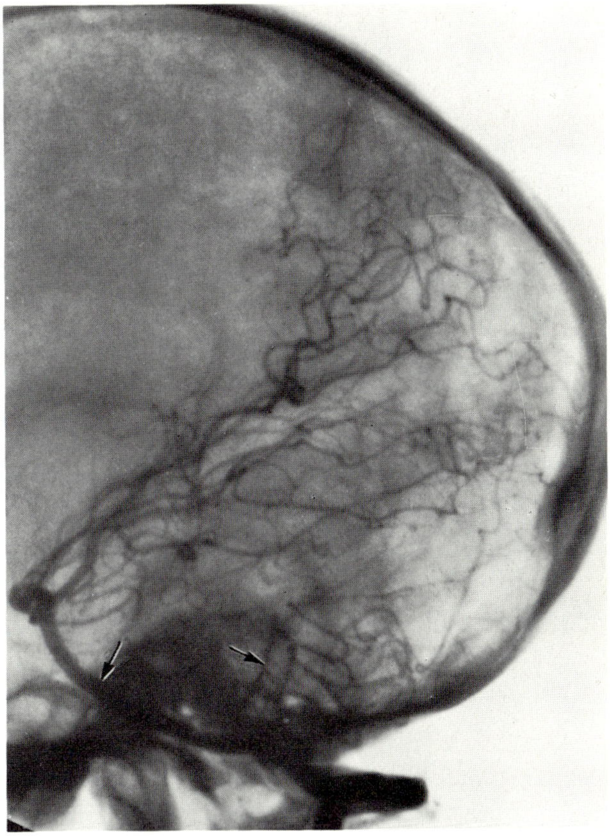

Fig. 5.
Vascular displacement by a cerebellopontine meningioma

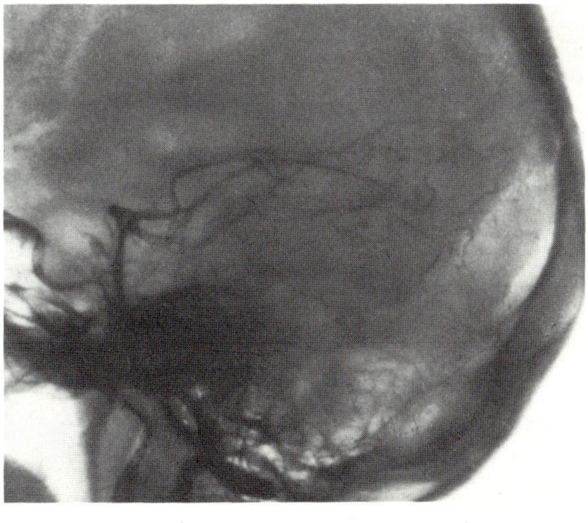

Fig. 6. The A. basilaris runs close to the clivus; the A. cerebelli superior is dislocated medially and is elevated

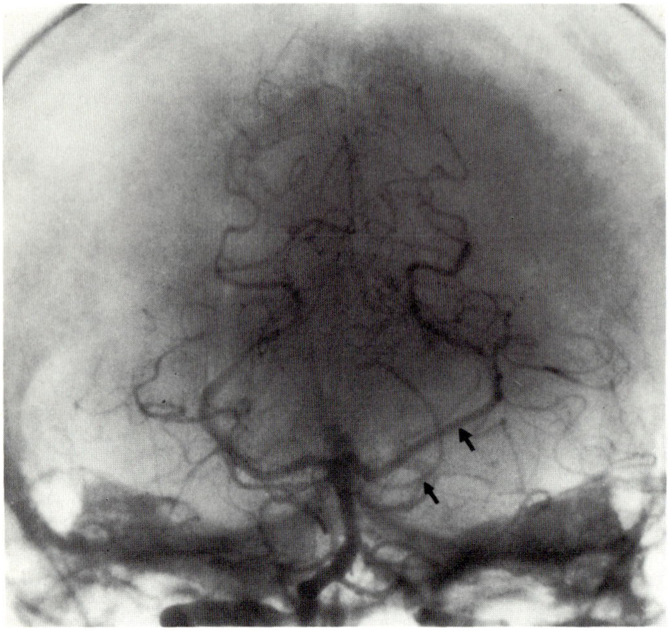

Fig. 7. Sagittal view: The A. cerebri posterior is lifted; the A. cerebelli superior is dislocated medially and its hemispheric branches are distended

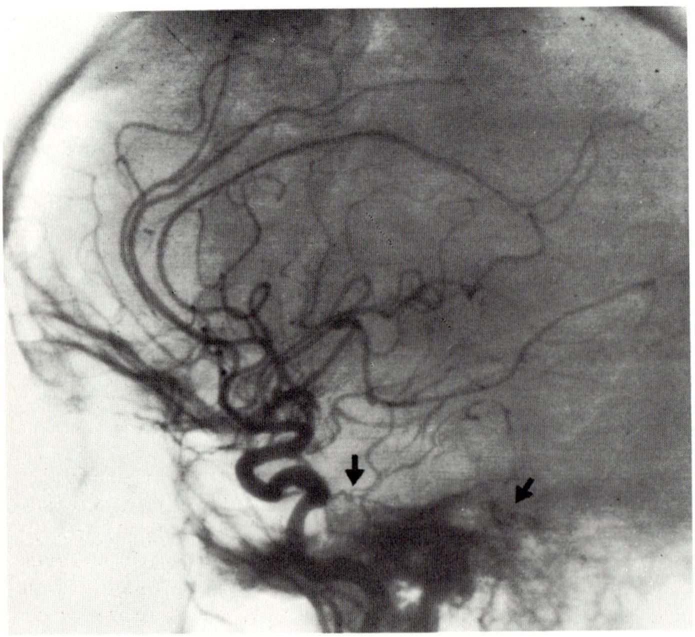

Fig. 8. Some small vessels orginating from the infraclinoidal part of the carotid siphon running towards the cerebellopontine angle

Intra- and Postoperative Complications in Cerebello-Pontine Angle Tumors and Their Relation to the Patients' Position, Type of Ventilation and Cranial Nerve Lesion

R. ENZENBACH, U. SWOZIL, A. v. MEER, E. JAUMANN, and R. SCHMIDT

During the past 8 years, 72 tumors of the cerebello-pontine angle were operated on. In Table I all cases are listed with regard to their histopathological diagnosis.

Table I. Histopathological findings in 72 cerebello-pontine angle tumors

histopathological diagnosis	number of cases
acoustic neurinoma	51
meningeoma	10
epidermoid	4
metastasis	2
LINDAU-tumor	2
melanoma	1
ependymoma	1
spongioblastoma of cerebellum	1

The relatively high incidence of intra- and postoperative complications is related to the difficulties inherent to the surgical approach to this part of the brain. Best known, in this regard, is the relation of the patients position during surgery and the intraoperative blood loss (Table II).

In the prone position, which was used in 9 cases during 1965 and 1966, the mean blood loss amounted up to 2500 cc. About the same quantity was lost in 12 patients in the lateral position with the trunk slightly elevated: 2480 cc, whereas, in the sitting position, intraoperative blood loss could be considerably reduced to a mean of 480 cc. In 26 patients, that is more than 50% of all cases who were operated on in the sitting position, no blood transfusion was required, and therefore the risk of hepatitis is considerably decreased, which according to GRUBER (1), occurs in 7-12% of all transfusions with a mortality rate of 10%. The superiority of the sitting position is thereby clearly demonstrated. Anyhow, the loss of time needed for fixation of the patient, is of no importance for an operation lasting about 4 hrs.

Table II. Blood loss as related to different positions during operation

number of cases	position	blood loss (in cc)
51	sitting	480 (100-1700)
12	lateral	2480 (350-9700)
9	prone	2500(1000-6000)

From the sitting position, however, air embolism may result as a serious complication. When introducing this position into our clinical practice, there were 2 such incidents. In one patient, air entered via an opened sinus during incision of the dura; in the other patient, air embolism occurred from a bone vein during trepanation. There were no more cases of air embolism, since intermittent positive pressure (IPP) ventilation has been applied throughout, from the incision of the skin until preparation of the tumor is started. When using this technique, there seems to be no need for an additional catheter, prophylactically introduced into the right atrium.

It has been, and still is, a matter of discussion between neurosurgeons and neuroanesthesiologists whether to use spontaneous breathing or artificial ventilation at the time of preparation of the tumor, particularly when the tumor lies close to the brainstem. When the patient is breathing spontaneously, there might be a rise of the endexpiratory CO_2- content up to 8%, thus leading to a concomittant increase of the cerebral blood flow which, in turn, may enhance the development of brain edema. Supporting the spontaneous breathing by manual assistance, on the other hand, is of little advantage only, because this will result in an intra-thoracic pressure rise. Moreover, it had been shown by OROSZ (2) many years ago, that irregulatories of the ventilatory stimulus are generally preceded by those of the circulatory system. Therefore respiratory disturbances seem to be of less significance during preparation of the tumor. In good agreement with this, we have never observed isolated intraoperative disturbances of the respiration without progressive disturbances of the circulatory system. For this reason, we have recently used controlled ventilation with positive-negative-pressure changes during the time of the tumor preparation. In addition, special attention is paid to cardiac function; including ECG control on an oscilloscope, acoustic signaling of the pulse frequency and monitoring of the arterial and venous blood pressure.

Cardiac arrhythmias were found to be the most often among the intraoperative complications, resulting in a drop of blood pressure in 17 patients, while in only 5 patients an increase of blood pressure was found.

All of the cardiac arrhythmias were found to occur during the preparation of the tumor. Most frequently, in 44 cases, bradycardia was found (Fig. 1); less often other forms of cardiac and circulatory disorders were detected: tachycardia - 8 cases -, extrasystoly presenting as sinus arrhythmia or ventricular premature contractions - 26 cases -, bigeminus - 9 cases -, or often combined forms - 36 cases (Fig. 2). With only one exception, all arrhythmias could be controlled within the time of the operation. Usually, a normalisation of the cardiac rhythm was found to occur after the tumor had been removed or could be obtained by drug therapy. However, when cardiac arrhythmias reoccurred during the early post-

Table III. Frequency of cardiac- and circulatory disorders in 72 cerebellopontine angle tumors

bradycardia	44
premature contractions	26
drop of blood pressure	18
bigeminus	9
tachycardia	8
rise of blood pressure	7
cardiac arrest	1
combined forms	36

operative course - 3 cases with tachycardia - this seems to be indicative of a poor prognosis. It should be mentioned that none of the 72 patients died during surgery. Intraoperative disturbances of heart and circulation by far outnumber the respiratory disturbances. There were only 3 instances with shortlasting episodes of cessation of respiration, during the time when supported spontaneous ventilation was used: an 8-year-old boy, operated on because of a spongioblastoma of the cerebellum, could be transferred on the 20th postoperative day in good condition, although he had been on a respirator for 6 days following the operation. The other case was a 64-year-old man with an acoustic neurinoma. He showed good recovery and could be discharged 33 days later. The third case, however, a 51-year-old woman, operated on for a metastasis, died on the 3. postoperative day from bleeding and brain swelling.

More specific problems, related to cerebello-pontine angle surgery, arise from those postoperative complications which are due to a partial or total - mostly transitory - palsy of the basal cranial nerves. Palsy of the facial nerve, being primarily of cosmetic interest, how to prevent it and how to restitute its function, has been the subject of many of the preceding papers. From the anesthesiological point of view, however, dysfunction of the vagal nerve is of much greater significance because impairment of swallowing and loss of sensibility of the glottis and the trachea may result in aspiration-pneumonia, which still represents a major problem during the postoperative course. Besides the cases of aspiration pneumonia, there is also one case with lung abscess in our material. On the other hand, since the sensibility of the glottis and the trachea is diminished, these patients tolerate tracheal intubation well for an extended period of time. The endotracheal tube ist not removed until the patient is fully responsive. In this material, we have never observed gulping or straining, which has to be carefully avoided in order to prevent bleeding. The patient is put in bed in an upright position, at least during the 1. postoperative day. In some cases, prolonged intubation, as described above, was continued for 2-4 days; in one patient for a total of 6 days. Tracheostomy, when necessary, is usually performed on the 1st postoperative day. Only in few cases, tracheostomy was performed following a period of prolonged intubation. Artificial ventilation is only required in patients showing signs of severe pulmonary dysfunction.

Another serious complication, as seen in 2 patients, is due to increasing stridor following extubation. In the 1st case, a 47-year-old man operated on a right-side acoustic neurinoma, a bilateral palsy of the recurrent nerve was found on the 8th postoperative day. The vocal cord on the right - the side of the operation - was diagnosed to be in the paramedian position with the left vocal cord being in the same position, revealing only slight movements (Fig. 3). The patient was immediately intubated with a nasal tube, thereafter a tracheostomy was made and artificial ventilation was applied for the next 20 days. During this time, there was a good restitution of recurrent nerve function, first seen on the contralateral side, later also on the side operated on. The patient could be decannulated on the 44th post-operative day. He was able to feed himself. The other case, a 49-year-old woman, had a plum-sized acoustic neurinoma on the left side. When the fully responsive patient was extubated postoperatively, she started to develop an increasing stridor early the next morning (Fig. 4). After the diagnosis of a bilateral paresis of the recurrent nerve had been established, a tracheostomy was performed. Again, in this patient - she is still in hospital - there is now good evidence of recovery of nerve function. Electromyographic study (EMG) of the sternocleidomastoid muscle revealed a complete loss of spontaneous activity and of fibrillation on the left side, indicating paresis of the accessory nerve. No pathological signs were found in the right side. These findings are strongly suggestive of an intraoperative involvement of the intracranial part of the vagal nerve, where both the vagal and the accessory nerve are closely joined. Involvement of the contralateral vagal nerve is probably best explained by postoperative brain swelling and subsequent shifting of the brain stem. In both patients, periods of bradycardia were observed during the operation which could be easily corrected by application of atropine (Fig. 5).

Conclusions

The advantage of the sitting position during posterior fossa surgery is well known. It was the aim of this report to focus the interest on postoperative complications in cerebello-pontine angle surgery. By using prolonged intubation or early tracheostomy, whenever required, and artificial ventilation, these complications can be treated successfully. Finally, careful pre- and postoperative evaluation of basal cranial nerve function is of paramount importance for early recognition and immediate treatment of certain postoperative complications.

REFERENCES

1. GRUBER, U.F.: Blutersatz. Springer-Verlag, Berlin-New York, (1968)

2. OROSZ, E.: Anaesthesist 14, 297-298 (1965)

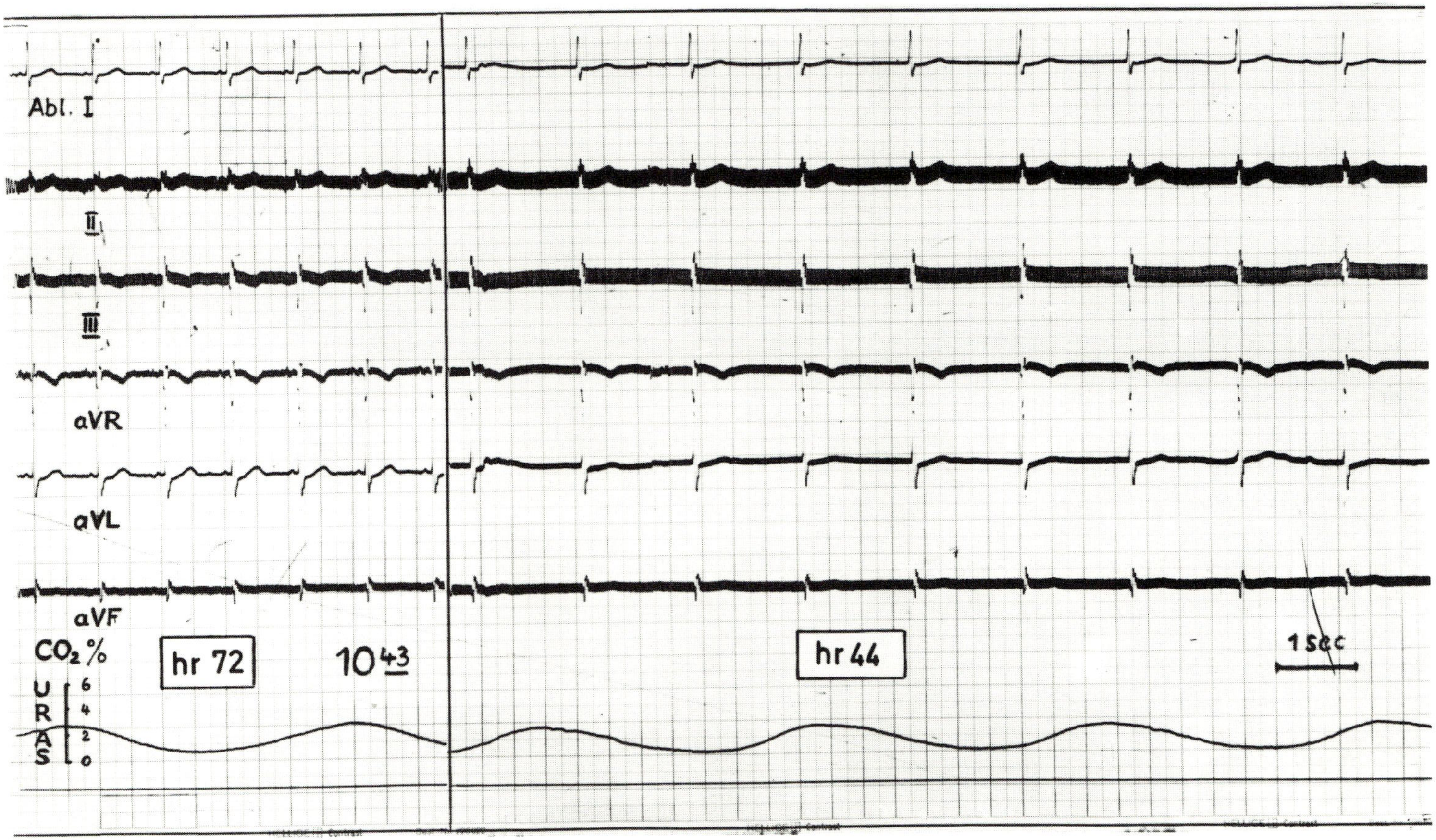

Fig. 1. ECG in standard recordings and respiratory CO_2-trace during removal of an acoustic neurinoma in a 58-year-old man

left part: normal heart rate (hr = 72/min); right part: bradycardia (hr = 44/min) during surgical manipulation of the tumor

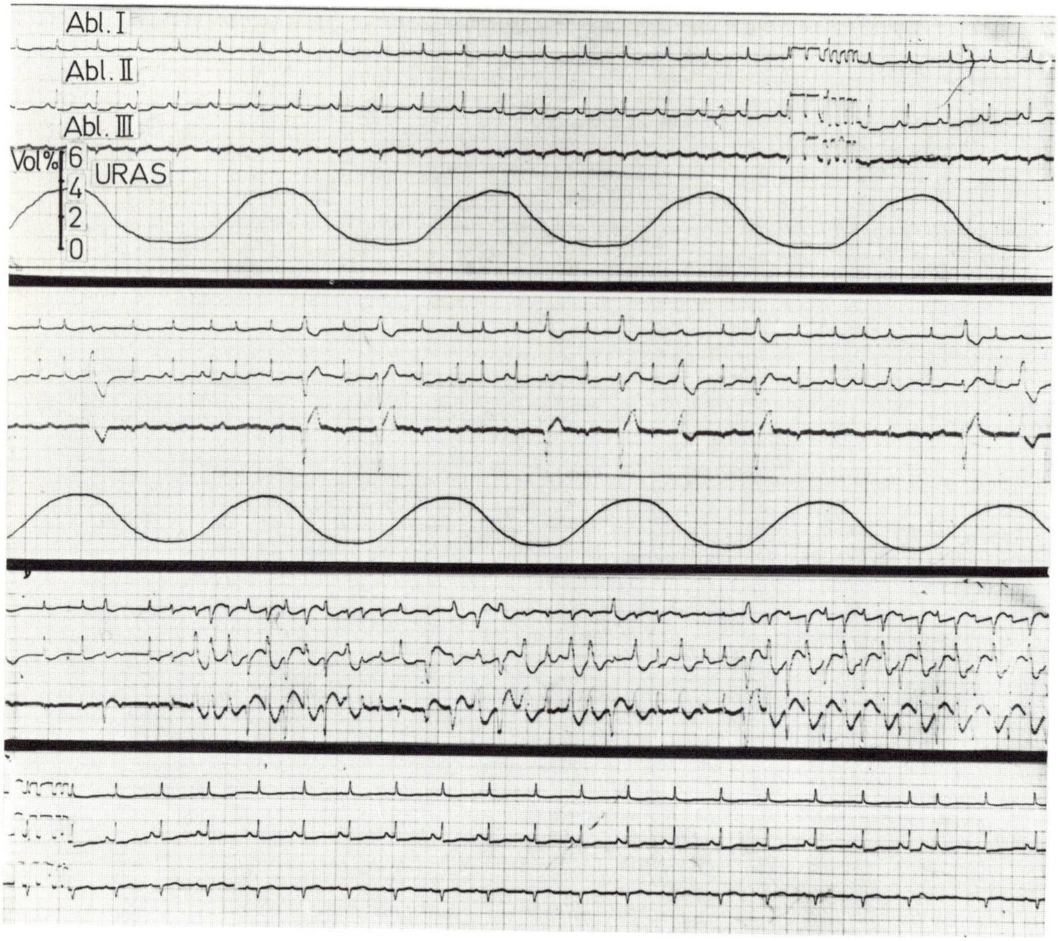

Fig. 2. ECG standard recordings and respiratory CO_2-trace during removal of an acoustic neurinoma in a 40-year-old man. Note the development of irregularities, starting with ventricular extrasystoles (second graph from top) and transition to manifestations of polytopic excitations (third graph from top) probably elicited by brainstem stimulation. Immediate and spontanous recovery at the end of the manipulations in the cerebello-pontine angle (lowest graph)

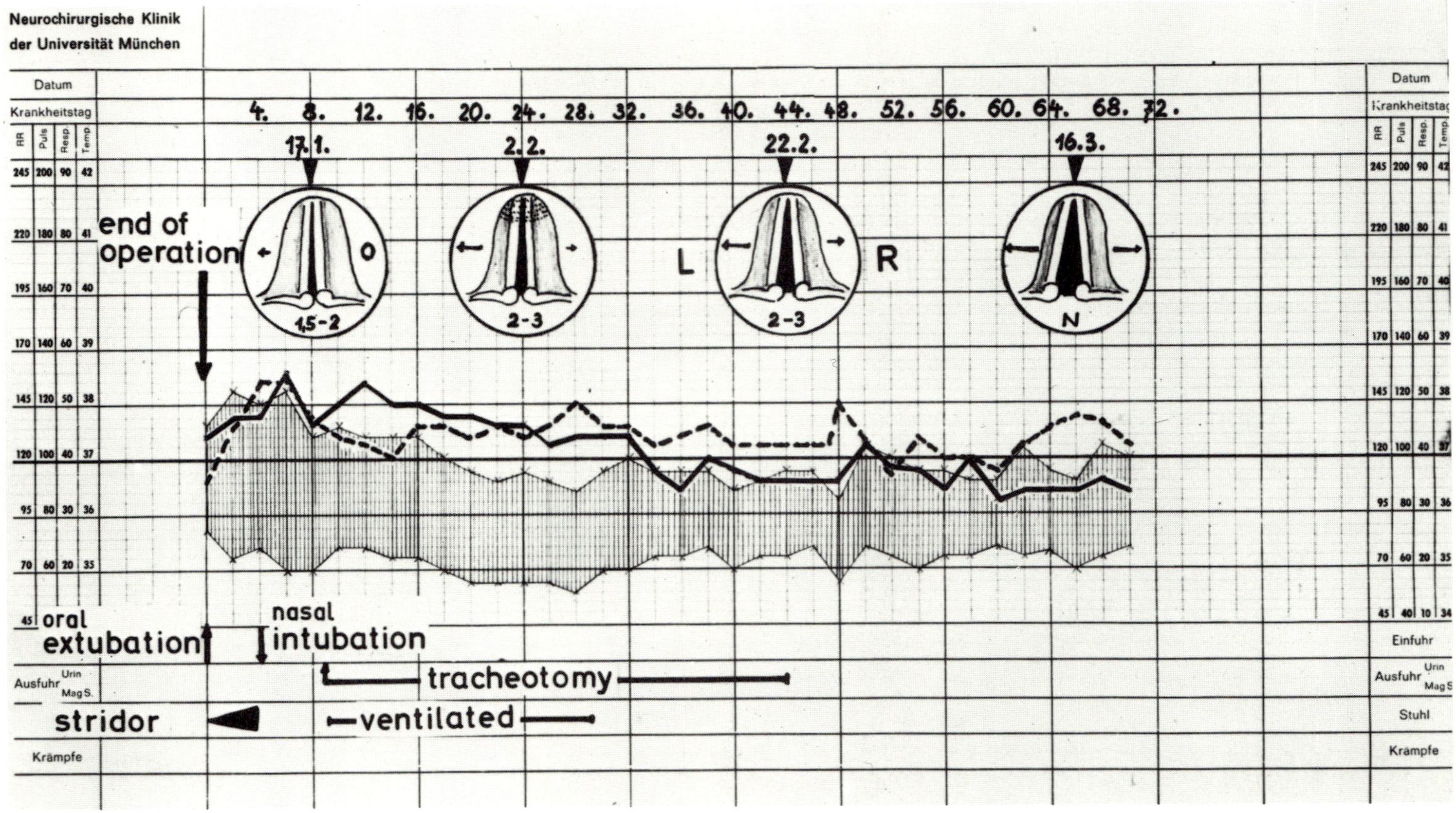

Fig. 3. Postoperative course of a 47-year-old man with acoustic neurinoma removal on the right side. Note the paramedian position of both vocal chords at the 8th pop. day. The width in between is approximately 1,5-2 mm. The vocal chord of the rigth side appeared completely paretic, whereas that of the left side showed a tendency to move. At the 24th day for 66th day the progressive recovery can be seen, first in the nonoperated side (left vocal chord), followed by the operated side. The anesthesiologic measures are shown at the bottom of this figure

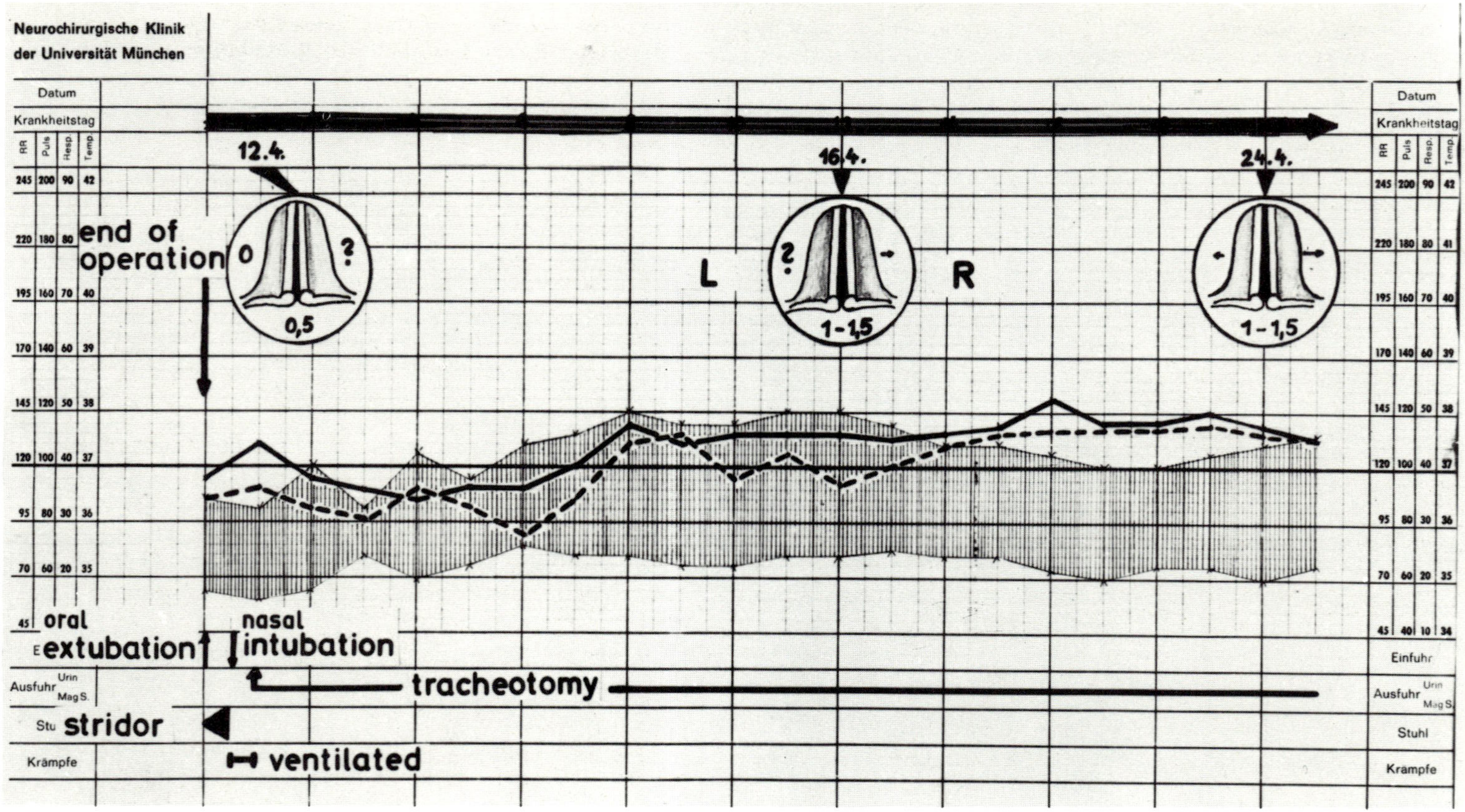

Fig. 4. Postoperative course of a 49-year-old woman with acoustic neurinoma on the left side. The bilateral vocal chord paresis developed already on the first pop. day. The glottis opened only for 0,5 mm, the left chord was completely paretic, the state of the contralatery chord was questionable. After 12 days, early symptoms of a recuperation can be detected, first from the right side, followed by the left side (operated)

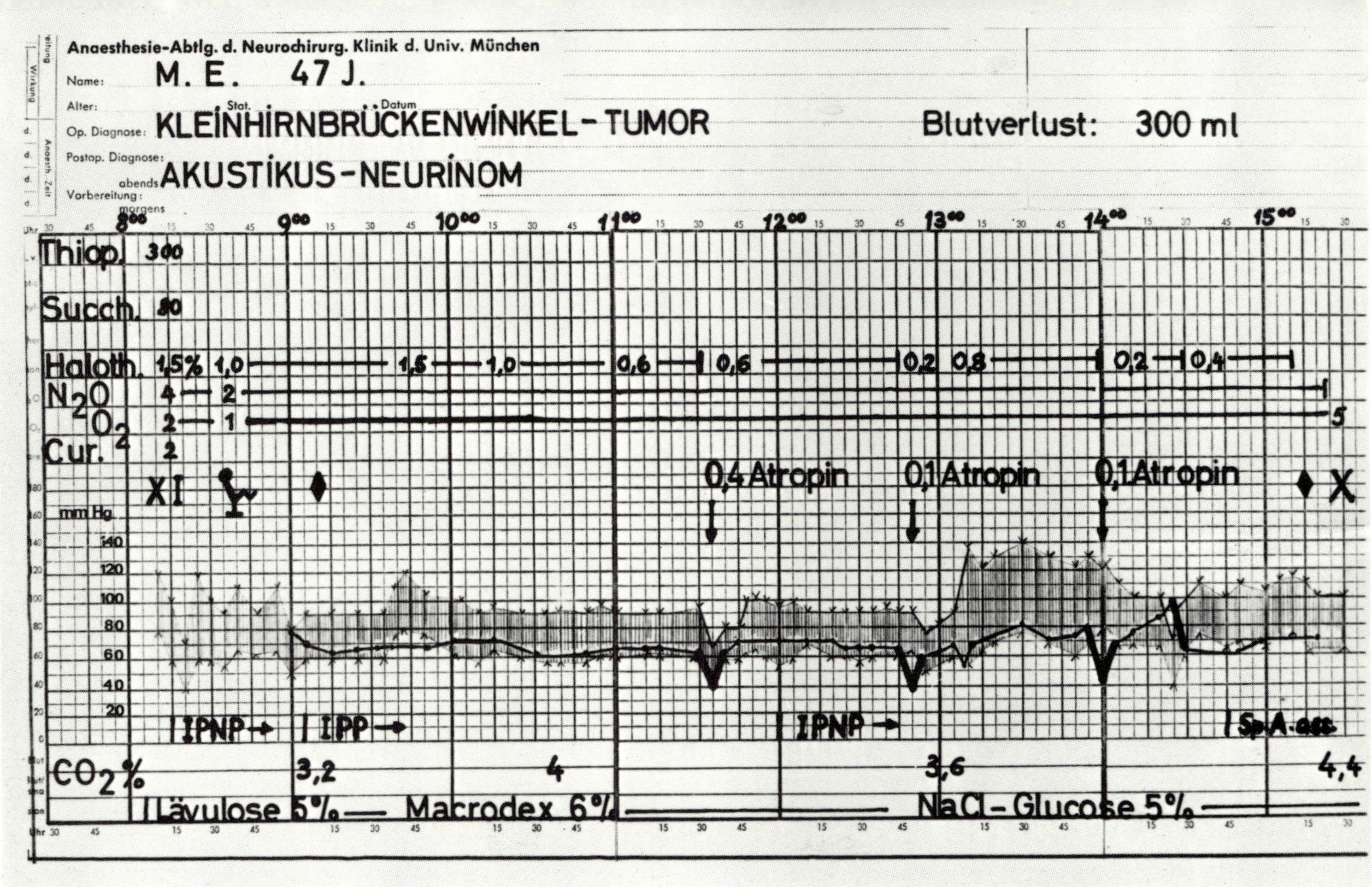

Fig. 5. Anesthesia protocol of the patient shown in Fig. 3 2 1/2 hours after begin of the operation a severe bradycardia combined with a drop of blood pressure developed, which was successfully treated by 0,4 mg Atropine. The same situation recurred three more times requiring the same treatment

Chapter VI.

Miscellaneous

Determination of the Size of the Third Ventricle Following Subarachnoid Hemorrhage by Echoencephalography

H. BÜCKING

Introduction

Cases of communicating hydrocephalus following subarachnoid hemorrhage (SAH) from rupture of intracranial arterial aneurysms were described as incidental in the earliest publications (1, 2).

When recognized, these cases probably were late sequelae with uncertain date of beginning and development.

For the first time KRAYENBÜHL 1948 (3), FOLTZ and WARD 1956 reported continuous clinical observations under control of repeated diagnostic investigations. Today the clinical features of this complication are well known (2, 5).

Method and case material

We used dynamic echoencephalography for serial measurements of third ventricular size following SAH (9). We studied 28 patients, ages between 18 and 71 years, up to 7 months following SAH, before and after operation, before and after shunting procedure, and inoperable cases. 118 measurements of the width of the third ventricle were obtained, i.e. at least 2 to 10 in an individual case. The selective case material of 28 patients represents 40% of 70 patients with aneurysms seen during a 10 months' period at the Neurosurgical Department of the University of Zurich.

In the remaining cases preoperative echo measurements were normal. Random tests and the uncomplicated clinical course showed that further repetitions were not necessary. Enlargements of the third ventricle, at least 3 mm or more than the normal value for the age were considered pathologic.

Results

In 71% of the cases (20 cases) the width of the third ventricle exceeded 10 mm up to 16 mm.

Table Ia gives a postoperative view of the echoventriculograms (EVG) based on a measurement prior to operation. In some cases ventricular enlargement was present before the operation. In the first postoperative week transient enlargements occurred. In 5 cases the EVG remained normal. Maximal dilatations of the third ventricle were observed in 2 cases after 2 weeks at the earliest.

Maximal dilatations of the third ventricle occurred in the later period (Table Ib)

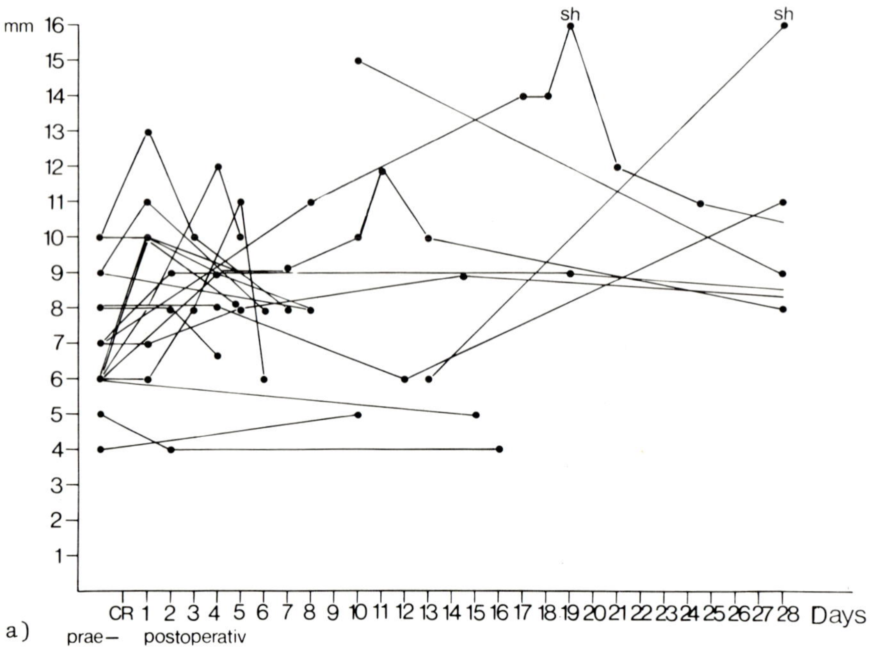

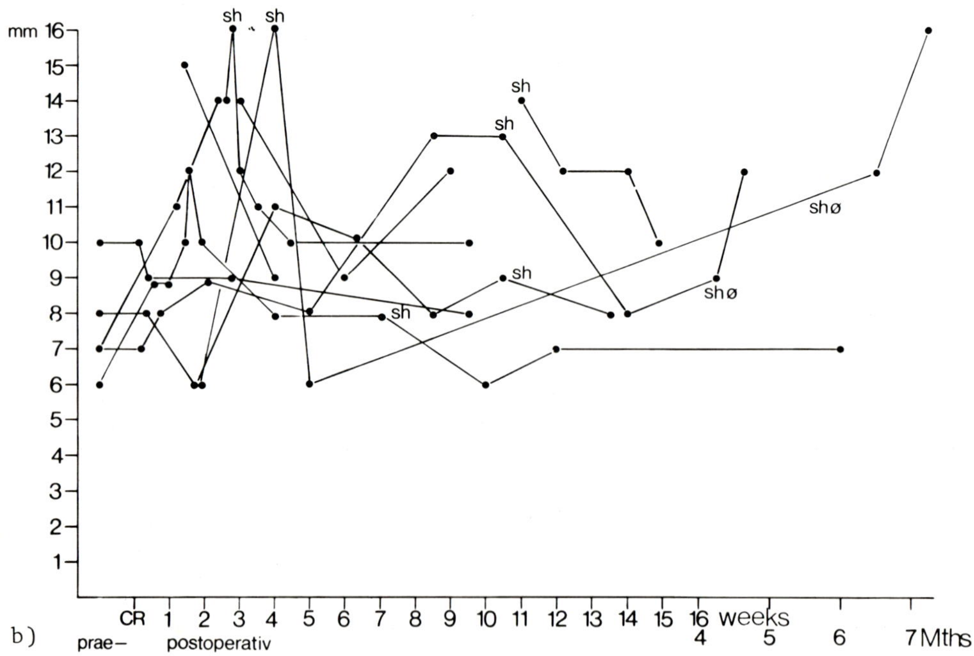

Table I. Measurements of the third ventricular width in mm a) during the early postoperative days b) in the late postoperative period
CR: craniotomy, SH: shunting procedure
First measurement prior to operation

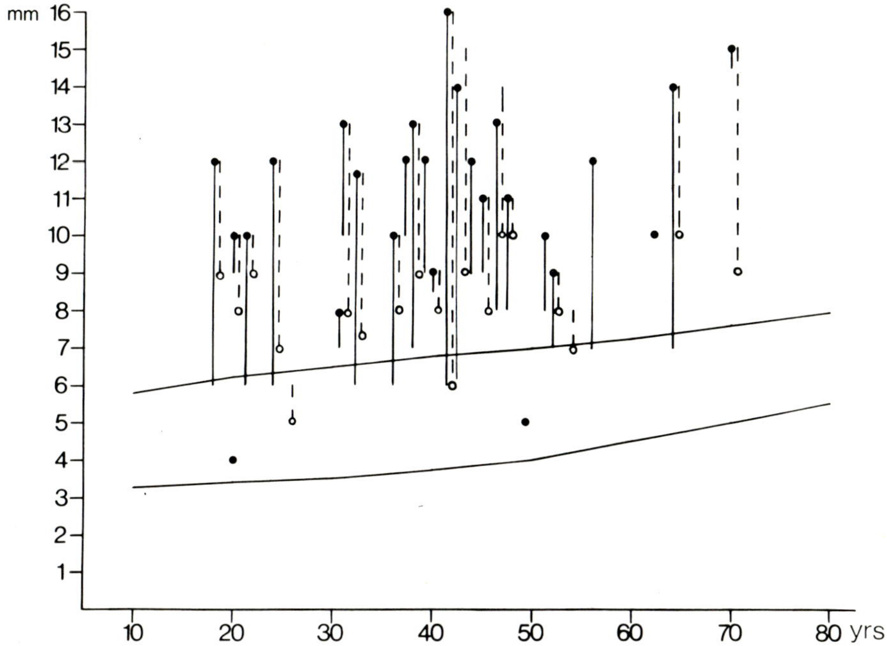

Table II. Measurements of the width of the third ventricle in mm, compared to the normal value of age. First measurement at the beginning of the line, maximal width during the course, reversal or last measurement. Two cases with repeated enlargement

from 3 up to 10 weeks after craniotomy. This complication of communicating hydrocephalus could be confirmed when the measurement was done in various intervals after the craniotomy.

Table II shows that in all ages the pathological results of third ventricular measurement exceeded the normal value of age (6).

In Table III all results are related to the date of the first or single SAH.

Different mental and neurologic dysfunctions which were not comparable with the delayed progressive brain organic syndromes (BOS) existed in 50% of the operated cases during and shortly after the SAH and prior to pathological EVG, but in all inoperable cases immediately.

The BOS in the late period is characterized by signs of mental deterioration like disorientation, impaired memory, decrease of mental and physical activity, reduction in consciousness, and accompanied by neurological dysfunctions like spastic paraparesis, akinetic mutism, ataxia and urinary incontinence. All patients did not necessarily have the whole complex of symptoms and the degree was moderate or severe. Mild symptoms might only consist of headache.

Pathological ventricular enlargements occurred with distinct intervals.

We have analysed intervals from 0 to 4 weeks and from 4 to 16 weeks, following the first SAH. Pathological EVGs at 0 to 4 weeks intervals were obtained in 8 cases. These ventricular dilatations were transient and concerned the early postoperative

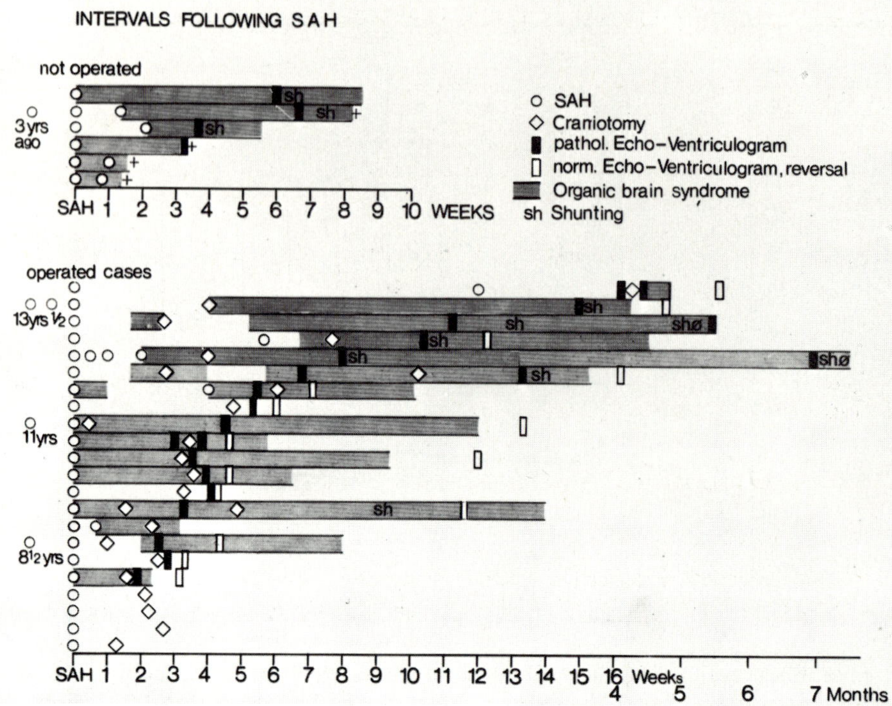

Table III. Measurements of maximal enlargement of the third ventricle at intervals following the first or single subarachnoid hemorrhage

period (Fig. 1). The patients had mild clinical signs or none. 5 moderate or severe BOS developed after an interval of 2 to 4 weeks from craniotomy, too. In 2 cases the diagnosis of communicating hydrocephalus was confirmed.

The incidence of single SAH was 12 of 13 patients in this group.

Pathological EVGs at long intervals from 4-16 weeks and more were measured in 9 cases (Fig. 2).

The distinct interval between craniotomy and these findings is obvious.

The incidence of multiple SAH in this group was 7 out of 9 patients. Complications in this group consisted of intracranial hematomas (55%) and cerebral angiospasms (30%). 8 cases at long intervals presented progressive BOS, 5 cases of a severe degree.

Course and duration of clinical signs and diagnosis

7 moderate or severe BOS, 2 at short and 5 at long intervals, advanced but then spontaneously improved within 4 to 8 weeks. Repeated lumbar punctures in special cases probably favored this course.

7 severe BOS of long intervals progressed and further diagnostic steps were done in order to confirm the diagnosis of hydrocephalus and abnormal cerebrospinal

fluid circulation. In 5 cases diagnosis was established by RIHSA cisternography, in 3 cases by pneumencephalography and in one case only by EVG and electro-encephalogram.

One confirmed severe hydrocephalus spontaneously improved.

Elevated cerebrospinal fluid pressures were measured in 7 cases 4 to 16 weeks following SAH, at the climax of pathological enlargement of third ventricular size and BOS.

Body temperature of septic type in some cases was present several weeks following SAH and preceded progressive clinical signs and pathological EVG.

Treatment with shunting procedure

6 cases were treated with ventriculo-atrial shunting procedure (PUDENZ-HEYER) which was performed from the 8th up to the 16th week following the first SAH. The BOS had a duration of 2 to 4 months or longer and were reversed after shunting procedure within 2 to 6 weeks. Normalisation of EVG often preceded.

Two cases were therapy - resistent.

Inoperable cases with and without shunting

In 3 out of 6 inoperable complicated cases the third ventricle was pathologically dilatated as the time interval increased (3-7 weeks) following SAH, and in no case earlier.

The severe BOS and neurological deficits existed immediately following the SAH and were superimposed by stupor, somnolence or initial coma. Three inoperable cases with rapid lethal course were complicated by severe cerebral vasospasm and intracranial hematomas.

D i s c u s s i o n

Communicating hydrocephalus following SAH is attributed to fibrosis of the leptomeninges in the basilar cisterns, in the cerebral sulci and the incisural region of the tentorium which results in obstruction of cerebrospinal fluid absorption.

Our ultrasonic investigations show that this process takes 4 to 16 weeks to develop following the first SAH, the shortest interval being 2 weeks.

If transient findings in the early postoperative period are neglected pathological EVG correlates in 23% (16 of 70 patients) with delayed progressive BOS and neurological dysfunctions. Seven advanced, moderate or severe BOS spontaneously improved. One case in advanced stage was lethal. Thus 11% (8 cases) remain, which presented pathological EVG and progressive clinical signs and in which the diagnosis of communicating hydrocephalus was confirmed. KAZNER and SCHIEFER in 1967 found a normal echoencephalogram immediately after SAH, but later in 43% the third ventricular size was 10 mm. HEIDRICH (7) mentions 54% enlargements of the third ventricle in 26 patients studied with pneumencephalography. GALERA (5) reports 30% hydrocephalic ventriculocranial index among 100 cases following SAH 3 weeks to 3 months , seldom up to 2 years.

In a recent study (8) the diagnosis of communicating hydrocephalus was made in 10% out of 280 patients with aneurysm, by combining various diagnostic procedures including echoencephalography.

Summary

We studied the changes in size of the third ventricle as an indication of developing communicating hydrocephalus following subarachnoid hemorrhage. This was determined by serial echomeasurements. Enlargements of the third ventricle occur at distinct intervals. Pathogenetic views of the underlying delayed process, establishment of diagnosis, spontaneous improvements and treatment are discussed.

REFERENCES

1. STRAUSS, I., J.H.GLOBUS and S.W.GINSBURG: Spontaneous subarachnoid hemorrhage. Arch.Neurol.Psychiat., Chicago 1932, 27, 1080-1130
2. SHULMAN, K., B.F.MARTIN, N.POPOFF and J.RANSOHOFF: Recognition and treatment of hydrocephalus following spontaneous subarachnoid hemorrhage. J.Neurosurg. 20, 1040-1049 (1963)
3. KRAYENBÜHL, H. and F. LÜTHY: Hydrocephalus als Spätfolge geplatzter basaler Hirnaneurysmen. Schweiz.Arch.Neurol.Psychiat. 61, 7-21 (1948)
4. FOLTZ, E. and A.A.WARD: Communicating hydrocephalus from subarachnoid bleeding. J.Neurosurg. 13, 546-566 (1956)
5. GALERA, R.G. and T.GREITZ: Hydrocephalus in the adult secondary to the rupture of intracranial arterial aneurysms. J.Neurosurg. 32, 634-641 (1970)
6. SCHIEFER, W. and E.KAZNER: Klinische Echoencephalographie. Springer, 1967
7. HEIDRICH, R.: Die subarachnoidale Blutung. G. Thieme Leipzig, 1970
8. YASARGIL, M.G., Y.YONEKAWA, B.ZUMSTEIN, H.STAHL and H.BÜCKING: Hydrocephalus following spontaneous subarachnoid hemorrhage; clinical features and treatment (in preparation)
9. BÜCKING, H. and R.HESS: Echoencephalographische und hirnelektrische Befunde nach Subarachnoidalblutung; Korrelation zur Klinik und Diagnostik in Fällen von Hydrocephalus (in preparation)

J.Un. 65 j. ♂ Reversal after shunting

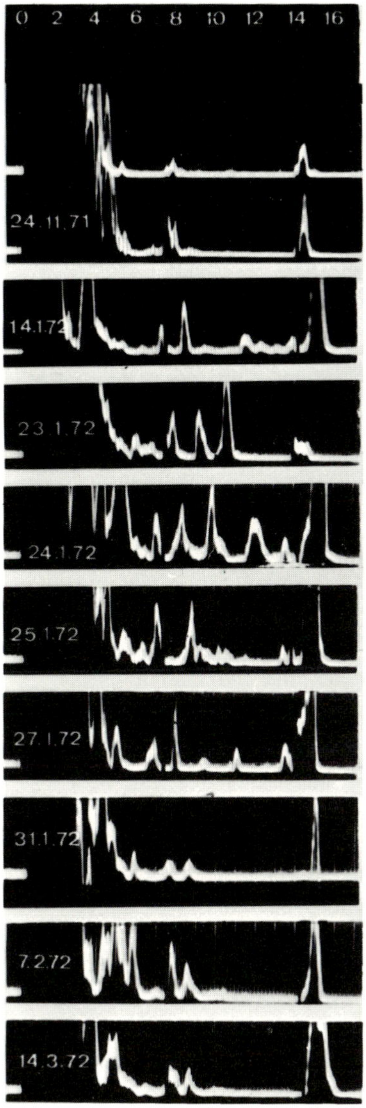

44 days before Op

17 days postop.

11 weeks interval
1. SAH-EVG

19 days-postop.

2 days after shunting

13 days after shunting

7 weeks after shunting

Fig. 1. Transient early postoperative enlargement of third ventricle

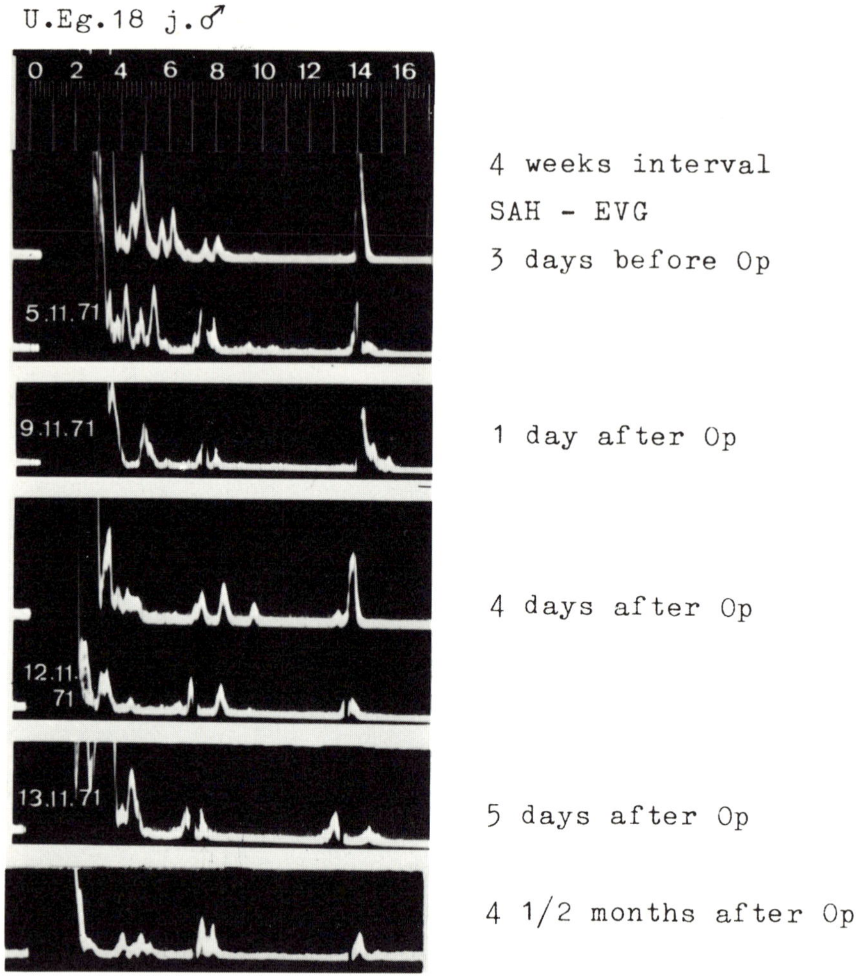

Fig. 2. Progessive enlargement of third ventricle

Experience with Ultrasonic B-Scan, Assessing the Ventricular System in Children and Adults

T. GRUMME

Two-dimensional echoencephalography was carried out for 1 year with four different equipments (Fa. KRETZ, ATOMICA, PICKER, KONTRON) and for the last 1 1/2 years with the KRETZ equipment only. Recording was performed according to the compound-scan. In children a 2 MHz- and in adults a 1 MHz-probe was always used: diameter 15 mm. Recording techniques: 1 Horizontally, 2.0-5.0 cm above the line from the lateral canthus to the external auditory meatus. 2. Vertically, at right angles to the line through the external auditory meatus, applying the probe over, or more in front of, or behind the ear. All pictures of the B-scan, which was done on different levels, were compared with the results of the A-scan as well as the pneumencephalographic findings. Our experience is based on 30 children and 20 adults.

Results

1. Children: In the majority of cases the third ventricle can be determined by horizontal and vertical scanning. Although B-scan gives a better optic impression, the A-scan succeeds better in determining accurately the width of the third ventricle (Fig. 1). The lateral ventricles can be represented as cavities in almost every case of extreme hydrocephalus. Medium sized dilatation fo the ventricular system can only be demonstrated in about one third of cases (Fig. 2 and 3). For the evidence of an asymmetrical hydrocephalus (Fig. 4) we found proportions similar to those observed in extremely and medium sized hydrocephalus as described above. A congruent presentation of normal ventricular system, as obtained by pneumencephalography, has not yet been achieved by this method.

2. Adults: The recordings of the normal and pathological ventricular system are not encouraging at the present time. In a few cases (namely patients with occlusive hydroecephalus) the third ventricle and parts of the lateral ventricle are demonstrated. Special probes either working on 1.5 MHz or having separated areas for ultrasonic wave transmission and reception did not influence these results.

Discussion

If two-dimensional echoencephalography is to replace air encephalography in appropriate cases, then the ventricles of the brain must be represented as real cavities. Single demonstrations of parts of the ventricular wall are not sufficient to make reliable, relevant statements on the brain ventricles. Apart from the optical gain, no conspicuous advantage is established as compared to the A-scan.

The good results observed with increasing ventricular width in children are explained by the favourable echo conditions. Figures 5 and 6 demonstrate the reasons why the normal ventricular system is not represented as a cavity under the present technical conditions: the echo conditions are extremely unfavourable. The shape of the normal ventricular system allows at most a partial outline in the region of the body and the anterior horn of the lateral ventricle, because an optimal angle of incidence for the ultrasound of about 90° can almost never be obtained.

The poor results in adults are additionally caused - and all authors agree in this respect - by the poor echo conditions with increased absorption of the ultrasonic energy by the cranium.

From comparative consideration of the literature available since 1963 and our own investigations, it appears that only better technical conditions and new probes, possibly containing several individual probes, will permit further development in the field of echoventriculography with the B-scan.

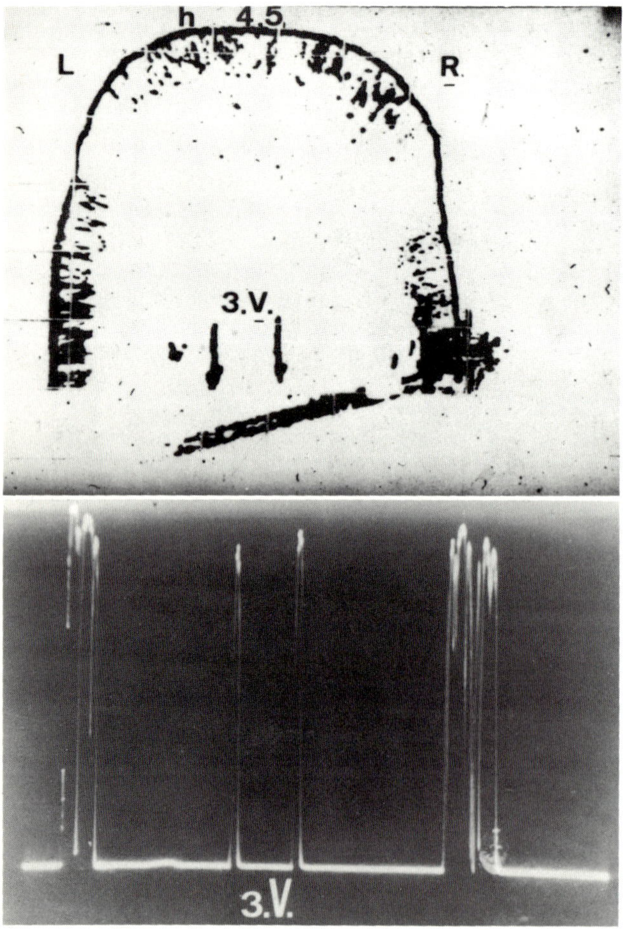

Fig. 1. The third ventricle; comparison between A-scan

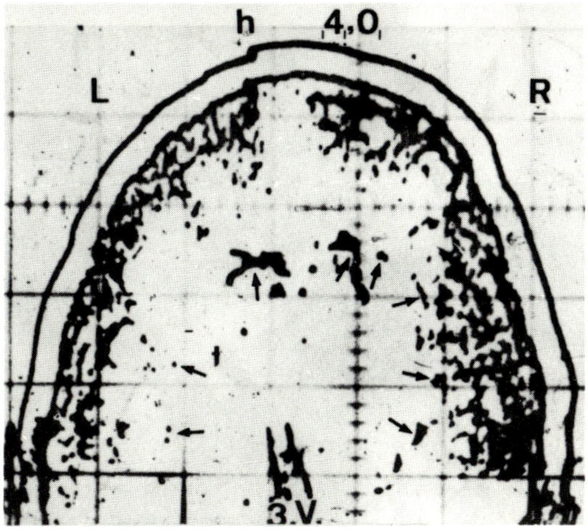

Fig. 2. Medium-sized hydrocephalus; horizontal cut

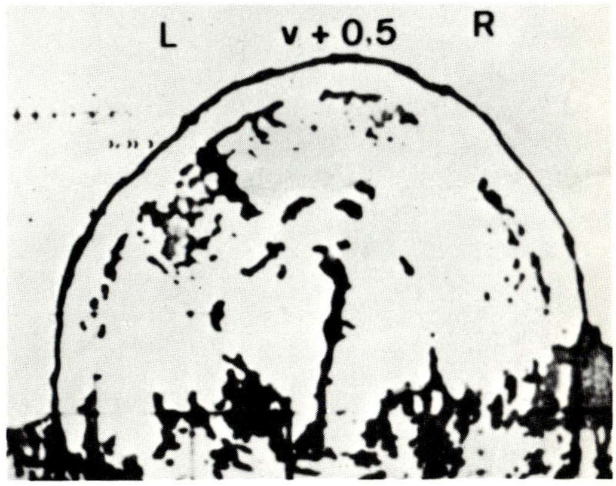

Fig. 3. Medium-sized hydrocephalus; vertical cut

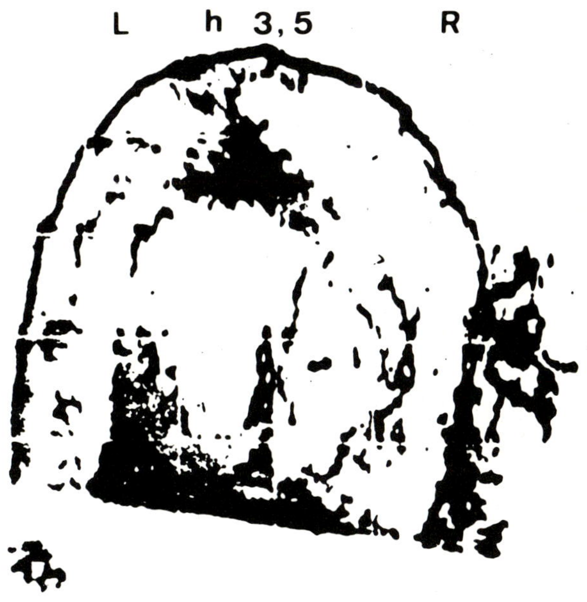

Fig. 4. Asymmetrical hydrocephalus; horizontal cut

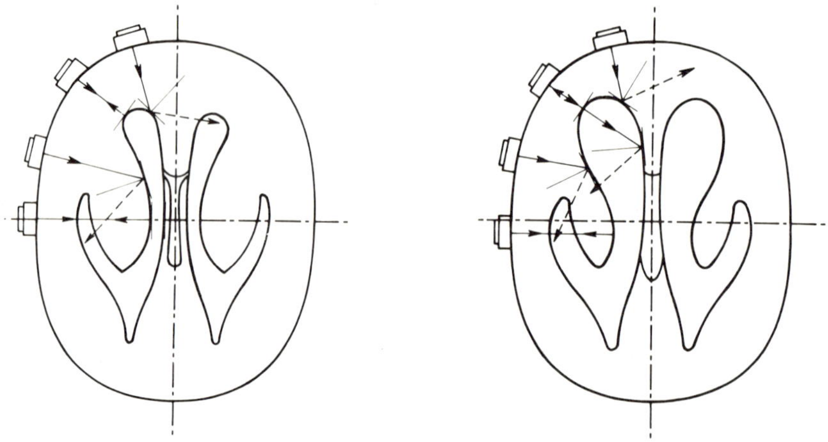

Fig. 5. Condition for ultrasound-reflexion in cases of normal and pathological ventricular system; horizontal cut

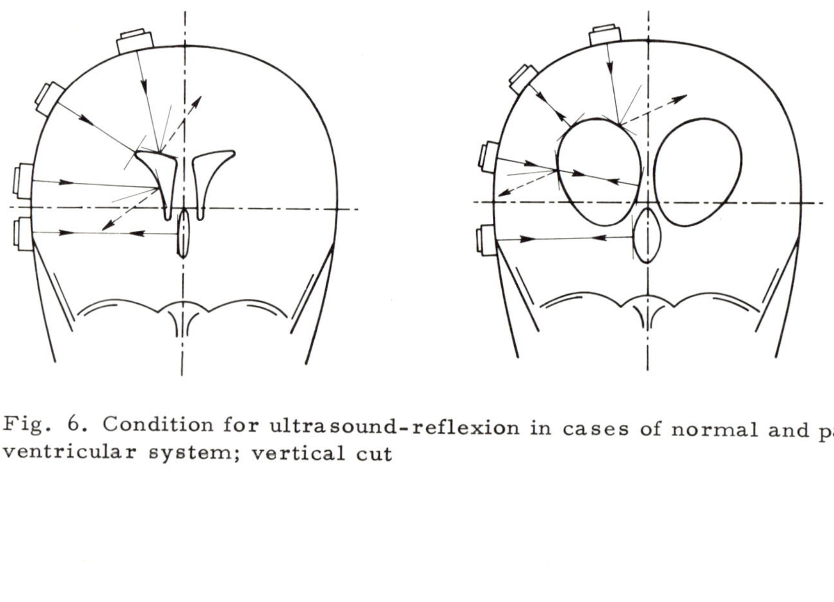

Fig. 6. Condition for ultrasound-reflexion in cases of normal and pathological ventricular system; vertical cut

Comparative Study of Computerized and A-Mode Midline Echoencephalography

E. HOPMAN, E. KAZNER, and B. VOGEL+)

A-mode echoencephalography has gained increasing clinical importance during the last few years for rapid orientation regarding the position of the cerebral midline structures. However, the number of those who master this technique is still small, since only constant training and control by neuroradiological findings leads to reliable results. Many attempts to standardize the A-mode technique failed (WHITE, 1970; WHITE and HUDSON, 1971). A constant adjustment of the ultrasonic apparatus or a constant application point of the probe cannot be expected. There is too much variation in the size and thickness of the skull and in the projection of the cerebral midline structures on the surface of the skull from individual to individual.

For some years, the development and perfection of computerized ultrasonic techniques has been in progress, with the aim of allowing an automated midline echo determination. Computerized ultrasonic equipment does not have an oscilloscopic screen. Instead of this, the position of the midline structures is displayed digitally. Over a period of one year, a midline computer++) was used clinically and the data were compared with the results of conventional A-mode technique and neuroradiological findings.

Principle of operation

As usual in A-mode technique, a 2-MHz probe is applied to the skull in the temporal region (Fig. 1). The computer at first searches for the so-called distal echo, originating from the scalp-air interface. This echo appears distal to the echo from the inner skull table-dura mater interface (end echo). From its position, the computer calculates the theoretical midline location. Then the gate for midline echo search is opened. The search for the midline echo is limited to 16 millimeters left and right of the theoretical midline. This limitation seemed to be suitable since shifts exceeding 16 mm are extremely rare. If the computer finds a single echo of high amplitude in the mid-gate, its position is read out in millimeters and displayed digitally. A 2-mm graduated scale indicates both the direction and magnitude of a given shift. After plotting the read-out data on a bar diagram the operator then re-cycles the computer to start the measurement cycle again. The measurement is repeated 30 to 50 times from either side of the skull. Multiple measurements result in a "histogram" which facilitates a rapid evaluation (Fig. 2). Each histogram represents a summation of echoes of high amplitude in the mid-gate. By the large number of readings erratic measurements of the midline position

+) technician

++) MIDLINER, PICKER ROENTGEN GMBH, 4992 Espelkamp

are minimized. If no large echo is found by the computer, or if two or more large echoes are found simultaneously in a single reading, the computer recycles and starts the search for the distal echo again.

In comparison with the conventional technique, this method has the advantage that operator bias is eliminated. The physician or the technician who also can perform this investigation, may concentrate upon the application of the probe; the necessity to control the screen and adjust the apparatus is abolished. Maximal objectivity can be reached, if one person applies the probe without optical control of the digital display, while a second operator makes the readings. This procedure accelerates the investigation considerably. The duration of the investigation is 5 to 10 minutes with one operator and only 3 to 4 minutes with two operators.

Results

The comparative study included 530 patients with various intracranial diseases (Table I) during the last twelve months.

Table I. Computerized echoencephalography - results in 530 patients with intracranial disease

Histogram	Number of patients	Midline Reading-Out	
		correct	incorrect
Normal Midline Position	382	379	3
Midline Displacement	114	108	6
Uninterpretable, Technically insufficient	34 (6.4%)		
Total	530	487 91.9%	9 1.7%

Primarily we were interested in the reliability of the midline computer in the presence of a midline displacement. Fig. 3 shows an example of a midline shift in the histogram. The midline complex is displaced by about 6 millimeters from right to left. The maximum values from right and left overlap. This finding corresponded completely with the A-mode echogram and the carotid angiogram.

In 117 patients with a midline shift of 2 mm or more in the computer echogram or in the A-scope, the midline echo measurements of both methods were compared. The diagram in Fig. 4 shows a close correlation of measurements. Only in patients with slight shifts did false computer-readings occur (6 false positive and 3 false negative, see also Table I and II). In 105 from the 117 patients, the ultrasonic findings were checked by contrast medium investigations. In all these cases the

Table II. Computerized echoencephalography - incorrect and unsatisfactory results (43 cases = 8.1 per cent)

Histogram	Number of patients
False positive midline shift	6
False negative midline shift	3
No response	10
Unilateral response	7
Technically insufficient uninterpretable	17
Total	43

ultrasonic measurements could be confirmed. In 12 patients the neuroradiological control was not necessary. These had postoperative follow-up measurements to observe the decrease of the preoperatively existent midline echo shift. From a total of 111 midline displacements in the A-mode echogram, the computer detected 108 (97.3%). The above-mentioned 3 patients with false negative midline echo reading-out showed only slight shifts in the conventional echogram (2.0 to 2.5 mm) as a result of receding brain edema after intracranial surgery. The preceding trepanation with alterations of structures, necessary for the determination of the distal echo, may be the cause for this failure. However, in patients with intact bony skull we could not observe false negative computer measurements. In the presence of scalp swelling, it is uncertain, whether or not, erroneous measurements can occur as in the A-mode technique, since after some technical failures in head-injured patients with subgaleal hematoma - there were only sporadic responses - we no longer employed the midline computer in such cases. The false positive results in half of the cases also concerned patients with trepanation defects. In two cases, the maximum midline reading-out was at 2 millimeters, a borderline value. Only once did the histogram show an unexplained midline displacement of 4 millimeters.

The reliability of the computer measurement, as evaluated by the team after a short period of training, is underscored by the fact, that in all cases with questionable midline measurement in the A-mode echogram, the computer was used to clarify the situation. As an example, the histogram of a 68-year-old man is reproduced (Fig. 5). It shows a marked displacement of the midline complex from right to left. During the A-mode investigation, it was doubtful whether a midline shift or a ventricular dilatation was present. The patient had a glioblastoma in the right temporal lobe.

Secondly, we were interested in the possibility of determining the width of the third ventricle using the midline computer. The breadth of the midline complex in the histogram and the width of the third ventricle are doubtless related. The histogram in Fig. 6, for instance, shows a small midline complex. The width of the third ventricle in the A-mode echogram was 4 to 5 millimeters in this case.

In 44 patients of our series, a dilatation of the third ventricle could be found, using the A-mode technique (width of the third ventricle 8 mm or more). In 7 patients, the computer echograms were technically insufficient or not interpretable. A markedly dilated third ventricle obviously often leads to such an unsatisfactory result (Fig. 9). The interpretation of the A-mode echograms of these patients caused no problems. In 17 patients only the midline came out in the histogram. In the remaining 20 patients, an approximate determination of the third ventricle width was possible. If the third ventricle is about 8 millimeters in diameter, often only a single 8 mm wide midline complex is to be seen in the histogram. From 10 to 12 millimeters, separate bars can be plotted from the lateral walls of the third ventricle. Fig. 7 and 8 show histograms in the case of hydrocephalus. In Fig. 7, only the ventricular walls are displayed. In Fig. 8 beneath the ventricular bars, the midline complex is demonstrated. Reliable results among the 44 patients with hydrocephalus represented only 45 per cent of the patients examined by means of the midline computer. This points out thatcomputerizedechoencephalography is not a very useful technique in detecting ventricular dilatation.

The total of unsatisfactory or false measurements using the computer was 8.1 per cent (Table II). However, the false positive and false negative midline shifts have been discussed. In 10 cases, even with maximum amplification, no response was detected; in 7 further cases, only unilateral response was obtained. Seventeen cases proved to be technically insufficient oruninterpretable. Fig. 9 for example shows such a histogram of a child with extreme hydrocephalus. All uninterpretable histograms resulted from patients with intracranial anomalies.

Conclusions

In the comparative study in patients with supratentorial space-occupying lesions leading to a displacement of the midline structures, computer echography of the cerebral midline proved to be a significant simplification with respect to conventional A-mode echography. This procedure can also be performed by a technician without special training, and still results in a midline determination of very high reliability. The method is less adaptable to the determination of hydrocephalus or patients with lesions in the midline region.

REFERENCES

1. GALICICH, J.H. and J.B. WILLIAMS: A computerized echoencephalograph. J.Neurosurg. 35, 453-460 (1971)

2. WHITE, D.N.: Ultrasonic encephalography. Queen's University, Medical Ultrasonic Laboratory Publication, Kingston/Canada 1970

3. WHITE, D.N. and A.C.HUDSON: The future of A-mode midline echoencephalography. Neurology (Minneap.) 21, 140-153 (1971)

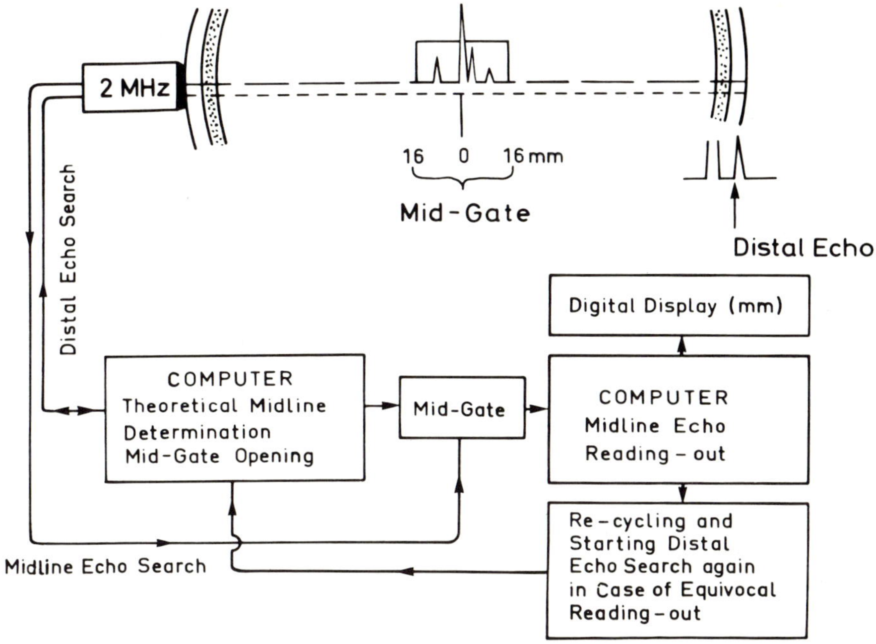

Fig. 1. Principle of computerized midline echoencephalography (after GALICICH and WILLIAMS, 1971)

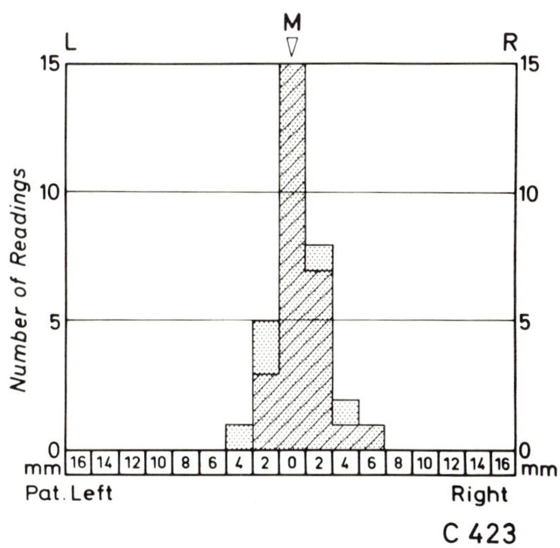

Fig. 2. Computer echogram (=histogram) showing normal midline position

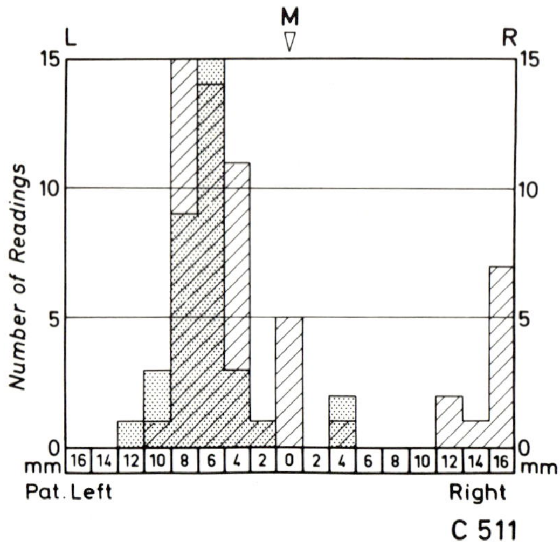

Fig. 3. Histogram of a patient with an intracerebral hematoma in the right parietal lobe. The midline complex is markedly shifted from right to left

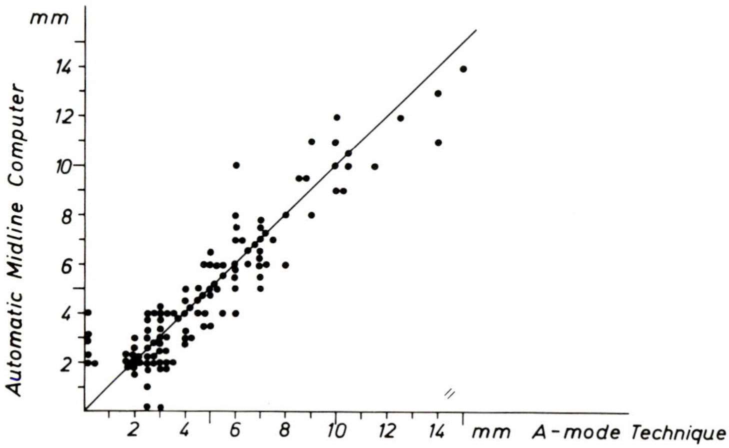

Fig. 4. Comparison of midline shift in A-mode and computerized midline echo-encephalography (n = 117). Close correlation between the results of both methods

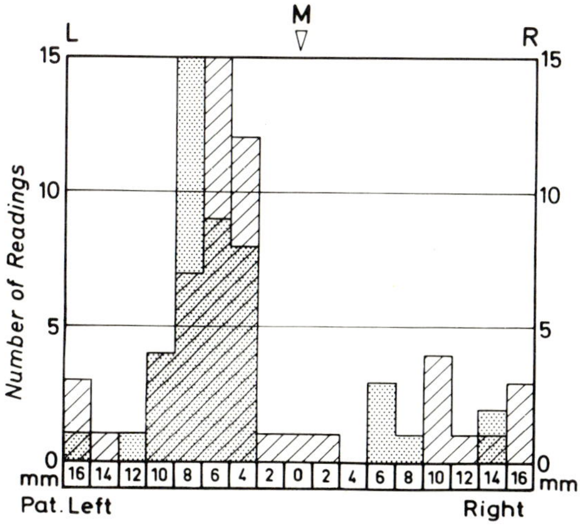

Fig. 5.

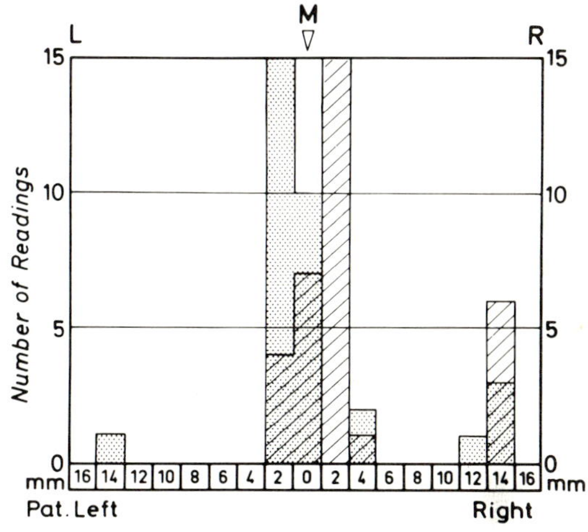

Fig. 6.

Fig. 5. Unequivocal midline shift in the histogram of a patient with questionable findings in the A-mode echogram

Fig. 6. Four-mm wide midline complex in a patient with a small third ventricle

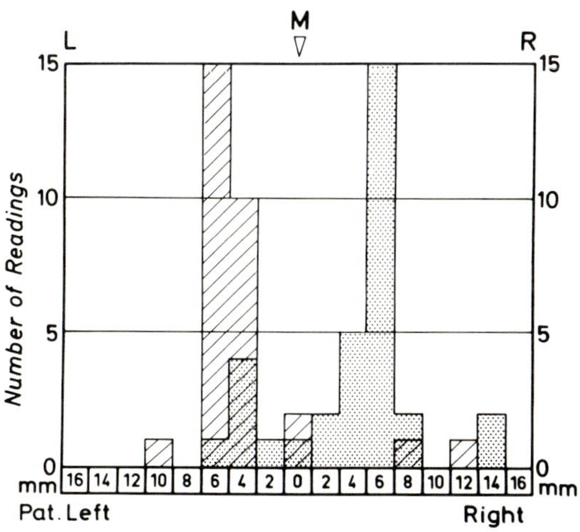

Fig. 7.

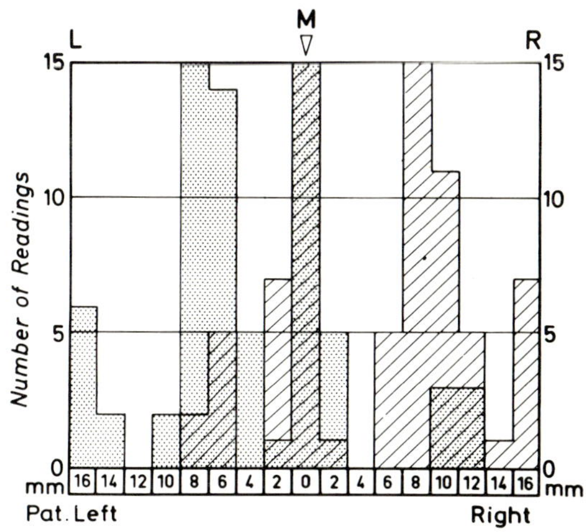

Fig. 8.

Fig. 7. Histogram of a patient with marked dilatation of the third ventricle. The two bars at 6-mm left and 6-mm right originate from the lateral walls of the enlarged third ventricle

Fig. 8. Histogram of a patient with marked dilatation of the third ventricle. Beneath the bars from the walls of the third ventricle at 6/8-mm left and 8/10-mm right the real midline is displayed

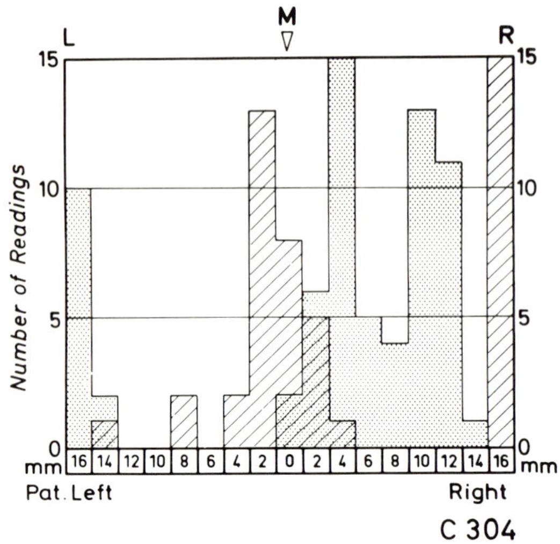

Fig. 9. Uninterpretable histogram of a child with a highgrade hydrocephalus. In the A-mode echogram the third ventricle was 25 mm in diameter

Scintigraphic Findings with Cerebrovascular Lesions

W. WALTER

Individual scintigraphic examinations and, in particular, follow-up series of cerebrovascular lesions are valuable in the differential diagnosis and the prognosis of these lesions. The scintigrams performed on 185 cases at our clinic in the last 4 years may be grouped as follows:

1. Spontaneous intracerebral hematomas
2. Cerebrovascular lesions (grouped into acute symptomatology and chronic symptomatology)
3. Vascular occlusions
4. Arteriovenous angiomas with and without hematoma
5. Saccular aneurysms with and without hematoma
6. Subarachnoid hemorrhage with or without demonstrable vascular malformation and with or without demonstrable so-called vascular spasms
7. Av-cavernous sinus fistulas
8. Cerebral venous thromboses
9. Brain contusions
10. Chronic subdural hematomas

The examinations were carried out in the Nuklear Medizinisches Institut (Head: Prof. Dr. F. Wolf) with 99^{m} technetium.

In the differential diagnosis between encephalomalacia and space-occupying lesions, the follow-up scintigrams are particularly important. In the case of typical scintigraphy during follow-up, a tumor can be excluded. However, few cases show a concentration of activity for several months. In several cases, craniotomies were performed because of the persistent suspicion of tumor. Here extensive areas of encephalomalacia were found which revealed a picture of total tissue necrosis at the histological examination. In the case of vascular occlusions the follow-up observations showed a typical scintigraphic finding. The extent and the amount of concentration of activity almost always corresponded to the degree of neurological deficit or to the seriousness of the clinical picture. Cautious prognoses can be set here if the slight concentration of activity quickly decreased at the follow-up scintigraphic examination. This is particularly true for partial occlusions of the middle cerebral artery. Here the scintigram often shows signs of increased local perfusion (luxury perfusion) which are also apparent in the angiogram, indicating poorer oxygen utilization.

In our experience, hemorrhagic encephalomalacia leads to earlier and more marked concentrations of activity in the scintigram. This was particularly notable in 3 cases of cerebral vein thrombosis that had led to a massive hemorrhagic infarct. A concentration of activity was visible within the first 24 hours.

The spontaneous intracerebral hematomas are best seen in the scintigram between the 6th and 10th day. In a few isolated cases craniotomies were not performed since the clinical status improved and the follow-up scintigram showed a decrease and normalization of the scintigraphic finding. Approximately 40 % of the intracerebral hematomas did not lead to pathological concentrations of activity. Here the scintigram was probably performed too late or too early. However, the concentration of activity is partly dependent on the time interval between injection and scintigraphic examination. Occasional cases of hematoma that were not recognized in the scintigram at first showed a positive finding after an interval of 3 hours following injection. The few cases of cavernous sinus aneurysms appear as increased concentrations of activity at the base of the skull in the scintigram. Particularly remarkable was the fact that the carotid ligations led to a complete normalization of the clinical symptomatology on the one hand and to normalization of the scintigraphic finding which had been pathological at first.

Of special interest are the scintigraphic findings in cases of subarachnoid hemorrhage with so-called vascular spasms. Previously (WALTER and SCHÜTTE 1964) it was pointed out that such vessel spasms occurred more frequently together with severe neurological deficits and prolonged disturbances in consciousness. In all cases of subarachnoid hemorrhage with aneurysms and pronounced vascular spasms in the angiogram, pathological scintigraphic findings appeared in the corresponding perfusion area. During the follow-up period an increase or decrease in pathological activity in the scintigram was accompanied by an improvement or worsening of the neurological status and the state of consciousness. These scintigraphic findings

Table I. Results of scintigraphic investigations of 185 patients. ▨ positive, □ negative, F examination too late, S examination too early

Spontaneous intracerebral hematomas	13	FFFF SSSS 8	
Arterial occlusions	13	4 without neurological deficit	
Vascular lesions (chronic stage, more than 3 months)	22		
Vascular lesions (acute stage)	18		
Arteriovenous angiomas	11 (with hematoma)		
Saccular aneurysms	9 (with hematoma)	19 (without hematoma)	
Subarachnoid hemorrhages	11 aneurysm with spasm	3 spasm without aneurysm	20 SAB without aneurysm & without spasm
A.v.Sinus cavernosus fistula	3		
Venous thromboses	2		
Brain contusions	6 1 to 14 days	9 more than 2 weeks	
Chronic subdural hematomas	12	2	

were also found in occasional cases of subarachnoid hemorrhage where the angiogram had failed to show an aneurysm. The previously mentioned opinion that such spasms can lead to circulatory disturbances which can in turn cause reversible or non-reversible brain tissue damage, has been confirmed by these scintigraphic and angiographic comparative investigations. Further confirmation was achieved by the cases which were autopsied. Here it could be demonstrated unequivocally that the scintigraphic finding and the corresponding neurological status could not be explained by an intracerebral hematoma, but rather by hemorrhagic softening in the perfusion area of the spastic vessels. Subarachnoid hemorrhages due to aneurysms but without such spasms of the vessels all showed a negative scintigram. The relatively small number of contusions is included here because the histopathological substrate of the contusions may strongly resemble that of a hemorrhagic infarct. Acute contusions lead to marked scintigraphic findings chiefly within the first 8-10 days. In cases of contusions over 4 weeks old, the scintigram did not show any changes. Here too, the follow-up examinations of individual cases showed that an improvement in the patient's condition, i.e. a decrease in the neurological deficit was accompanied by a decrease in the pathological concentration of activity in the scintigram. All but two of the chronic subdural hematomas showed the well-known typical, sickle-shaped concentration of activity. We could not explain this negative finding.

An improvement in the diagnosis of cerebrovascular lesions with the help of brain scintigrams will be achieved through the use of regular follow-up examinations.

The findings mentioned here, some of them only as small groups are intended to stimulate larger series so that a typical scintigraphic pattern can be worked out for the various vascular lesions in the future.

Surgical Treatment of a Carotid-Cavernous-Fistula Without Interruption of the Carotid Circulation

B. KONTOPOULOS and H. PENZHOLZ

The surgical treatment of carotid-cavernous-fistulas is always particularly difficult if the intracranial collateral circulation is insufficient. This is not a rare problem as proven by an increasing number of recent publications. This report concerns a case in which, as we think, we found a good solution for this surgical problem and want to compare our procedure to other possibilities presently under discussion.

The pathophysiology and the clinical picture of the carotid-cavernous-fistula are well known. In 1809 TRAVERS reported the first cure of this disease by the ligature of the common carotid artery on the neck. Since the beginning of this century a more radical elimination of the fistulas was tried by an additional ligature of the internal carotid artery at the neck which was later completed by a simultaneous intracranial ligature of the internal carotid artery by HAMBY and GARDNER in 1933. Since there have always been recurrences following this procedure to occlude the fistula, the complete embolization of the carotid siphon was tried after a previous intracranial clipping of the internal carotid artery and the subsequent ligature of the internal carotid artery at the neck. This procedure, also developed by HAMBY and GARDNER, aimed at combining the advantages of the technique of muscle embolization, reported by BROOKS in 1930, with the methods of carotid ligature. For a long time until present it remained the standard operation for eliminating a carotid-cavernous-fistula without relapse.

The main disadvantages of these methods are the definite occlusion of a carotid artery and the necessity of an additional intracranial operation. At least to avoid the disadvantage of an additional intracranial operation it was tried to modify the already mentioned method of embolic occlusion of the carotid siphon, so that an occlusion of the middle cerebral artery would seem to be impossible, even without a previous intracranial clipping of the internal carotid artery. To our knowledge SERBINENKO was the first who solved this problem by tying a piece of muscle to a thread of a certain length. KOSARY, KRAYENBÜHL, GRUNERT chose similar ways. Unfortunately these methods also lead to a definite occlusion of the carotid artery and are not useful in cases with insufficient collateral circulation. With BROOKS' method and an adequate choice of a piece of muscle of a certain size the occlusion of the fistula must become possible without an interruption of the carotid circulation.

In our case we were forced to try this procedure because of an extraordinarily insufficient collateral circulation. A 58 years old patient suffered a head injury during a motor-bicycle accident in 1970. He was admitted to the hospital because of a deteriorating vision of the right eye and a noise in his head in december of the same year. On admission we found a left exophthalmus and a pulse synchronous noise.

The tentative diagnosis: carotid-cavernous-fistula was proven by arteriography.

The noise disappeared under compression of the carotid artery at the neck, but the patient became aphasic and displayed a hemiparesis within 10 seconds. It could be proven that there was no collateral circulation either via the anterior communicant or the posterior communicant artery by angiography of the right carotid artery with simultaneous compression of the left carotid artery and by left retrograde brachial angiogram. In this extraordinary situation the attempt to use the following operative technique seemed to be justified: we measured the distance between the carotid bifurcation and the fistula on the angiogram considering the factor of enlargement. The distance was 13, 1 cm. On January 8th, 1971, we exposed the bifurcation of the left carotid artery under local anesthesia. A round piece of muscle with a diameter of at most 3 mm was prepared, marked with a clip and fixed to a thread (4xO). The thread was marked with a knot at the 13, 1 cm limit. After this careful preparation the embolization was performed in a typical way via the external carotid artery. The critical phase of the operation was the short-term cross-clamping of the internal carotid artery for 21 seconds. The aphasic and hemiparetic symptoms, which - as expected - occurred after a cross-clamping for 10 seconds, disappeared following restoration of the circulation. The immediate disappearance of the pulse synchronous noise was the sign of successful occlusion of the fistula, as proven by an intraoperative angiogram.

Our intention to maintain the circulation of the carotid artery was successful. The thread was fixed at the 13, 1 cm-mark at the bifurcation of the carotid artery, and the artery was sutured.

Fourteen days following surgery the patient was again able to work. Now, twenty-eight months later he is free of symptoms and completely restored.

At the beginning of this year two published papers seem to confirm the described method. Both authors likewise used small emboli fixed to a thread of a certain length. OHTA (1973) used polyurethan foam, BLACK (1973) used muscle and obtained an occlusion of the fistula maintaining the circulation of the carotid artery. RIECHERT and PARKINSON chose the direct approach to the cavernous sinus to maintain the carotid circulation.

REFERENCES

1. BLACK, P., S. UEMATSU, M. PEROVIC, and A. E. WALKER: Carotid-cavernous fistula: a controlled embolus technique for occlusion of fistula with preservation of carotid blood flow. J. Neurosurg. 38, 113-118 (1973)
2. BROOKS, B.: Discussion. Trans. South. Surg. Ass. 43, 176-177 (1931)
3. GRUNERT, V. und M. SUNDER-PLASSMANN: Beitrag zur chirurgischen Therapie der Carotis-cavernosus-Fisteln. Acta Neurochir. 25, 109-114 (1971)
4. HAMBY, W. B.: Carotid-Cavernous Fistula. Springfield, III: Thomas 1966
5. HAMBY, W. B. and D. F. DOHN: Carotid-cavernous fistulas: report of thirty-six cases and discussion of their Management. Clin. Neurosurg. 11, 150-170 (1964)
6. HAMBY, W. B. and W. J. GARDNER: Treatment of pulsating exophthalmos with report of two cases. Arch. Surg. 27, 676-685 (1933)

7. KOSARY, I.Z., M.A.LERNER, M.MOZES and M.LAZAR: Artificial embolic occlusion of the terminal internal carotid artery in the treatment of carotic-cavernous fistula. Technical note. J.Neurosurg. 28, 605-608 (1968)

8. KRAYENBÜHL, H.: Treatment of carotid-cavernous fistula consisting of a one-stage operation by muscle embolization of the fistulous carotid segment. In: Micro-vascular surgery. Ed. by R.M.P. Donaghy and M.G. Yasargil. Stuttgart, Thieme 1967, p. 151-167

9. OHTA, T., S.NISHIMURA, H.KIKUCHI and M.TOYAMA: Closure of carotid-cavernous fistula with polyurethane foam embolus. J.Neurosurg. 38, 107-112 (1973)

10. PARKINSON, D.: Carotid cavernous fistula: direct repair with preservation of the carotid artery. J.Neurosurg. 38, 99-106 (1973)

11. PARKINSON, D.: A surgical approach to the cavernous portion of the carotid artery: anatomical studies and case report. J.Neurosurg. 23, 474-483 (1965)

12. PARKINSON, D.: Transcavernous repair of carotid cavernous fistula: case report. J.Neurosurg. 26, 420-424 (1967)

13. RIECHERT, T.: A new surgical method for treatment of pulsating exophthalmos. Progr.Brain Res. 30, 445-449 (1969)

14. SERBINENKO, F.A.: Okkliuziia ballonom kavernoznogo otdelf sonnoi arterii kak metod lecheniia carotidno-cavernoznykh soustii. Vopr.Neirokhir. 35 (6), 3-9 (1971)

15. SERBINENKO, F.A.: Kateterzatsiia i okkliuziia magistral' nykh sosudov golovnogo mozga i perspektivy razvitiia sosudistoi neirokhirurgii. Vopr. Neirokhir. 35 (5), 17-27 (1971)

16. TRAVERS, B.: A case of aneurysm by anastomosis in the orbit, cures by ligation of the common carotid artery. Med.Chirurg.Trans. 2, 1-16 (1811)

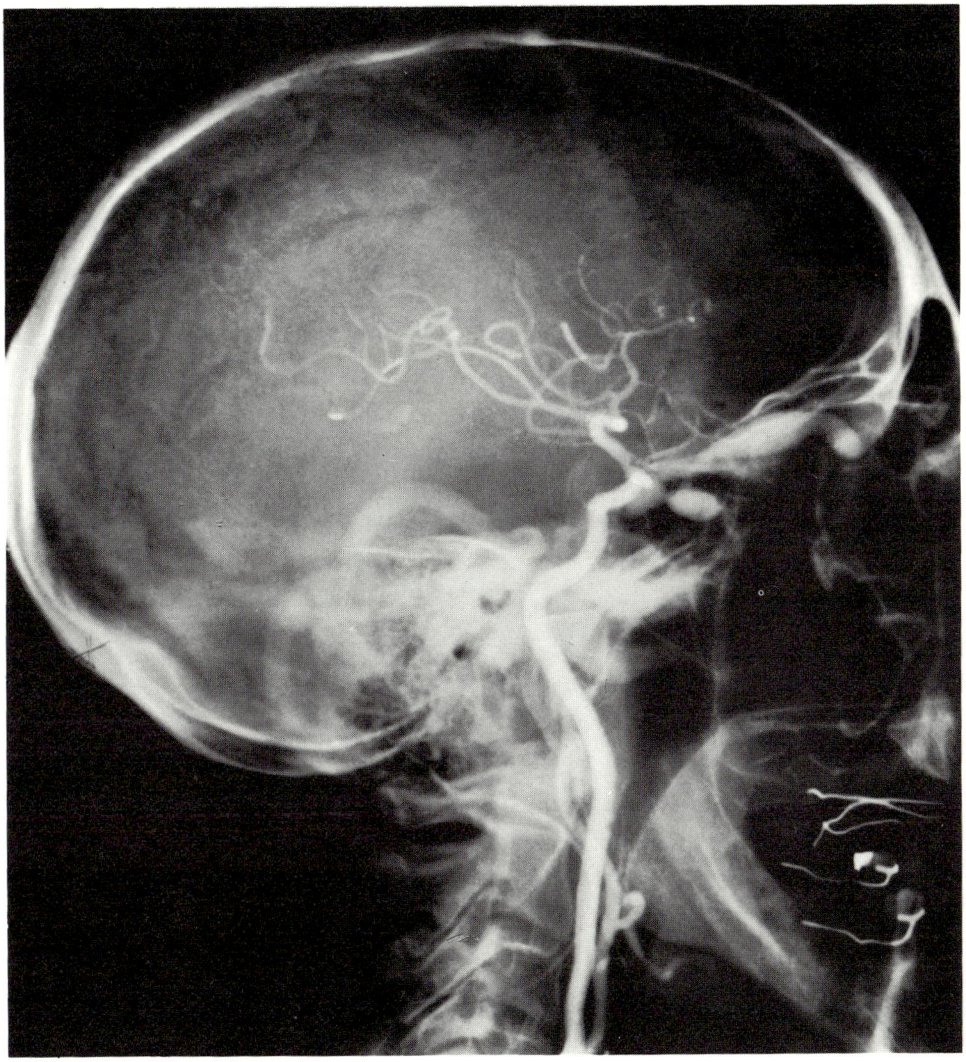

Fig. 1. Preoperative right carotid angiogram

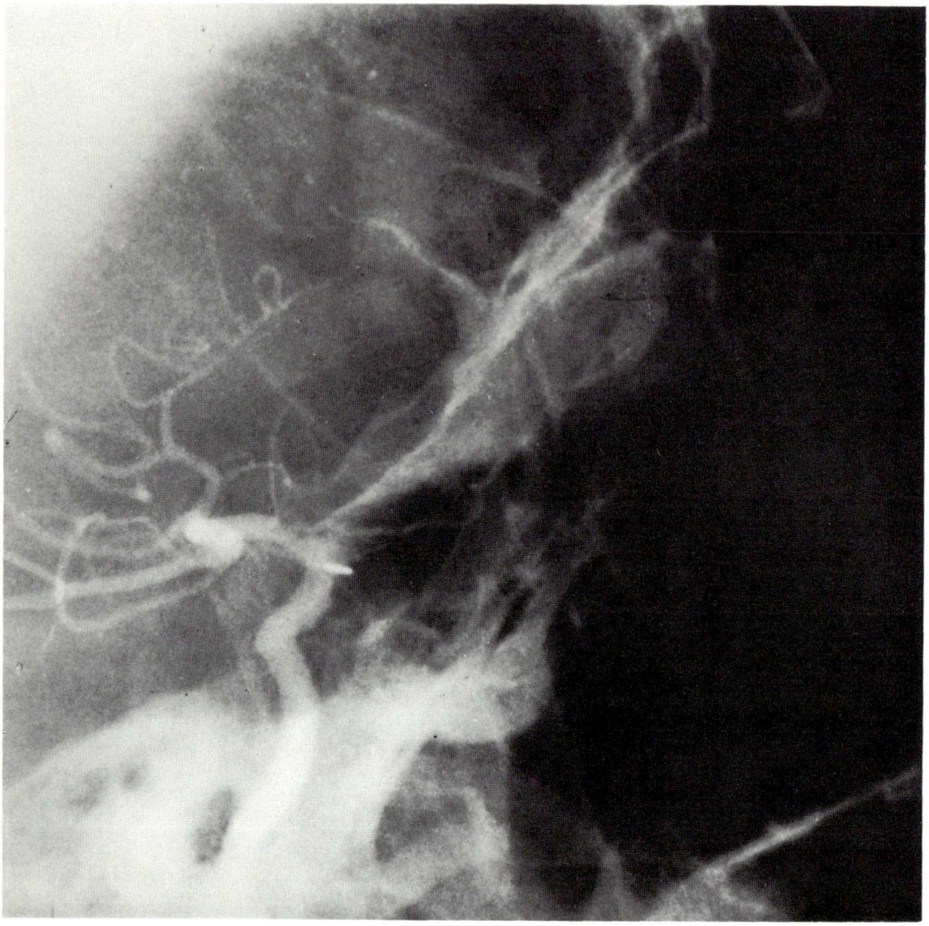

Fig. 2. Intraoperative right carotid angiogram following successful muscle embolization.

The Therapy of Extracranial Arteriovenous Malformations of the Carotid-Vertebral Circulation

R. WÜLLENWEBER, J. WAPPENSCHMIDT, and E. LINS

Extracerebral arteriovenous malformations occurring as isolated angiomas of the skull or dura mater (4, 6, 7, 9, 11, 14, 17) can be treated by ligature, complete removal or circumcision of the dura mater, thus presenting hardly any therapeutical difficulties. The angiomas of the orbita can normally be cured by complete removal as well (8).

However, completely different circumstances are found in cases of extracerebral angiomas of the carotid-vertebral circulation located in the soft tissues of the face and neck and frequently draining through the cerebral sinus (1, 2, 3, 5, 10, 12, 13, 15, 16).

Heavy subjective complaints, such as pulse-synchronous bruit, severe neurological and psychical disturbances can be observed, caused by a deficient cerebral blood flow. While hemorrhages occur seldom, a progressive cardial insufficiency is frequently seen due to the chronic overload of the right heart. Since a complete removal is not possible in these cases on account of the extension and localisation of the vascular malformations, the only therapy likely to provide success is the ligature of all afferent vessels.

Case reports

Case 1: 41 years old man with papilledema, severe cerebellar symptoms and tinnitus. Following ligature of the ext. carotid artery and all other afferent vessels with dissection of the neck-muscles, craniotomy and circumcision of the dura there was an improvement for some months (Fig. 1a). One year later all symptoms reappeared and the angiograms showed a shunt with cerebral circulatory insufficiency (Fig. 1b). The patient died suddenly of acute cardiac failure.

Case 2: Similar clinical findings and angiographic results in an 8 years old girl, who died after a cardiac arrest before any operation could be done.

Cases 3 and 4: Two patients, who suffered only from a pulse-synchronous bruit were operated on by ligature and partial extirpation of the angiomas located in the skull, the neck muscles and the bone. The symptoms disappeared only for some weeks, then the tinnitus recurred.

As demonstrated by the above examples, ligature of the afferent vessels improves the clinical state only for a short time, since new anastomosis develop and reopen the shunt. If the pulse-synchronous noise is the only symptom of the vascular malformation, operations with a higher risk are not indicated. But in cases with severe neurological disturbances as well as progressive heart insufficiency all attempts that promise improvement are justified. Therefore in 2 other cases we tried to occlude the angiomas by ligature of the afferent vessels combined with embolization by small plasticspheres and muscle pieces.

Case 5: 47 years-old man suffering from a growing tumor in the jaw-angle and a pulse-synchronous noise. Angiographic findings: arteriovenous malformation supplied by the external carotid and vertebral arteries (Fig. 2a). Following ligature of the occipital artery the angioma was embolized by sylastic spheres from the ext. carotid artery, which was ligated following this procedure. As confirmed by the angiographic (Fig. 2b) control, the angioma was completely occluded and the swelling disappeared. But the noise recurred some months later in less severe form, so that the ligature of the contralateral occipital artery became necessary.

Case 6: 35 years-old man suffering from an angioma of the cheek, growing to a monstrous swelling within 3 years. A pressure-ulcer caused by a dental prothesis eventually led to massive hemorrhage into the oral cavity. Following ligature of the ext. carotid artery, the occipital artery and other arteries of the opposite side of the face, the brachial artery angiogram (Fig. 3a) showed that the ext. carotid artery and the angioma filled through small arteries from the neck region. So the ext. carotid artery was exposed once more and embolized with plastic spheres and small muscle pieces until the vascular malformation was occluded (Fig. 3b). After this operation the swelling diminished but a complete recovery could not be obtained.

Conclusion

The therapy of the extracerebral arteriovenous malformations of the carotid-vertebral circulation by ligature of the afferent vessels combined with embolization by sylastic spheres and small muscle pieces might improve the operative results known so far. Using plastic spheres we did not succeed in occluding the angiomas completely, since no progressive thrombosis could be seen. Therefore it is suggested to perform embolization with materials of higher adhesive properties, for instance by roughening the surface of the spheres and impregnating them with thrombin.

Summary

Arteriovenous shunts supplied both from the carotid and vertebral circulation cause cardiac disturbances as well as cerebral circulatory deficiency.

The assessment of the extension and location of the angioma can be very difficult and in some cases it is only possible by subtraction and large angiographic series. Following ligature of afferent vessels new anastomosis always appear. In most cases an extirpation of the malformation - located in the dura mater and the soft tissues of the face and scalp - is impossible.

In 6 cases we tried to exclude the malformation from the circulation by ligatures in different steps, but the long term results were bad. Therefore in our opinion the only successful treatment may be the ligature of as many afferent vessels as possible combined with an embolization using sylastic spheres and small muscle pieces.

REFERENCES

1. CAROLL, C.P.H. and R.K.JAKOBY: Neonatal congestive heart failure as a presenting symptom of cerebral arteriovenous malformation. J.Neurosurg. 25, 159-162 (1966)

2. CLOETE, G.N.P., L.J.NEL and F.A.K. van WYK: Arteriovenous fistulae of the verbebral vessels. S.Afr.Med.J. 42/11, 253-256 (1968)

3. ISFORT, A.: Zur Behandlung der extrakraniellen Angiome. Chirurg 33, 433-436 (1962)

4. ISFORT, A.: Spontane Hirnblutungen. Schering AG, Berlin (1967)

5. KRAYENBÜHL, H. and M. YASARGIL: Die vasculären Erkrankungen im Gebiet der A. vertebralis und A. basilaris. Stuttgart, Thieme 1957a

6. KRAYENBÜHL, H. and M. YASARGIL: Das Hirnaneurysma. Series chirurgica der Documenta Geigy. Basel, Geigy 1958

7. LAINE, E., P.GALIBERT, C.LOPEZ, J.DELAHOUSSE, J.M.DELANDTS-HEER et J.L.CHRISTIAENS: Anévrysmes artério-veineux intraduraux de la fosse postérieure. Neuro-Chirurgie 9, 147-148 (1963)

8. MAUERSBERGER, W.: Zur Klinik, Diagnose u. Therapie der retrobulbären Angiome und Gefäßgeschwülste. Inaug.Diss. Bonn 1973

9. OLIVECRONA, H. and J. LADENHEIM: Congenital arteriovenous Aneurysms of the Carotid and Vertebral arterial systems. Berlin-Göttingen-Heidelberg: Springer 1957

10. PECKER, Mm. J., J. et A.JAVALET: Deux nouveaux cas d'anévrysmes artério-veineux intraduraux de la fosse postérieure alimentés par la carotide externe. Neuro-Chirurgie 11, 327-332 (1965)

11. RÖTTGEN, P.: Venöses Angiom der Dura. Zbl.Neurochir. 3, 87-99 (1938)

12. SHUMACKER, H.B. jr., R.L.CAMPBELL and R.F.HEIMBURGER: Operative treatment of vertebral arteriovenous fistula. J.Trauma 6, 3-19 (1966)

13. STORRS, D.G. and R.B.KING: Management of extracranial congenital arterio-venous malformations of head and neck. J.Neurosurg. 38, 584-590 (1973)

14. TÖNNIS, W. and H. LANGE-COSAK: Klinik, operative Behandlung und Prognose der arteriovenösen Angiome des Gehirnes und seiner Häute. Dtsch. Z. Nervenheilk. 170, 460-485 (1953)

15. VERBIEST, H.: Extracranial and cervical arteriovenous aneurysms of the carotid and vertebral arteries. Report of a series of 12 personal cases. John Hopkins Med.J. 122/6, 350-357 (1968)

16. VOGELSANG, H.G.: Die arteriovenösen Angiome im extrakraniellen Carotis- und Vertebralisbereich. Dtsch.Z.f.Nervenheilk. 184, 83-97 (1962)

17. van der WERF, M.A.J.M.: Sur un cas d'anévrisme artérioveineux intraduraux bilatéral de la fosse postérieure chez un enfant. Neuro-Chirurgie 10, 140-144 (1964)

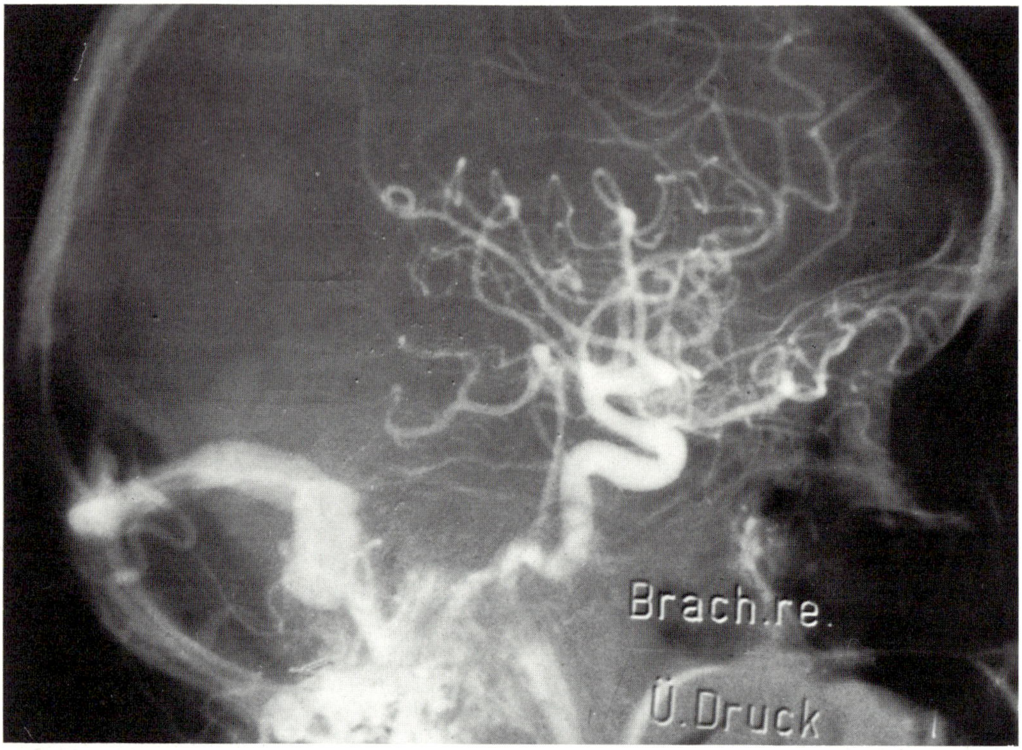
Brach.re.
Ü.Druck

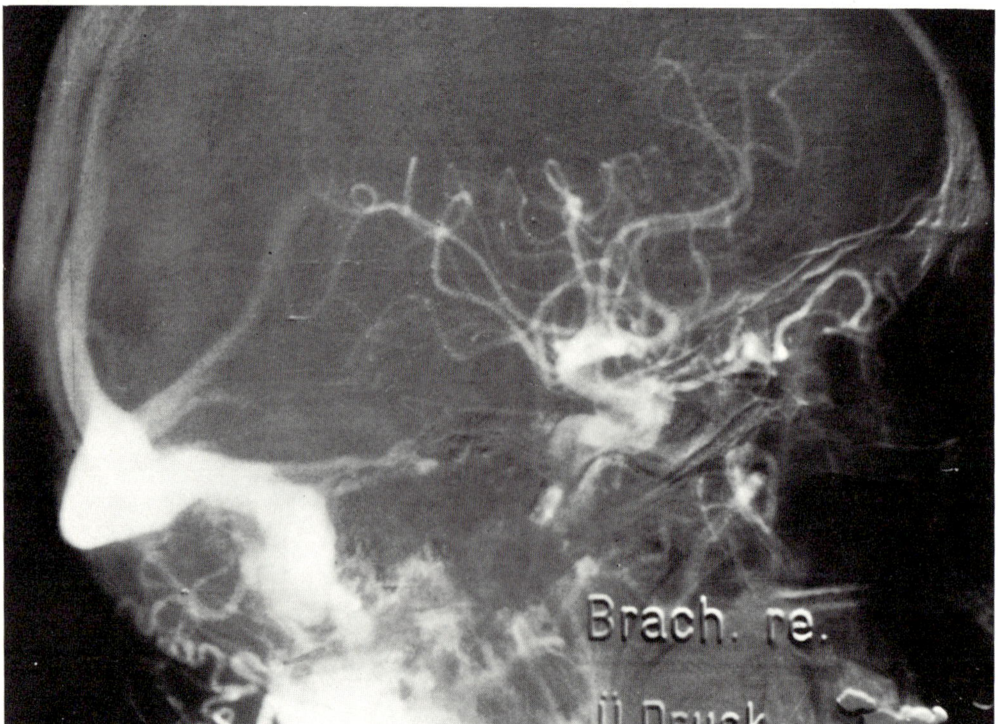
Brach. re.

◀Fig. 1a. Brachial artery angiogram after ligature of the ext. carotid artery and all other afferent vessels

◀Fig. 1b. Angiogram of the same case one year later

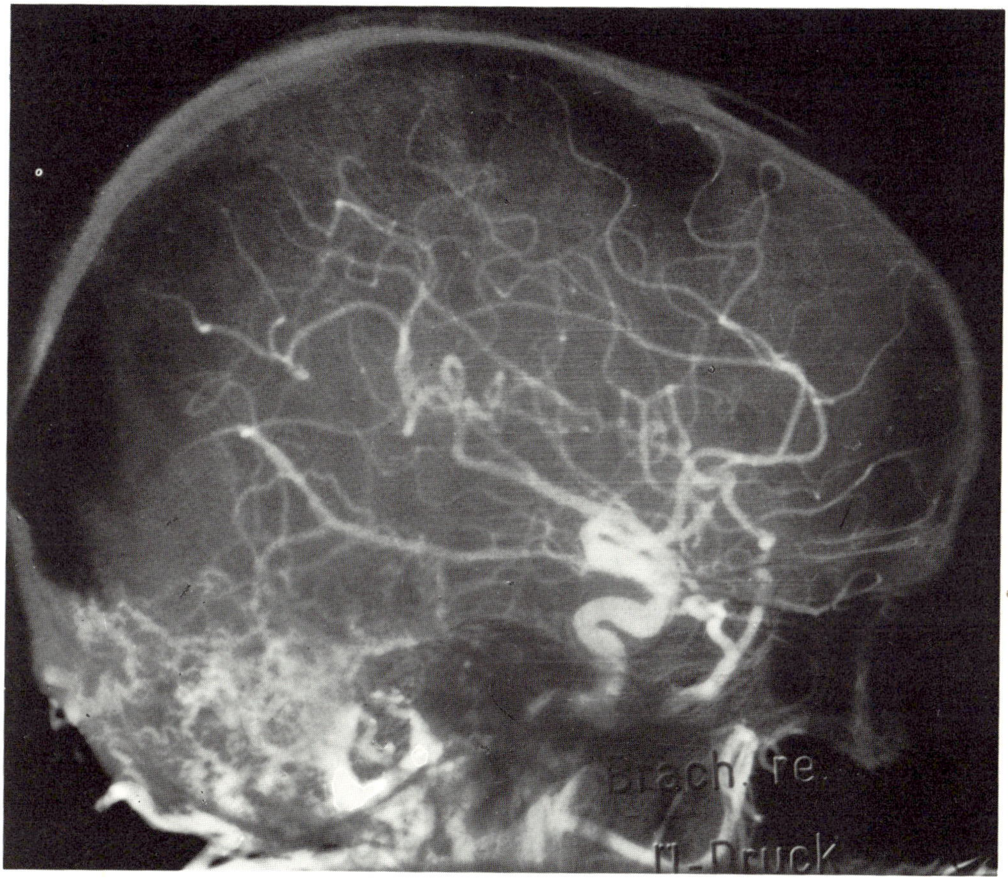

Fig. 2a. Brachial artery angiogram in a case of arteriovenous malformation

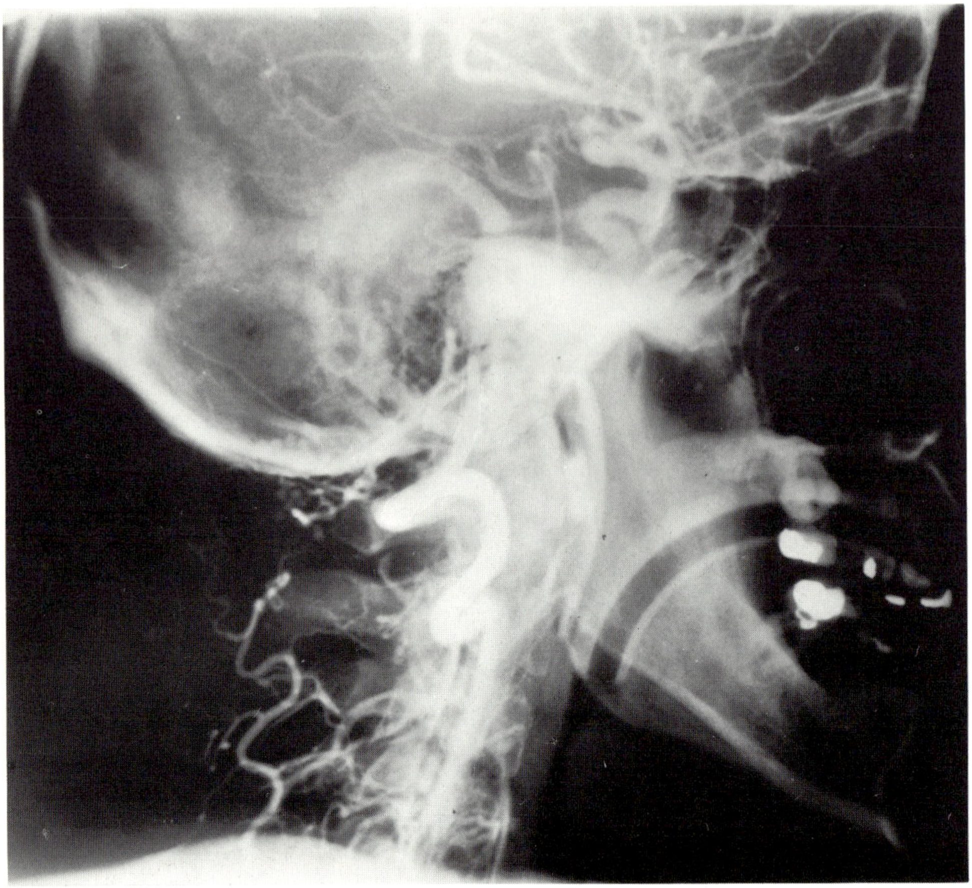

Fig. 2b. Control angiogram following ligature and embolization of the ext. carotid artery

Fig. 3a. Brachial artery angiogram following ligature of the ext. carotid artery, ▶ showing the filling of the angioma with contrast medium

Fig. 3b. Control angiogram following embolization. The plastic spheres can be ▶ seen in the region of the angioma

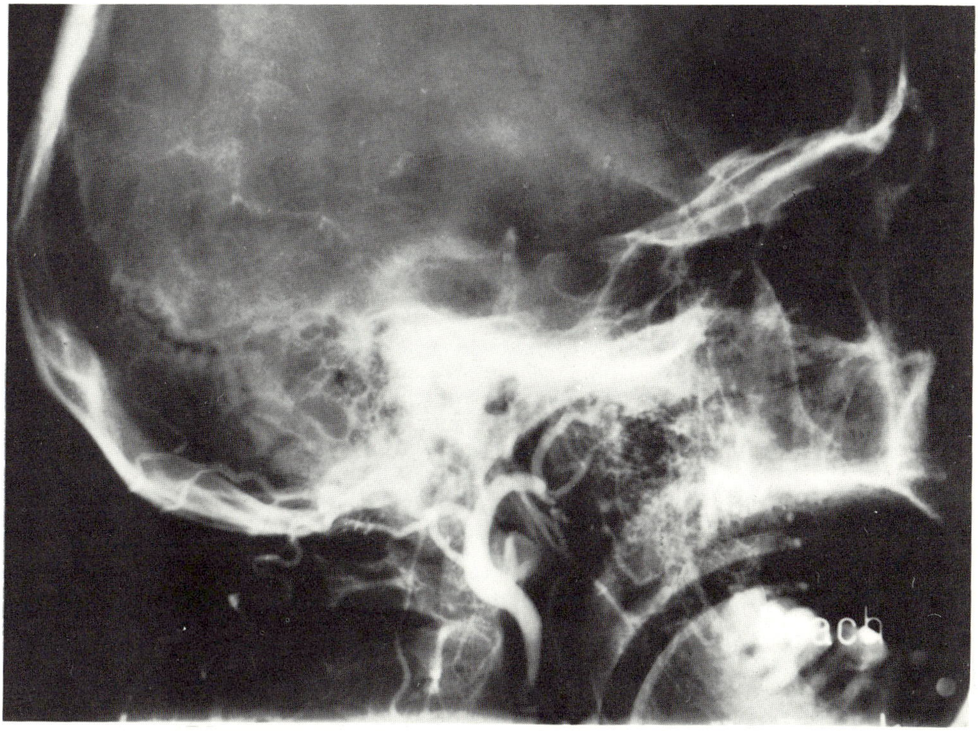

Fig. 3a.

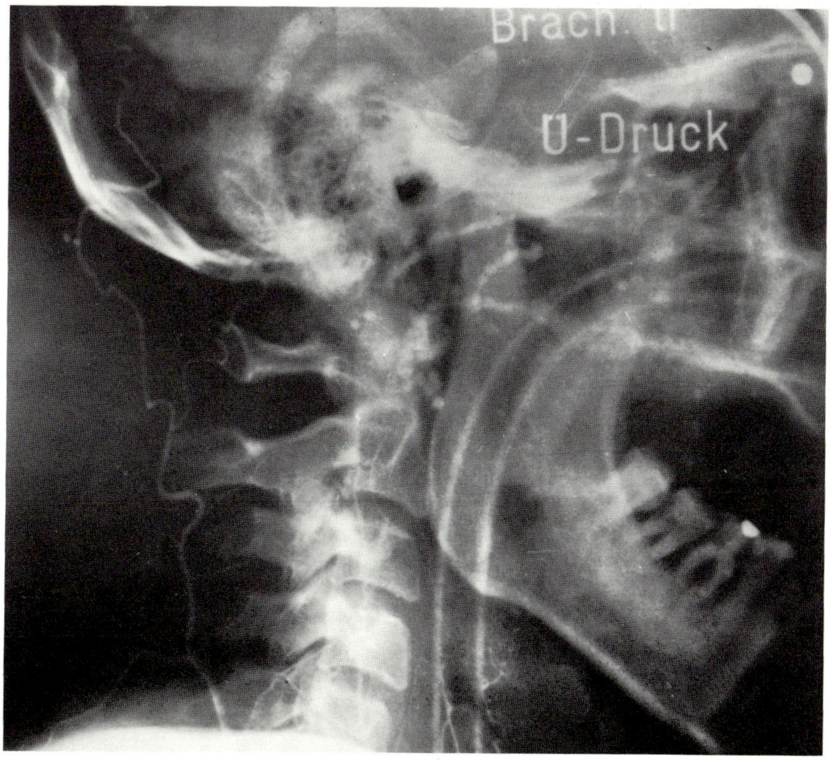

Fig. 3b.

Clinical, Morphological and Pathogenetic Consideration on the So-Called "Temporal Lobe Agenesis Syndrome"

T. KOLBERG, R. WÜLLENWEBER, and F. GULLOTTA

ROBINSON has tried in numerous papers (1955, 1958, 1964) to outline a syndrome consisting of large defects of the temporal lobe with widening of the middle fossa. In the opinion that these lesions were developmental in origin, he designated the state as "temporal lobe agenesis syndrome".

Six such cases observed in the Neurosurgical Clinic in Bonn, led us to some critical considerations about the clinical signs, morphological features and pathogenesis.

Own cases (see table): Of our 6 cases only one was female. The age varies between 2 1/2 and 57 years. The clinical signs were rather heterogenous, however, focal epilepsia was seen most frequently. In 2 cases subdural hematomas led to admission.

The angiography (Fig. 1) showed a widely bow-shaped dislocation of the middle cerebral artery upwards and towards the midline with an almost vertical origin from the internal carotid artery. The middle fossa appeared avascular. The anterior cerebral artery was not, or only slightly, dislocated towards the other side. This angiographic constellation indicates a loss of substance in the temporal brain. The frontal films show the local bulging and thinning of the temporal bone. Plain skull X-rays of the skull base, frontal stereoscopic and tomographic X-rays, show the widening of the middle fossa anteriorly and downwards with elevation of the lesser sphenoidal wing as described by ROBINSON (1955, 1958). This is an expression of pathologic pressure conditions in the region.

In all cases, except in those with subdural hematomas we found at surgery (Fig. 2) a thickening of the arachnoid underneath the dura mater, which appeared normal. Underneath the visceral capsule of the subdural hematoma, a second independent membrane appeared; this was identic to the thickened and hypervascularized cyst wall found in the other cases. Sometimes rests of cerebral tissue or molecular layers were macroscopically seen adherent to the hypervascularized membrane. Following incision of this thin membrane a large defect appeared, mostly in the temporal lobe, sometimes in the temporo-frontal brain (2 cases). The defects contained cerebrospinal fluid of normal composition and were mostly smoothwalled, their walls being vascularized. In one case septa were seen. Medially one could see parts of the wall of the temporal horn and the basal ganglia. Only once there was communication with the temporal horn of the lateral ventricle.

Histological examination (Fig. 3) showed a small stripe of cerebral tissue (molecular layer) underneath the thickened and fibrotic arachnoid in all cases.

Table I. Summary of clinical, surgical and histological findings of our patients

		SYMPTOMS	SURGERY	HISTOLOGY
I	♀ 51 y	Sens. aphas. Sopor Delta focus	Fibrotic arachnoidea Temporal lobe defect Defect ground pale, smooth	Thickened arachnoidea with rest of brain tissue
II	o 57 y	Hemiparesis Desorientn. Delta focus	Subdural haematoma, 2nd membrane over temporal and basal frontal lobe defect, defect ground pale, strings	Under haematoma capsule 2nd inner hypervascularized membrane with rets of brain tissue
III	o 15 y	Focal epil. Delta focus	Hypervascularized membrane over temporal and basal frontal lobe defect. Defect ground pale, smooth	Fibrotic, hypervascularized leptomeninges with rest of molecular layer.
IV	o 2 1/2 y	Retarded talk begin. Emotional outbursts.	Hypervascularized membrane over anterior temporal lobe defect. Defect ground pale, smooth	
V	o 18 y	Focal epil. Delta focus	Hypervascularized membrane over anterior temporal lobe defect. Defect ground pale, smooth	Fibrotic, hypervascularized leptomeninges with thin rests of molecular layer.
VI	o 17 y	Papilloed.	Subdural haematoma, 2nd membrane over temporal defect ground pale, smooth. Communic. with temp. horn.	Under haematoma capsule 2nd inner hypervascularized membrane with rest of molecular layer

Discussion

Our morphological findings correspond to those seen in porencephalic cysts, that is, defects of the immature brain due to vascular processes. Therefore, we cannot agree with ROBINSON. These lesions have, in fact, nothing to do with a developmental origin. Moreover, the suggestion of ROBINSON (1958) that an agenesis of the temporal lobe should lead to a widening of the middle fossa can hardly be understood or accepted. In these cases the developing or already developed temporal lobe has undergone an injury. The arachnoidal casts, which sometimes are also discussed as possible pathogenetic factor (TÖRMÄ and HEISKANEN 1962; KARVOUNIS et al. 1970; AGUILHERA et al. 1970), can be excluded by the histological examination; in those cases, in fact, the membranes consist only of thickened arachnoid without brain tissue. Furthermore, there always is a stronger displacement of the anterior cerebral artery. Arachnoid cysts can, of course, produce atrophy of the underlying brain on the base of local pressure; covering a porencephalic defect, an arachnoidal cyst can be found as well. But the porencephalic defect itself, is always of vascular origin.

The topographic extension of the brain defects lead us to suppose that they are of venous rather than of arterial origin; concluding proofs, however, could not be found in the angiographic studies. It should not be forgotten that following such vascular lesions in the immature brain, a large collateral oedema appears, destroying the adjacent areas and thereby confusing the original topography of the lesion.

The additional observation of subdural haematomas -certainly of secondary origin- also presented by ROBINSON and others, could be an interesting point. It permits the opinion that in these cases there may have been a high venous fragility.

Summary

Clinico-morphological investigations on 6 cases of so-called "temporal lobe agenesis syndrome" (ROBINSON) have shown that this syndrome is not maldevelopmental in origin, but due to vascular processes in immature brain, that is porencephalic defects.

REFERENCES

1. AGUILHERA, F., M. B. BLAZQUEZ, and S. OBRADOR: Quistes arachnoideos silvanos (Agenesia del lobulo temporal). Revista Espagnola de oto-neuro-oftalmologia y neurocirurgia, 28, 187-197 (1970)
2. KARVOUNIS, P. C., J. C. CHIU, K. PARSA and S. GILBERT: Agnesis of temporal lobe and arachnoid cyst. New York Medical Journal, 2349-2353 (1970)
3. ROBINSON, R. G.: Intracranial collections of fluid with local bulging of the skull. Journal of neurosurgery, 12, 345-353, (1955)
4. ROBINSON, R. G.: Local bulging of the skull and external hydrocephalus due to cerebral agenesis. British Journal of Radiology, 31, 691 (1958)
5. ROBINSON, R. G.: The temporal lobe agenesis syndrome. Brain, 88, 87-106, (1964)
6. TÖRMÄ, T. and O. HEISKANEN: Chronic subarachnoidal cysts in the middle cranial fossa. Acta Neurologica Scandinavica, 38, 166-170 (1962)

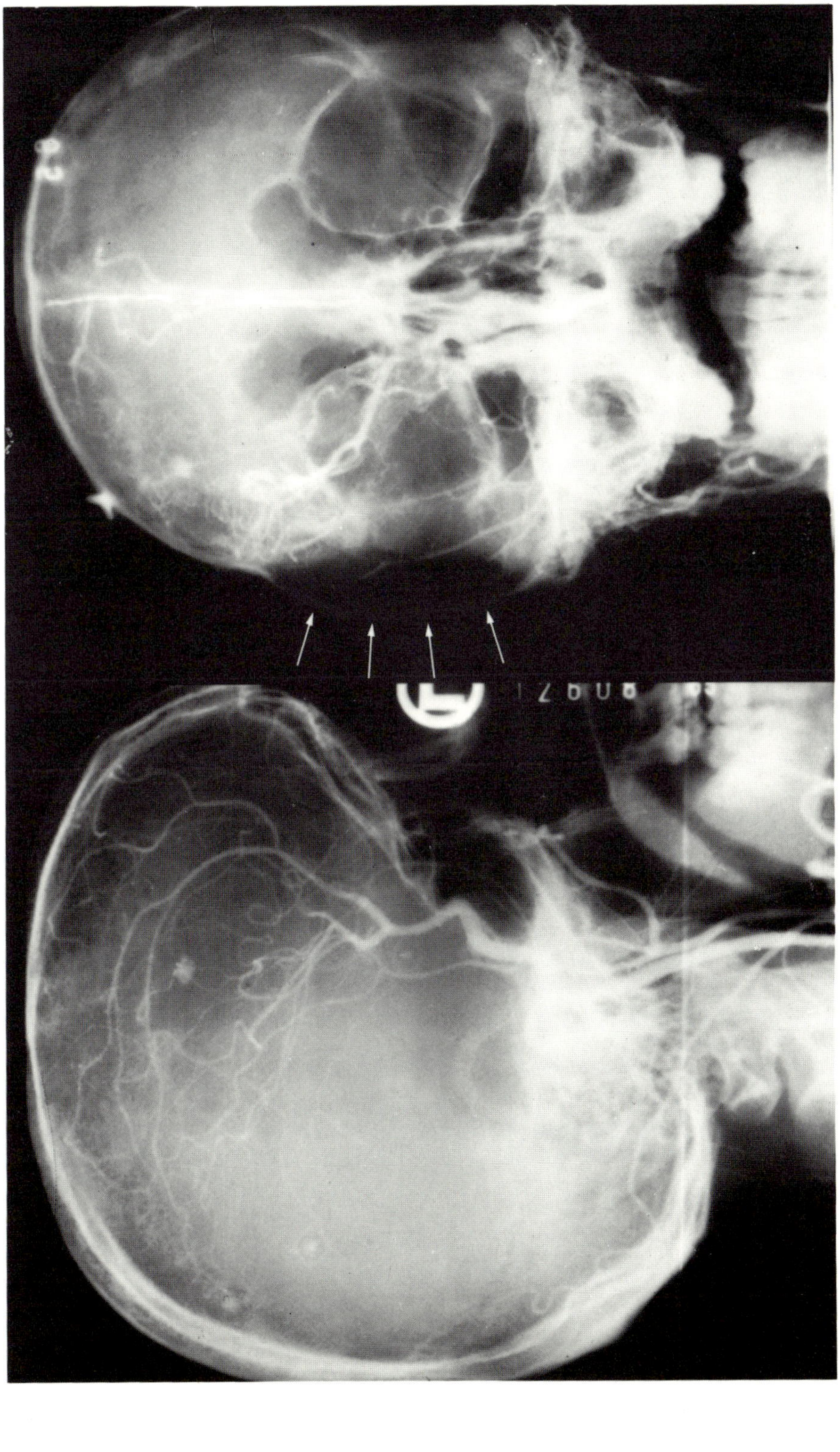

Fig. 1 Cerebral angiography. Elevation and dispacement of the middle cerebral vessels. Avascularity in the temporal region. No displacement of the anterior cerebral vessels. Local bulging of the temporal bone (arrows)

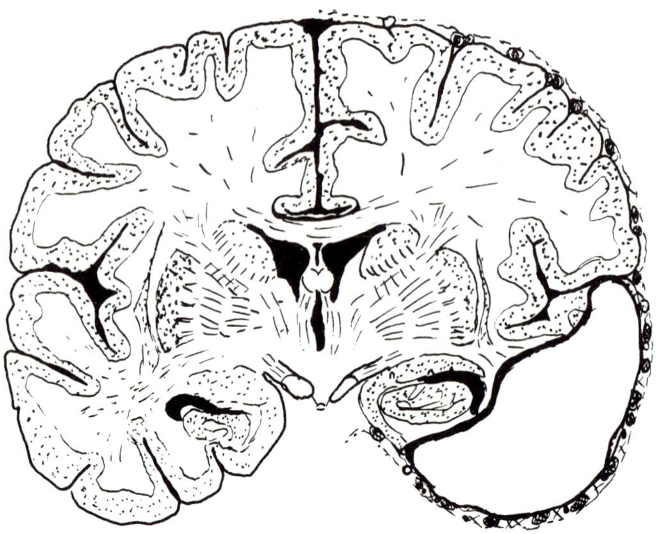

Fig. 2 Schematic representation showing the operative findings in frontal section. Note the hypervascularity of the outer cyst wall and the topographic correspondence with the temporal white matter

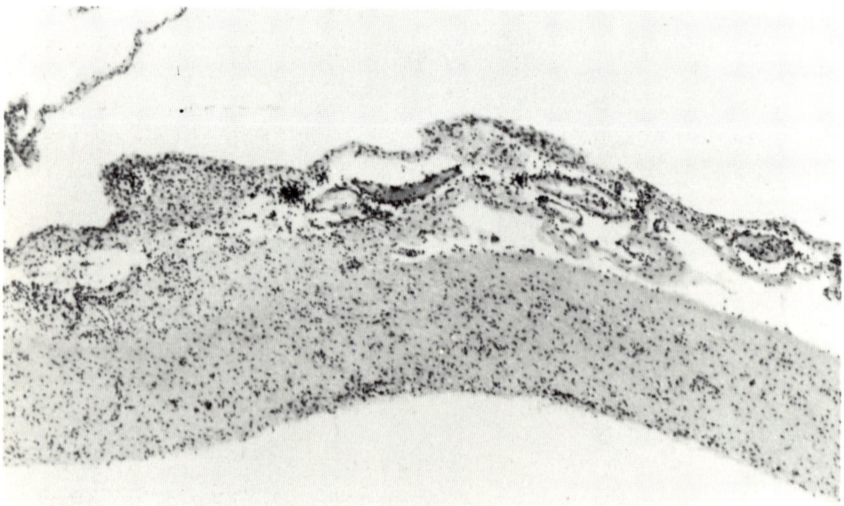

Fig. 3 Histological section of the membrane, showing the thickened arachnoid with remnants of cerebral tissue beneath

The Bilateral Orbita-Round-About-Osteotomy and -Swivelling in Morbus CROUZON

W. ENTZIAN

The dysostosis cranio acialis (M. CROUZON) is often parallelled by a diverging position of the osseous orbitae. Consequently the visual axes diverge as well, stereoscopic binocular vision cannot be acquired and these patients can look severely disfigured. Different operative methods have been suggested and applied (TESSIER; CONVERSE).

Case report

The 12 years old school girl had a symmetric diverging position of the orbitae because of pathological broad midline structures of the nasal bone and ethmoidal cells. The interpupillary distance was increased to 82 mm, the angle of strabismus was approximately 20°. In early childhood a fist correction of the nasal bone had been performed. The girl did not have any other malformation (including the findings of cerebral angiography, pneumencephalography and EEG) and she showed good abilities at school.

The time for surgery was chosen at this age, because growth of the osseous structures of the face and orbitae can be considered to be almost concluded. Surgical indication was posed only for cosmetic reasons - although there are numerous known complications.

Performance of the operation

The round-about mobilisation of both osseous orbitae was aimed, so that by swivelling each pupil should be translocated medially by 9 - 10 mm. - Bifrontal skin flap, which is divided in the midline down to the tip of the nose. A bifrontal bone flap is reflected following an absolutely horizontal sawing line closely above the orbitea, because after the swivelling they should be fixed to this frontal bone flap (1 in fig. 1); epidural approach to the anterior fossae and osteotomy closely along the margin of the small sphenoid wings (2 in fig. 1); osteotomy of the lateral orbital wall (3 in fig. 1) along the zygomaticosphenoidal suture down to the sphenomaxillar fissure; osteotomy of the zygomatic arch (4 in fig. 1); resection of an osseous wedge-shaped segment of the frontal and sphenoid bones. This osseous segment (5 in fig. 1) was according to the calculations frontally 10 mm broad, was located between the untouched olfactorial groove and the medial orbita wall, reached downwards to the nasal cavities whose roofs were opened, and reached backwards to the mentioned sphenoidal osteotomy. The osteotomy of the maxillar

+) Indication, planning and performance of the operation were done together with Prof. Dr. Krüger, Director of the Kieferchirurgische Universitätsklinik Bonn

cavity was done through an infraorbital incision and from the nose (6 in Fig. 1). There is no need to make an osteotomy of the fragile basal and medial orbital wall (7 in Fig. 1). The fulcrum of the swivelling manoeuvre was the untouched area of the optic canal and the superior orbital fissura. Afterwards the orbitae are fixed to the remaining midline structures of the nose, to the reimplanted frontal skull flap and by inserting a piece of rib into the osteotomy of the maxillar arch. - Intraoperatively it was controlled, that the pupillar distance was normalized to 65 mm. Finally a piece of rib was inserted into midline skull defect that resulted from the extirpation of an ossified place of attachment of the falx.

The operation was done by both the facial-maxillar surgeons and the neurosurgical team - sometimes working simultaneously. The procedure lasted for little more than seven hours.

Postoperatively high antibiotic protection was applied. No inflammatory complication and no paralysis of any cranial nerve or any other neurological defect occurred. The ophthalmological follow-up shows an over-function of the M. obliquus -inferior and a hypofunction of the M. obliguus-superior of the left eye. The angle of strabismus is reduced down to 4°. If the girl will be able to learn stereoscopic vision - possibly after a strabismus-corrigating operation - is uncertain.

Comparison of pre- and postoperative X-ray films show the effect of the orbital swivelling (Fig. 2 and 3).

The pathological broad ethmoidal cells have disappeared and the normalization of the topography of the medial orbital walls can be clearly recognized. - The cosmetic effect (Fig. 4) concerning the position of the orbitae and the bulbi seems reasonable as well; the back of the nose being still broad will be corrigated in a final step later on by a facial-maxillar manoeuvre.

Summary

The operative proceeding according to TESSIER and CONVERSE for a bilateral orbital swivelling in a 12 years old girl with M. CROUZON is reported. The operation was done because of cosmetic reasons, the position of the orbitae could almost be normalized, no complication occurred.

REFERENCES

1. TESSIER, P.: The scope and principles-dangers and limitations and the need for special training. Orbito-cranial surgery. Transaction fo the 5th International Congress of Plastic and Reconstructive Surgery, p. 903, Butterworth 1971

2. CONVERSE, J.M. and D. WOOD-SMITH: An atlas and classification of Midfacial and cranio-facialosteotomies. Orbito-cranial-Surgery. Transaction of the 5th International Congress of Plastic and Reconstructive Surgery, p. 931, Butterworth 1971

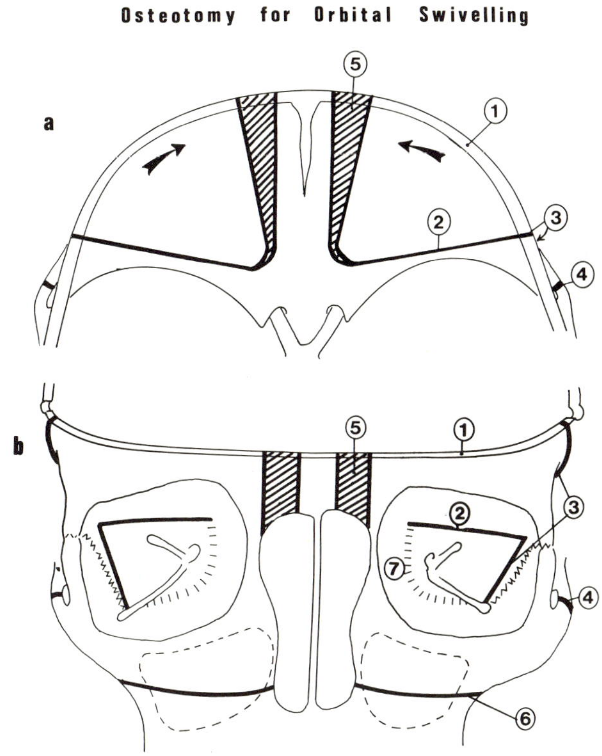

Fig. 1a and b. Frontal and upside views for the round-about-osteotomy and swivelling of the orbitae after resection of the pathological broad sphenoid cells (4) in a case of M. CROUZON. No osteotomy necessary for the fragile floor and medial wall (7) of the orbitae.

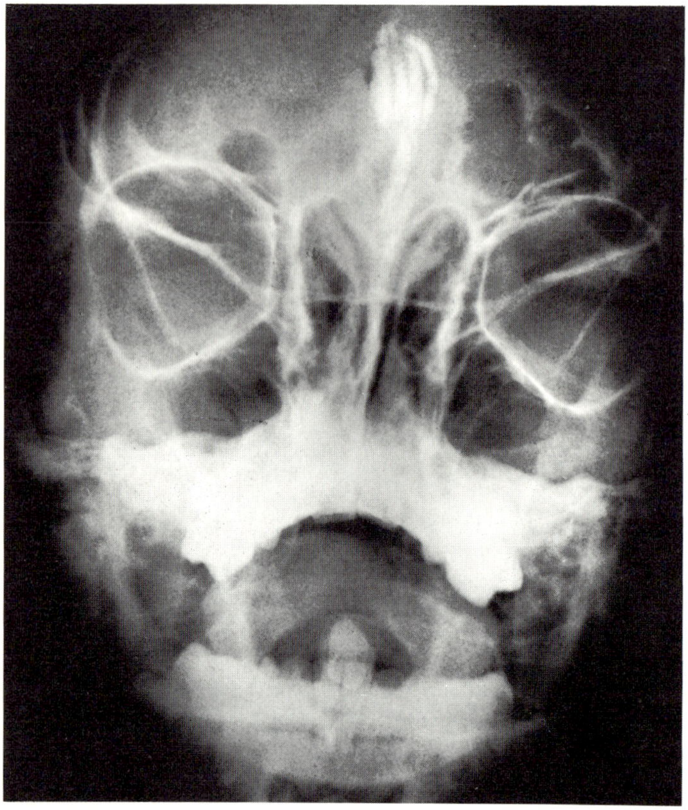

Fig. 2a and b.
Pre- and postoperative X-ray films of the nasal and orbital region show the normalized relation between nasal midline structures and orbitae. The extension of the sphenoid cells is normalized

Fig. 2a.

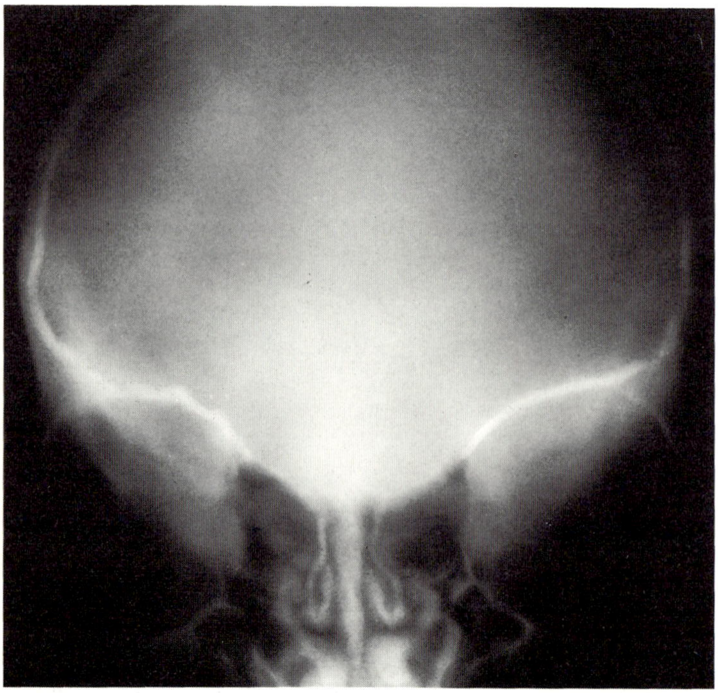

Fig. 3a and b.
Pre- and postoperative tomography show medial swivelling of the orbitae, recognizable by the normalized position of the medial orbital walls

Fig. 3a.

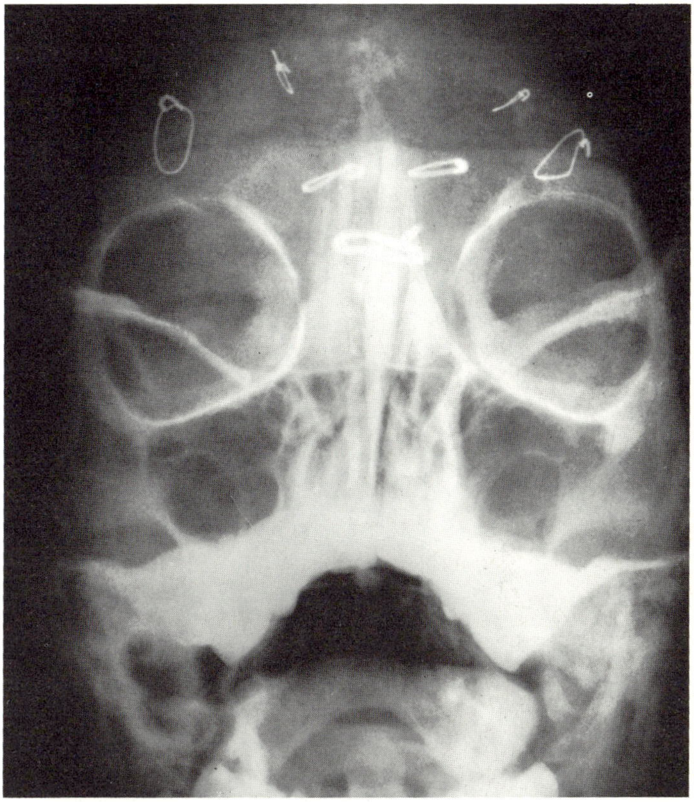

Fig. 2b.

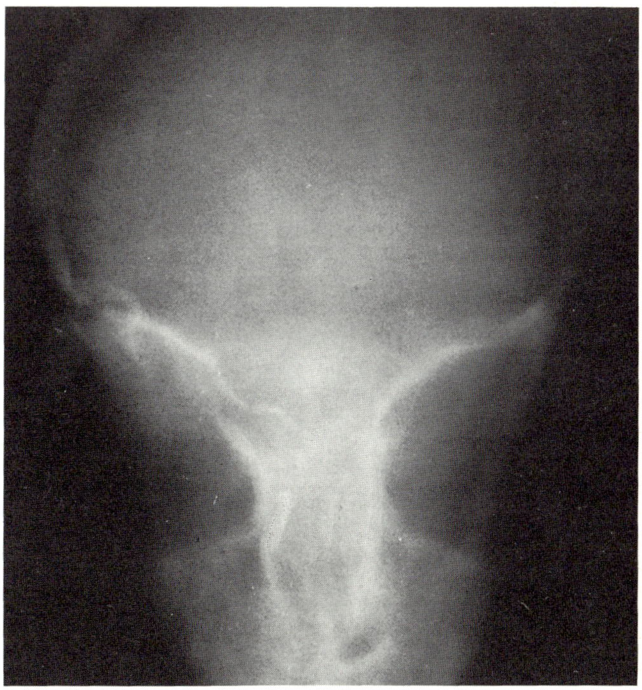

Fig. 3b.

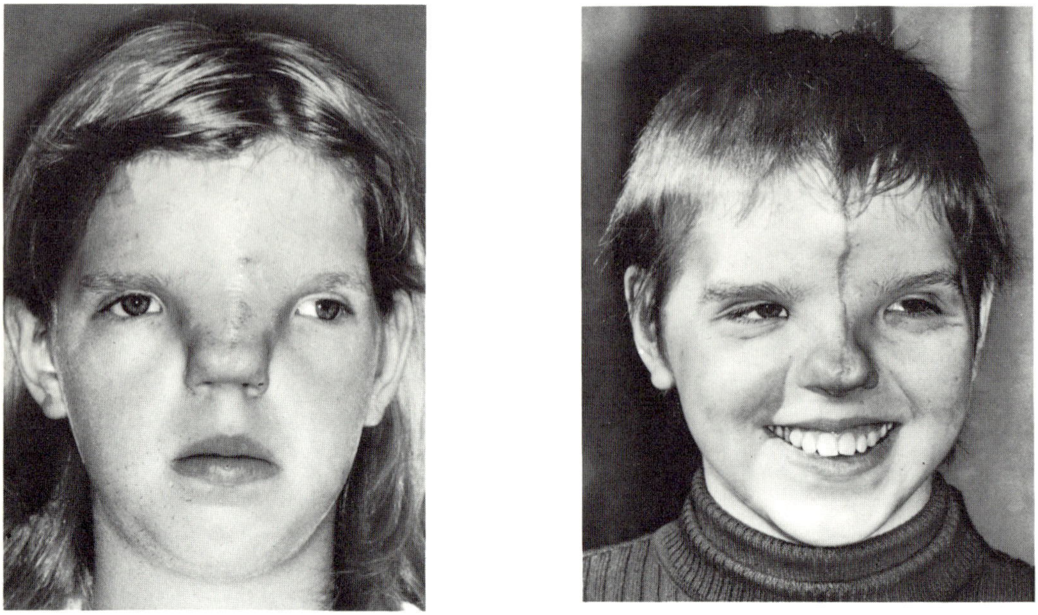

Fig. 4a and b. 12 years old girl before and after orbital swivelling with normalization of pupillar distance from 82 to 65 mm

Retrolabyrinthine Section of the Posterior Root of the Fifth Nerve (Abstract)

W. E. HITSELBERGER and J. PULEC

Over the last five years the authors have carried out selective section of the posterior root of the fifth cranial nerve on 30 patients. In the past it has been recognized by neurosurgeons that selective section of the posterior root as advocated by Walter DANDY is a better method of surgical approach to the problem of tic doloureaux than the conventional subtemporal gasserian ganglion operation advocated by FRAZIER. The reason for this is that the incidence of recurrence of tic pain is considerably lower. Additionally, selective section of the nerve in the posterior fossa is usually associated with preservation of touch sensation over the face and preservation of the corneal response. The reason, this procedure has not been carried out in general neurosurgical practice in spite of its obvious advantages is because of the associated morbidity and mortality in any suboccipital surgery.

Recently with the advances made in temporal bone surgery, primarily initiated and encouraged by Dr. William HOUSE, the authors have devised a technique whereby going through the temporal bone the posterior root can be exposed without the associated morbidity of a conventional suboccipital craniotomy. This approach entails the use of an operating microscope and high speed drills. In this way, there is increased lighting and magnification as well as more precise control of neurologic and sensory structures in the temporal bone. The procedure is carried out through a mastoidectomy. The bone is removed over the sigmoid sinus and forward to the posterior semicircular canal. This then exposes the dura between the sigmoid sinus and the posterior semicurcular canal. The dura is then opened. The opening is no more than a centimeter in length. The surgeon then is enabled to go along the face of the petrous ridge to the posterior root of the fifth nerve. This nerve lies anterior and superior to the seventh and eighth nerve complex. The motor root lies on the anterior surface of the fifth nerve in the posterior fossa and is usually not seen. The trigeminal root is clinically oriented superiorly to inferiorly with the first division fibers being superior and the third division fibers being inferior and the second division fibers lying in between. Appropriate section to the nerve is carried out depending on the distribution of the patient's pain. This procedure has the morbidity of a mastoid procedure instead of a suboccipital craniectomy.

This operation has been carried out on 30 patients over the last five years. In four patients the cerebellopontine angle tumors were encountered in the operative field and explained the patient's tic. The tumors were removed. In 20 patients with typical tic doloureaux section of the fifth nerve has resulted in complete disappearance of the pain with preservation of touch and motor function of the fifth nerve in every case. In six patients with atypical facial neuralgia the results have been excellent in two. In three patients some relief of the pain was obtained but not completely. In another patient the results of surgery were unimpressive and despite a block to pinprick over the involved area the patient still complained of her preoperative atypical facial neuralgia.

In summary, this operation is an extension of DANDY's work on the posterior root of the trigeminal nerve for tic doloureaux. The microsurgical approach to the fifth nerve through the temporal bone has several obvious advantages.

1. The morbidity of this procedure is the morbidity of a mastoid operation instead of the morbidity of a suboccipital craniectomy.

2. This procedure can be carried out on elderly patients. In our own series a patient aged 72 was operated on with no surgical problems. The fact that the patient is supine eliminates many of the positional causes for postural hypotension and air embolization making the procedure much less dangerous than the conventional operations that use a sitting position.

3. Anesthesia control of the patient is much better again because of the supine position that is utilized. This position is the standard position for all temporal bone surgery and approaches to the cerebellopontine angle.

4. The obvious advantages of the posterior root section with preservation of light touch, the motor root are inherent in the procedure.

5. This procedure is to be preferred over the long-term management of tic patients with the toxic drug Tegretol in the authors' opinion. It is a procedure that is readily adapted for the use of otologists and neurosurgeons that are trained in the team approaches to the temporal bone.

The authors will show movies to illustrate the various approaches. They will go into the results of the surgical procedures and be glad to discuss any phases of this approach to tic doloureaux with members of the association.

Supraspinal Pain Control by Dorsal Column Stimulation: A Possible Neuronal Interaction at the Level of Mesencephalic Reticular Formation

W. WINKELMÜLLER and H. DIETZ

Pain sensation is always a conscious phenomenon. For perception of a sensory stimulus the convergence of specific pain afferents and unspecific, respectively reticular, impulses in the same sensory cortical area is necessary. Pain sensation can be abolished by general anesthesia which blocks the unspecific projection system or by surgical interruption of the specific pain afferents. This oligosynaptic pathway can be surgically interrupted at the spinal level by chordotomy or by stereotactic lesion in the nucleus ventrocaudalis parvocellularis (V. c. pc.) of thalamus.

Recently SHEALY and NASHOLD introduced a more physiological method for handling pain by stimulating the dorsal funiculi. This treatment is based on the gate-theory of MELZACK and WALL (1965). It is assumed that stimulation of beta-fibers within the dorsal funiculi inhibits the activity of the slower pain conducting C-fibers at the first spinal synapse.

The phenomenon of pain control by dorsal column stimulation is investigated in 6 own cases. The level of pain blockade is discussed including electrophysiological and pharmacological observations.

The implantation of a dorsal column stimulator was carried out in 6 patients with chronic, intractable pain. The results of pain control by this method were rather different: 4 patients who suffered neuralgic pain by tumor compression of different localization became nearly completely relieved and were taken off strong analgetics. In one patient with metastasis of a rectum carcinoma, the radicular pain sensation could be suppressed but not the localized pain caused by osseous metastases. Dorsal column stimulation had no effect in a patient with phantom limbs following complete traumatic paraplegia. This patient achieved pain relief for the first time by stereotactic thalamotomy.

The question arises if such a selection of pain interruption should rather be localized at the central level of pain management than directly at the entrance of pain information in the spinal cord. The centripetal influence of dorsal column stimulation with various frequencies has been investigated by means of EEG recordings. We observed that 25 to 150 c/sec stimuli suppress spontaneous alpha activity. (Fig. 1). During the desynchronized phase in the EEG a discrete bilateral mydriasis could be noticed. Accordingly, we assume that a polysynaptic unspecific activation by dorsal column stimulation is induced in the reticular formation.

The impulses ascend in the dorsal funiculi to the nucleus gracilis and cuneatus and reach the V. c. pc. of thalamus by the crossing lemniscus medialis (Fig. 2). According to electrophysiological investigations of FRENCH et al. (1953), collaterals terminate at reticular nuclei in the midbrain level and establish contact to the ascending activating system. At this level an interaction between noci- and proprioceptive afferents is possible because the spinothalamic tract also sends collaterals to the reticular gray.

HAGBARTH and KERR (1954) as well as KING et al. (1957) demonstrated that the midbrain reticular formation exerts a tonic control on pain afferents. Stimulation of this structure - producing an arousal reaction in the EEG - reduce the size of potentials evoked by pain in the sensory nuclei of thalamus and in the cortical projection area. Also, the diencephalic forerunners of the reticular activating system (medial thalamic nuclei, pallidum, putamen and caudate) have a suppressing influence on nociceptive stimuli (LONG, 1959). On the contrary, the cortical potentials evoked by pain become more localized and increase if the mesencephalic reticular formation is blocked by barbiturates or by coagulation. In this case, painful stimuli cannot reach the level of consciousness.

The pharmacological pain control with potent neuroleptica seems to affect the unspecific side of pain transmission too. Parallel to our clinical observations we studied the influence of Haloperidol on the unspecific activating system of cats: low frequent stimuli in the mesencephalic reticular formation produce unspecific phenomena (spindling and recruiting) in the ECoG (Fig. 3). 100 c/sec stimuli elicit a desynchronisation in the ECoG and an increase of arterial blood pressure. Following the application of Haloperidol the unspecific responses in the ECoG are inhibited and the blood pressure increase is blocked.

Thus the inhibition of pain projection is achieved pharmacologically by suppression of reticular afferents and by activation of the same system following dorsal column stimulation.

Thus pain perception is highly modulated by the degree of consciousness mediated by the diffuse projection system. The dorsal column stimulation cannot exert such an influence at the spinal level but more readily in the higher integrative midbrain.

REFERENCES

1. FRENCH, J.D., M. VERZEANO and H.W. MAGOUN: An extralemniscal sensory system in the brain. Arch. neurol. 69, 505-517 (1953)
2. HAGBARTH, K.E. and D.I.B. KERR: Central influences on spinal afferent conduction. J. Neurophysiol., Springfield 17, 295-307 (1954)
3. KING, E.E., R. NAQUET and H.W. MAGOUN: Alterations in somatic afferent transmission through the thalamus by central mechanisms and barbiturates. J. Pharmacol. Exper. Therap. Baltimore 119, 48-63 (1957)
4. LONG, E.G.: Modification of sensory mechanisms by subcortical structures. J. Neurophysiol. 22 412-427 (1959)
5. MELZACK, R. and P.D. WALL: Pain mechanisms: a new theory. Science 150, 971-973 (1965)
6. NASHOLD, B.S. and H. FRIEDMAN: Dorsal column stimulation for pain: a preliminary report on 30 patients. J. Neurosurg. 36, 590-597 (1972)
7. SHEALY, C.N., J.T. MORTIMER and J.B. RESWICK: Electrical inhibition of pain by stimulation of the dorsal columns: preliminary clinical report. Anesth. Analg. Curr. Res. 46, 489-491 (1967)

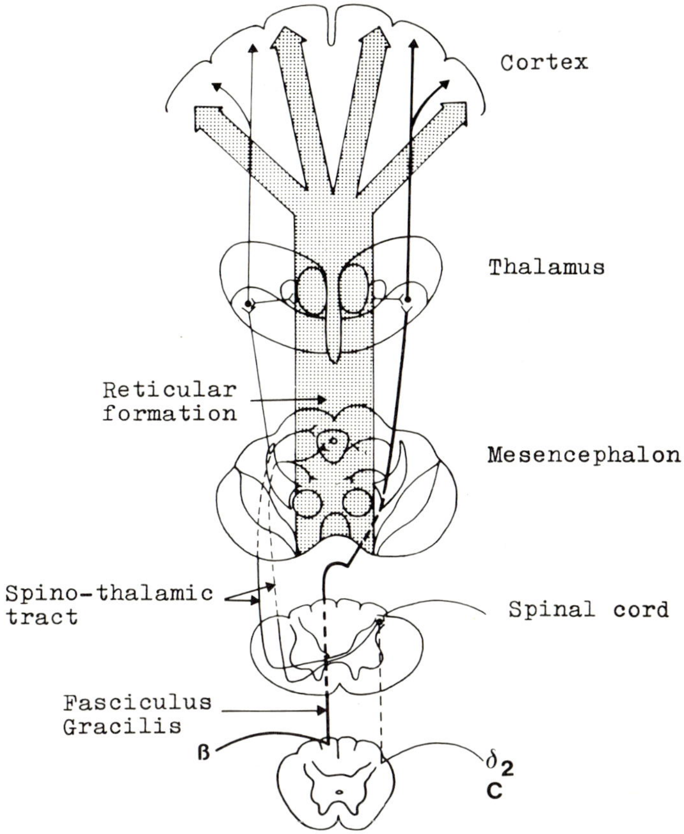

Fig. 1. Diagram of the major pathways concerned with noxious (C-fibers) and tactile stimuli (β -fibers). The unspecific activation of sensory cortex is set up by collaterals contacting to the ascending diffuse projection system at midbrain level

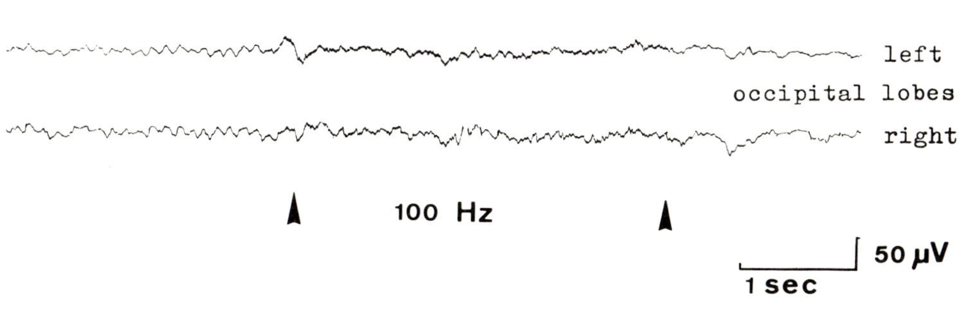

Fig. 2. Spontaneous alpha-activity in the EEG is reduced by 100 c/sec stimulation of the dorsal funiculi

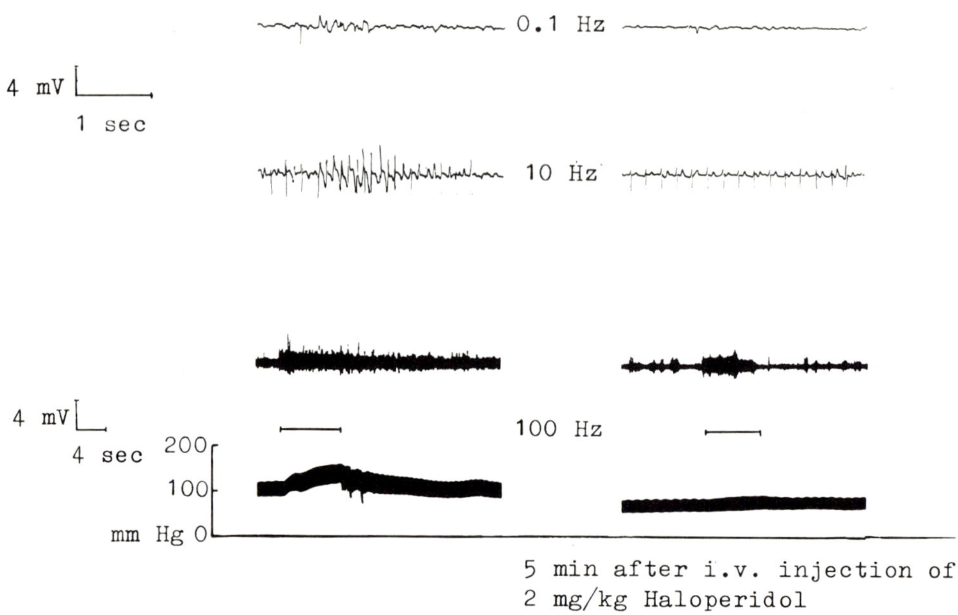

Fig. 3. Midbrain induced unspecific responses in the ECoG (Spindling and Recruiting) as well as blood pressure increase are blocked following the application of Haloperidol (right)

Osseous Instability in Cranio-Vertebral Dysplasia (Abstract)

W. SEEGER and A. L. AGNOLI

A short motion picture on a case of assimilation of the atlas associated with residual occipital vertebralization. It will be shown - with the aid of X-rays, drawings and a clay model - that additionally to the associated malformations, the instability of the clivus due to cleft formation between the jugular foramina, endanger the statics of the cranium should a suboccipital decompression be performed. The authors will demonstrate the anomalies in course of the vertebral artery and of the medulla, and will briefly discuss stabilizing measures.

Lumbal Dermal Sinus with Lateral Sinus Opening (Abstract)

K. DÜNNEBEIL and P. RUNGE

It is well known, that recurrent meningitis in childhood is most likely caused by an open communication between the central nervous system and the environment, constituting a congenital dermal sinus. The opening is generally located in the dorsal medial line. A careful inspection of the skin is necessary, because the sinus opening is usually tiny.

We have operated on a child with dermal sinus who had suffered from recurrent meningitis, and in whom the very small opening was located exceptionally lateral to the dorsal medial line. The dermal sinus extended medially in a transverse direction and terminated in a dermoid cyst in the subdural space. Furthermore, the child had vertebral anomalies, which probably can be explained by the same teratogenetical mechanism as the dermal sinus.

The rare lateral location of the sinus opening led to diagnostic difficulties in this case.

Hematomyelia with Paraplegia Following Coarctation of the Aorta

T. TZONOS

In cases of coarctation of the aorta neurological findings from the side of the spinal cord need not occur if a network of collateral vessels has developed. Cases of coarctation of the aorta with neurological findings are rare in literature. These neurological findings consist of pain and cramps, "going to sleep" (TYLER et al.), a partial BROWN-SEQUARD syndrome (HERRON et al.), as well as incomplete (CHRISTIAN et al.) and complete paraplegia with urinary insufficiency (HABERER, HENNING et al.). In lighter cases the pathogenesis of these neurological findings can be explained as a result of direct pressure of the collateral vessels on the spinal cord, or of ischemia. Neurosurgical treatment has not yet been reported.

In the case here reported, a fifty-year-old man with a hitherto unrecognized coarctation of the aorta suddenly developed an almost complete paraplegia of the lower extremities. When admitted to the hospital sixty hours later, he had pink spinal fluid and the Durolyopaque-myelogram showed a complete stop at the level of D 1/2 (Fig. 1). Laminectomy was performed immediately. The paravertebral muscles showed dozens of thick arteries, evidently collateral vessels, later demonstrated by angiography (Fig. 2). The spinal cord was edematous and sanguinous. Its ventral side was of blue-black colour. No fluctuation and no angiomatous malformation was seen. The ligamenta denticulata were cut through, the dura closed with insertion of a graft. Eight hours after the operation the patient could already move his legs again and showed further neurological improvement.

In this case, we assume that a hemorrhage from the arteria spinalis anterior or from an aneurysm, caused the symptoms. Possibly the spinal artery was patent. We think, the good result obtained, is due to laminectomy. The hemotomyelia and the edema of the spinal cord would probably have led to myelomalacia. The coarctation has since been corrected and the patient recovered well.

REFERENCES

1. CHRISTIAN, P. and W. NODER: Akute Rückenmarkssyndrome bei Isthmusstenose der Aorta als Folge eines pathologischen Kollateralkreislaufs über die A. spinalis ant. Zschr. Kreislaufforsch. 43, 125-131 (1954)

2. HABERER, H.: Ein Fall von seltenem Collateralkreislauf bei angeborener Obliteration der Aorta und dessen Folgen. Z. Heilkunde 24, 26-38 (1903)

3. HERRON, P. W., E. L. FOLTZ, F. P. PLUM, R. A. BRUCE and K. A. MERENDINO: Partial BROWN-SEQUARD-Syndrome associated with coarctation of the aorta. Review of literature and report of a surgically treated case. Amer. Hearth J. 55, 129-134 (1958)

4. TYLER, H.R. and D.B.CLARK: Neurologic complications in patients with coarctation of aorta. Neurology (Minn.) 8, 712-717 (1958)

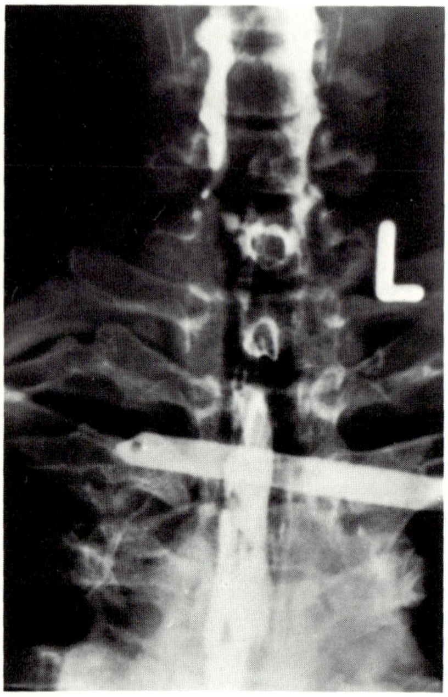

Fig. 1. Complete stop D 1/2

▼ Fig. 2. Colateral vessels demonstrated by angiography

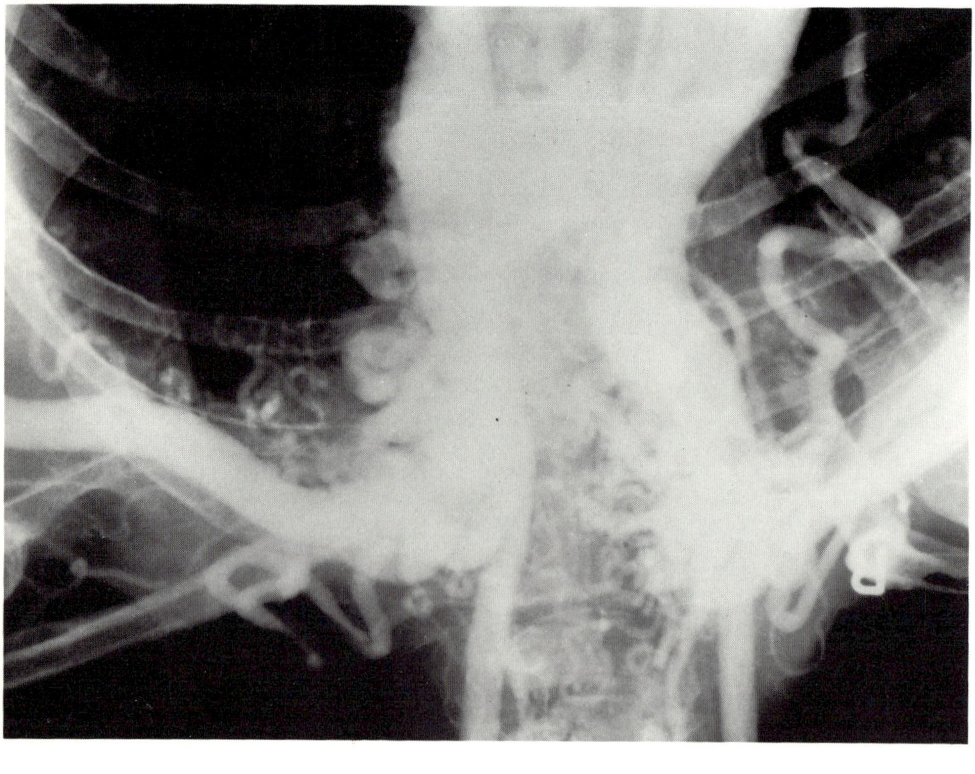

Spontaneous Subarachnoid Hemorrhage Due to Spinal Vascular Malformations

J. Wappenschmidt, E. Lins, and R. Wüllenweber

The number of vascular malformations in the spinal canal, diagnosed intra vitam has increased considerably following the application of spinal angiography. This circumstance has also provided a greater amount of information on the spinal causes of spontaneous subarachnoid hemorrhages. Because of the non-characteristic symptoms in such cases, the source of hemorrhage is frequently not recognized until the disease has progressed to an advanced stage.

Our material comprises seven angiomas and two true saccular aneurysms in the spinal subarachnoid space. Six of these cases had the clinical picture of a spontaneous subarachnoid hemorrhage. Two angiomas showed obvious signs of spinal compression even before the hemorrhage. In these it was not difficult to identify the source of hemorrhage. In cases such as these, subarachnoid hemorrhages have a bearing on the differential diagnosis, since they tend to narrow the broad spectrum of possible causes to two: vascular malformations or vascular tumors. There are four cases, however, that deserve particular interest. In these cases the initial symptom was recognized as an apoplectic subarachnoid hemorrhage, while localizing signs did not develop. Two of the cases were identified as angiomas of the cervical spinal cord.

In case No. 1 the spinal symptomatology had begun 15 months ago, and in the second case not until 5 years after the insult. In this latter case there was a combined epidural, vertebral, and spinal angioma.

The characteristic angiomatous vertebrae C 5 and C 6, with a reduced intervertebral space, and the constricted spinal canal, are shown in the plain lateral view of the cervical column. Myelography showed the intradural angioma, recognizable by the pathognomony of the stop at the C 3/C 4 level (Fig. 1).

Only the epidural angioma was removed during surgery, while the intradural angioma appeared to be inoperable. The following figure shows the arteriograms of the patient 4 years after a second subarachnoid hemorrhage had occurred, causing a 4 weeks disturbance of consciousness and a considerable deterioration of the neurologic state.

The illustrations provide a highly contrasting and homogeneous display of the vertebral as well as of the intradural angioma; the afferent vessels originate from the enlarged arteriae cervicalis ascendens and profunda (Fig. 2).

The afferent vessels and portions of the intradural angioma have been ligated in an additional operation. The control arteriogram shows a distinct reduction of the angioma (Fig. 3).

Subarachnoid hemorrhage without localizing signs was also the initial symptom in two cases of true saccular aneurysms in the upper cervical spinal canal. In both the violent pain in the nuchal and occipital regions, prodromal of the disturbance of consciousness, were interpreted as meningism, and cerebral angiographs were made assuming the existence of an intracranial vascular malformation. This appeared to be an appropriate measure since in the meantime misleading signs such as fundoscopic and EEG irregularities had been disclosed. The next figures show the arteriograms of the two patients, including the case already described, to demonstrate the approximate similarity of locations.

In the lateral views the aneurysms are located in the upper spinal canal between the occiput and the atlas, somewhat behind the dorsal aspect of the odontoid, and adjoining the ventrolateral circumference ot the spinal cord. In the sagittal views the aneurysm, in both cases, is projected to the right of the midline, no identification being possible as to whether the stalk originates from the inferior cerebellar artery, the vertebral, the first segmental artery, or from a persisting embryonic vessel (Fig. 4 and 5).

At surgery the origin of the aneurysm was described, in case No. 1, as being the vertebral artery, ventral from the roots of the accessory nerve and the first cervical root. In case No. 2 the aneurysm was found to be located immediately adjacent to the lower cerebellar artery which had to be occluded.

The control angiograms in both cases show the complete occlusion of the aneurysm, the vertebral arteries remaining open. In case No. 1 the only residual deficit consisted in a slight weakness of the sternocleidomastoid, while case No. 2 had Wallenberg's syndrome (Fig. 6). In conclusion we shall briefly describe a case of a tumor in the cauda region, which was admitted following two subarachnoid hemorrhages at short intervals, and showed severe disorientation of the patient. In this case, too, there had been no signs of spinal compression, which led us to plan a cerebral angiography first. Spinal diagnostics was resorted to because of a subsequently stated pain in the back, irradiating to both legs which had been present for two years.

In this case even the plain X-ray indicated the location of the tumor in the cauda region, showing a distinct excavation of the dorsal aspect of the second and third lumbar vertebrae. A complete stop was seen in the myelogram. A heavily vascularized ependymoma was disclosed at surgery (Fig. 7).

The above case histories and those described in the literature demonstrate that in a percentage of cases which cannot be exactly defined, spinal vascular malformation and tumors initially cause subarachnoid hemorrhage without focal signs. Not infrequently, however, the same can be ovserved in hemorrhages from intracranial sources. Therefore, the temptation is great to limit oneself to cerebral angiography, surgical disorders of the spinal region, which can lead to irreversible transverse section, if left to itself, remaining undetected.

It is simple enough, either to identify, or to rule out cervical vascular malformations. They very often tend to be hemorrhagic. Since the cervical spinal vascular system - similar to the vertebrobasilary system - can be visualized by brachial or subclavian arteriography, it is not difficult to examine, the cervical vessels additional to those of the posterior cranial fossa. Vascular diagnostic measures involving the thoracic and lumbar cord vessels, however, should not be applied unless a tumor has been excluded as the source of the hemorrhage by means of plain roentgenograms of the spinal column and positive myelography.

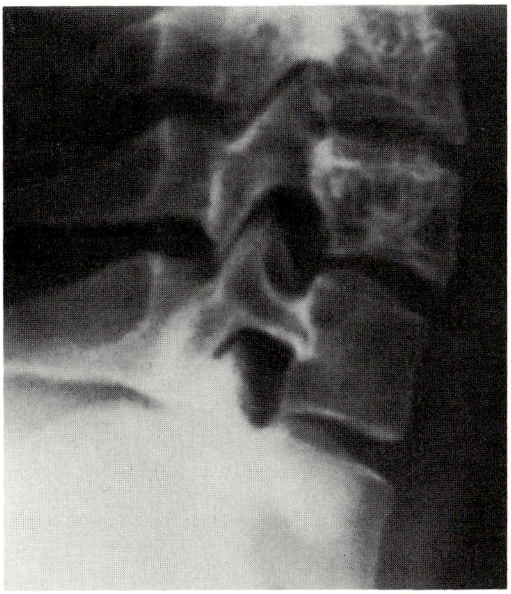

Fig. 1a.

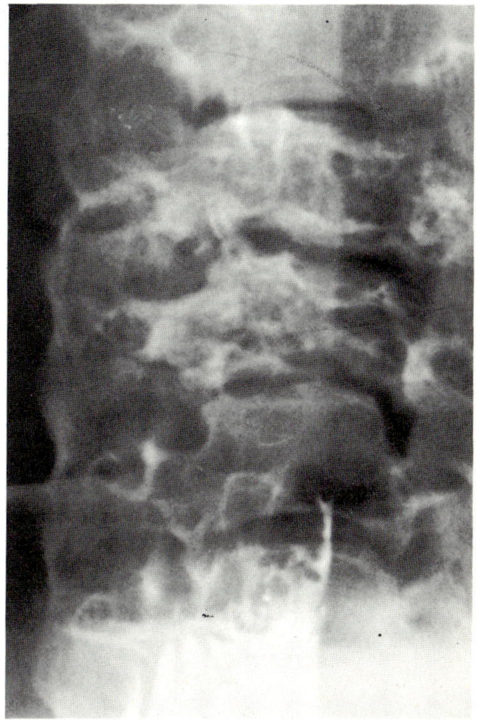

Fig. 1b.

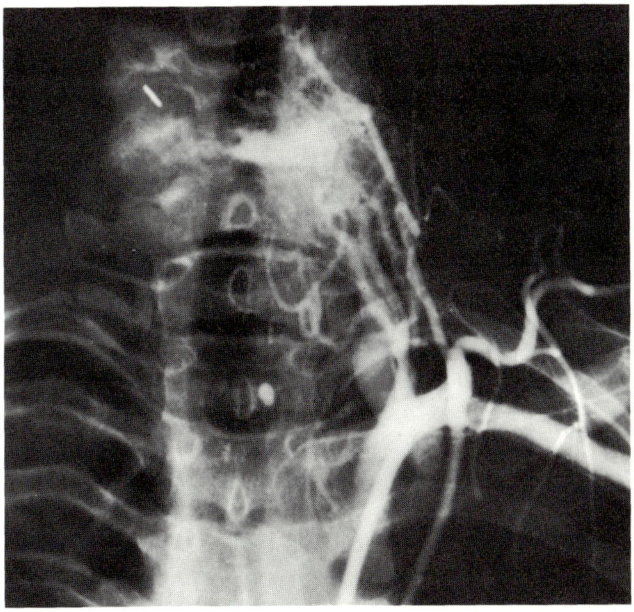

Fig. 2.

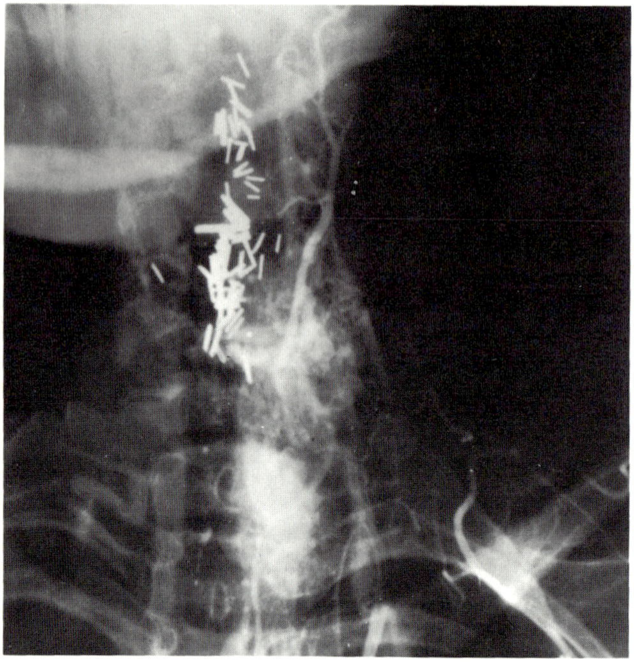

Fig. 3.

Fig. 4a. (left)
Fig. 4b. (right)

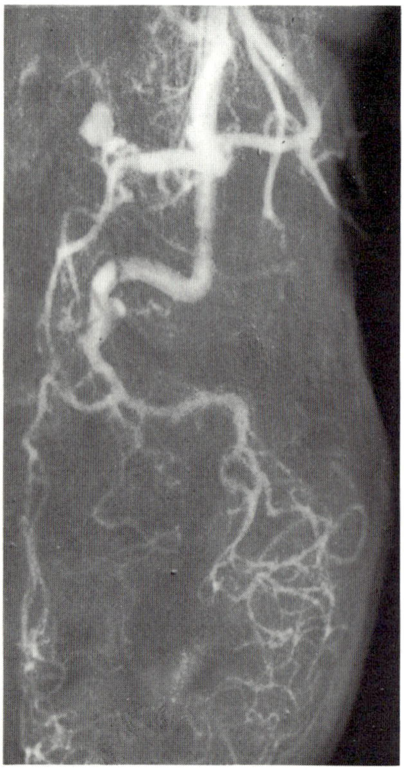

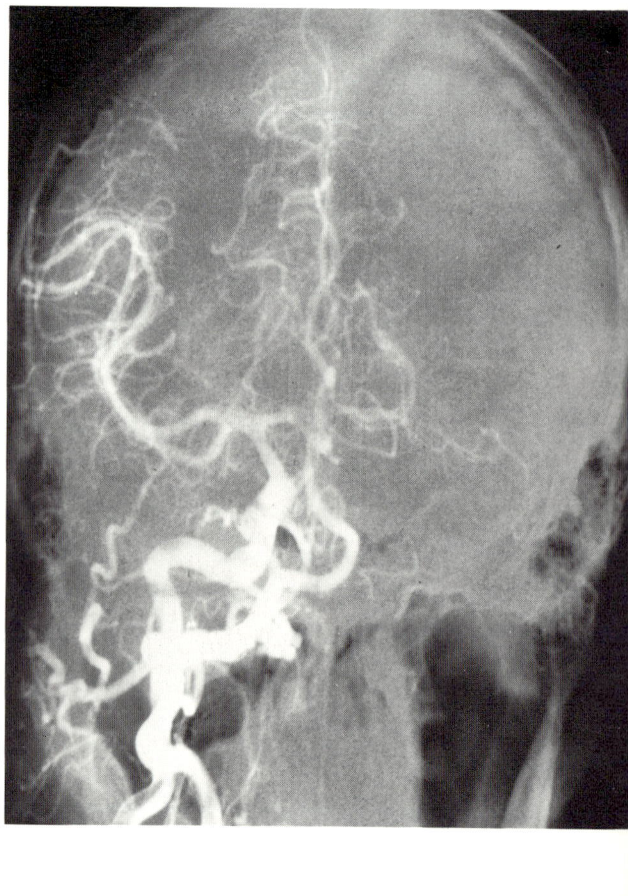

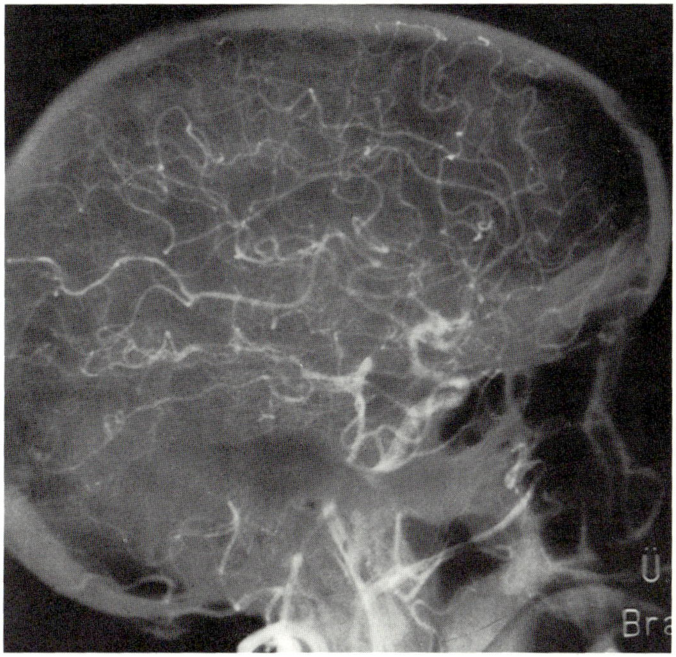

Fig. 5a.

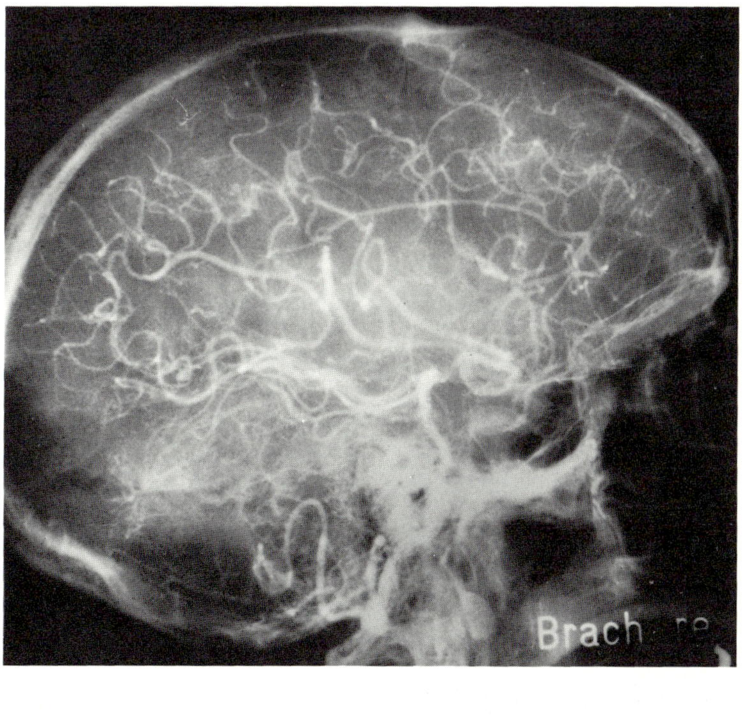

Fig. 5b.

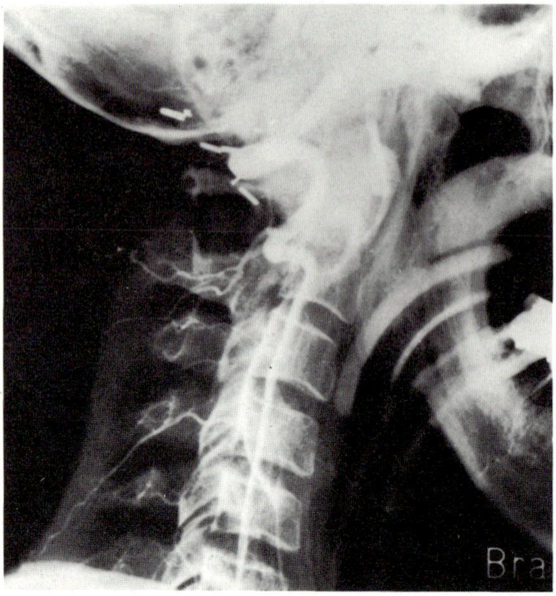

Fig. 6a.

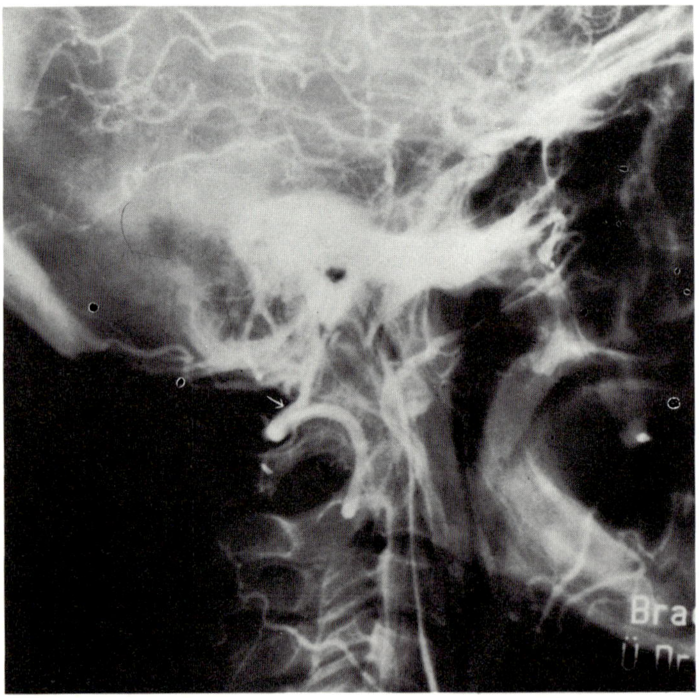

Fig. 6b.

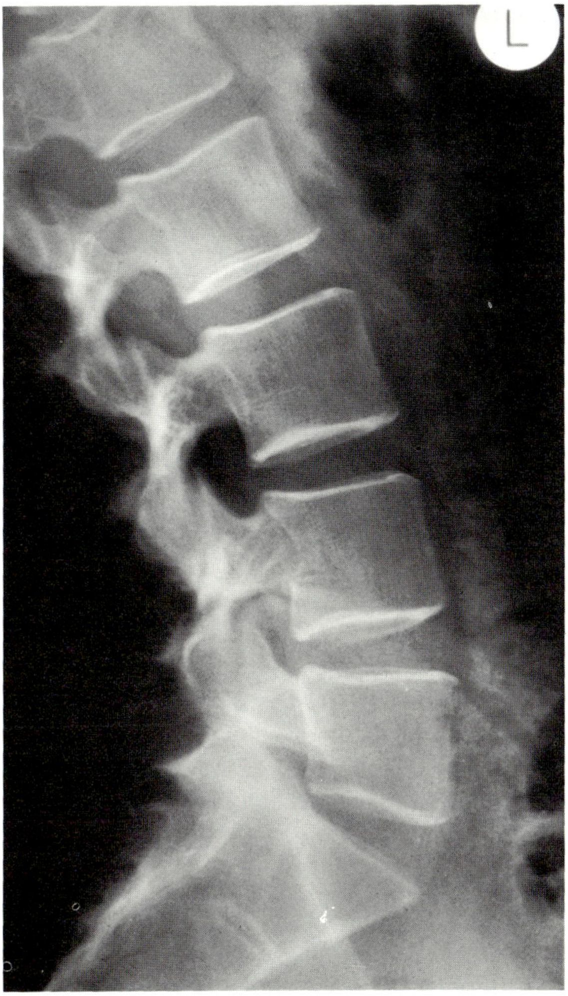

Fig. 7a.

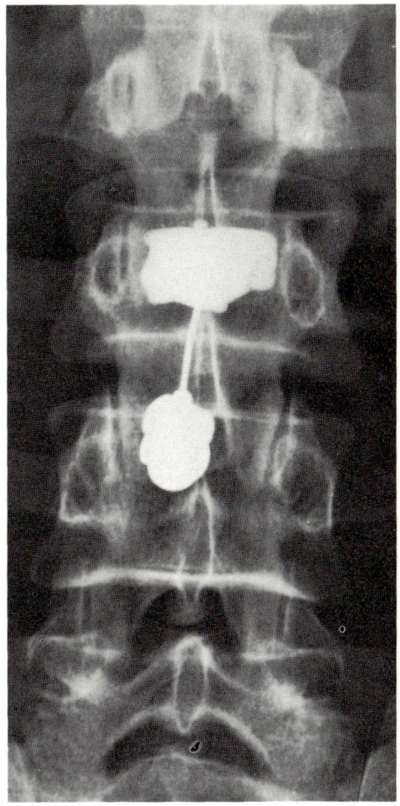

Fig. 7b.

Addendum

Presidential Remarks

"Behutsame Pflege des Alten
und frischer Wagemut für das Neue"

ADOLF BUTENANDT
(Nobelprize 1939)

In his opening lecture - not to be published in extenso - at the 24th Annual Meeting of the German Society of Neurosurgery in Mainz, 1973, the Society's President gave a brief review of the state of art of Neurosurgery, its present problems and its future tasks. The favorable perspectives as well as the possible dangers for the further development of our specialty were analysed in view of some historical data. The increasing importance of applied experimental and clinical research was stressed while, on the other hand, caution was recommended against the precipitous and uncritical fragmentation of Neurosurgery into subspecialties. Nevertheless, enough room must be left for the necessary developments. A strong recommendation was addressed to the German Government that the coming reforms in Public Health and hospital structure be determined by the patients' needs and not by the convenience of the Government organs or by utopic political ideologies.

Several jubilees were celebrated during the 24th Annual Meeting of the German Society of Neurosurgery. The 100th birthday of OTFRID FOERSTER was commemorated in the presence of members of his family.

The honorary members of our Society, WILHELM TÖNNIS and ARIST STENDER, celebrated their 75th, resp. 70th birthday. This is reason enough to pay reverence to the personalities and achievements of these two honorable men and co-founders of the German Society of Neurosurgery. Another marking feature of this year's Meeting was the bestowal of the OTFRID FOERSTER-Medal upon HUGO KRAYENBÜHL for his outstanding merits in the field of Neurosurgery.

KURT SCHÜRMANN

Board of the Deutsche Gesellschaft für Neurochirurgie 1972-1974:

President: Kurt Schürmann, Mainz
Vice-President: Helmut Penzholz, Heidelberg
Secretary: Wolfgang Schiefer, Erlangen
Treasurer: Horst Wenker, Berlin

Organizing Committee of the Annual Meeting in Mainz 1973:
Kurt Schürmann, Hans-Jürgen Reulen, Madjid Samii, Dieter Voth

In Memory of the 100th Birthday of Otfrid Foerster

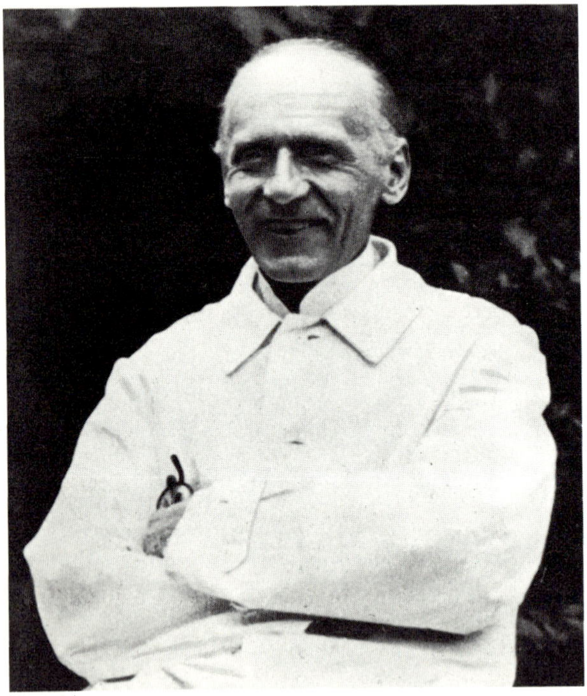

On November 9, 1973, we shall celebrate the hundredth anniversary of the day, on which Otfrid FOERSTER was born in Breslau as the son of Richard FOERSTER, professor of classical languages, archeology and eloquence. On this special occasion the German neurologists ought to remember this magnificent man with gratitude and veneration.

His life-work is of equal rank with that of his close friend, the great pioneer of modern neurosurgery, Harvey CUSHING. Both had come to neurosurgery from different directions, CUSHING from surgery, FOERSTER from neurology. Already as a student, FOERSTER had taken great interest in the lectures of the great neurologist in Breslau, WERNICKE, and after having finished his studies, he spent, on his advice, two years with DEJERINE in Paris and FRENKEL in Switzerland in order to work at therapeutic exercises for neurological patients. This led him to his first remarkable scientific work on "Therapeutic exercises for tabes dorsalis" (1901) which also reveals the two fundamental qualities which accompanied him through all his life: shrewd observation and analysis of neurological symptoms associated with a strong will to draw logical consequences for therapy, i.e. to be physician and scientist at the same time.

The fateful idea to use the scalpel for treating this kind of diseases rose from the observation that hemiplegia may take an atonic course in tabetics. The affection of the posterior roots characteristic for tabes, an "experiment of nature", encouraged him - also in moral respect - to dare the "experiment of operation": in 1908 he recommended to resect the posterior roots as therapy for spastic paralyses. One year later he introduced resection of the posterior dorsal roots for treating otherwise uninfluenced pain. These kinds of intervention, still known as "FOERSTER's operation" to-day, soon helped him to attain celebrity all over the world. These achievements, however, incited him to even more intensive research work. Both, most exact neurological examination before and after operation as well as electric stimulation of accessible nerve roots on the operating table, enabled him to compile a complete map of human dermatomes, which has not lost its significance until today. While initially FOERSTER had only been assistant and investigator to surgeons assuming a benevolent attitude toward him, he now became more and more an independently operating "neurological surgeon". With integrity and thorough indication, he transformed every operation into a permitted though audaciously directed and ingeniously performed experiment.

Surgery of the spinal roots was soon followed by surgery of the spinal cord itself. In 1913, he was the first in Europe to transect the anterolateral column for the relief of pain, and as early as 1917 he was able to report a successful total extirpation of an intramedullary tumor of the spinal cord. Any expert will know that under the conditions of that time, only a man who combined exact anatomical and physiological knowledge of the spinal cord with utmost manual skill, scrupulous attention and physical persistency, would succeed in this task.

During World War I, when innumerable soldiers were wounded, he became outstanding in the field of surgical tratment of peripheral nerve injuries. Almost 5.000 patients with peripheral nerve injuries went through his hands. He operated upon 775 of them most successfully. He mastered equally well the technique of covering too serious defects by means of autoplastic transplantations, and the indication to internal and external neurolysis. The most remarkable results of this gigantic work were his outstanding contributions to a handbook, the first on "Symptomatology and therapy of gunshot injuries of peripheral nerves" and the second on "Special physiology and special functional pathology of striped muscles", published in 1929 resp. 1937, which, to the present day, have lost nothing of their significance.

Towards the end of World War I and during the first years thereafter he dedicated himself increasingly to the operative treatment of patients with gunshot scar of the brain. Based on hundreds of stimulations of the cerebral cortex during surgical procedures resulted his classical works on epilepsy and "functional anatomy" of the cerebral cortex.

FOERSTER devoted the last two decades of his life increasingly to problems of brain tumors and the autonomous nervous system.

All these facts help to complete the picture of a remarkable man, scientist and physician. We have been able to mark only a brief review of those among his numerous achievements which were of decisive influence for the development of modern neurosurgery. His directive impulses to neurology, orthopedics and particularly to the rehabilitation of neurological patients can only be indicated here.

Above all, the memory of Otfrid FOERSTER should remind us of keeping awake the interest in his scientific bequest also among the young generation and of carrying on in his spirit for the benefit of science and the patient.

HELMUT PENZHOLZ

To the 75th Birthday of Wilhelm Tönnis

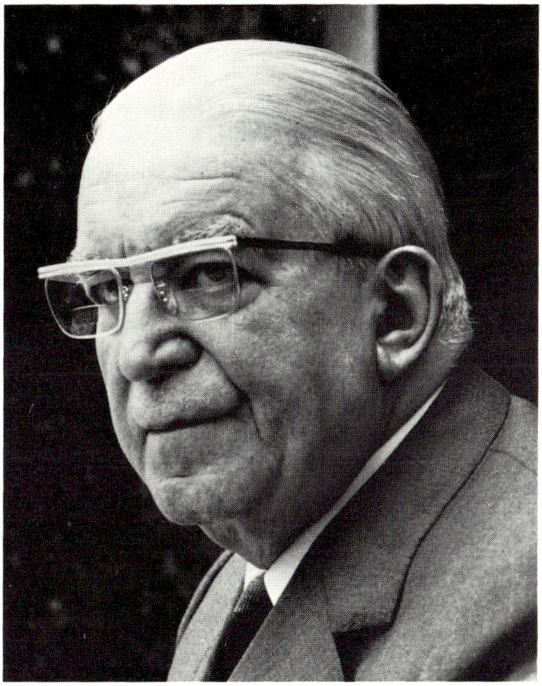

"Ehret Eure grossen Meister,
dann bannt Ihr gute Geister"

HANS SACHS (1494-1576)

It appears most appropriate to apply the above sentence by HANS SACHS chosen by WILHELM TÖNNIS to patronize the highest awards of the German Society of Neurosurgery, the FEDOR KRAUSE-Medal and the OTFRID FOERSTER-Medal to WILHELM TÖNNIS himself.

In the person of WILHELM TÖNNIS, on the day of his 75th birthday, June 16, 1973, we pay tribute to a veritable master of Neurosurgery. TÖNNIS made his acquaintance with Neurosurgery when he went to Stockholm 1932, to work with HERBERT OLIVECRONA as a Rockefeller-stipendiary. Thanks to his indefatigable clinical and scientific work he eventually convinced, in a few years, those who opposed to Neurosurgery as an independent specialty. As early as 1937, TÖNNIS became chairman of the first German Chair of Neurosurgery in Berlin. The systematic work at the bedside and in the operating theater was complemented by the straight collaboration with HUGO SPATZ, the Director of the Kaiser-Wilhelm-Institute for Brain Research in Berlin-Buch. This is a vivid example of the fruitful relationship between Brain Research and Neurosurgery. TÖNNIS became Head of the Division for Tumor Research and Experimental Pathology of the Brain of this Institute.

A period of widespread clinical and experimental research had begun with the birth of fundamental publications on intracranial hypertension, brain edema, cerebral circulatory diseases, tumors and vascular malformations of the brain. Due to his research and to his successful surgical activity TÖNNIS earned worldwide recognition within a few years. Thanks to his initiative, the "Zentralblatt für Neurochirurgie", the first neurosurgical journal in the world, was founded and is still related to his name. Although the Second World War imposed limitations on this fast and promising career, TÖNNIS dedicated his best efforts to the injuries of the brain, spinal cord and peripheral nerves. With almost incredible organisational ability he established the basic principles for the care of the injured from the moment of injury until their rehabilitation. Accumulated experience during this period constituted the base for the treatment of craniocerebral injuries for many years. Following the War, the places where TÖNNIS had worked, had been lost. 1946 TÖNNIS began the reedification-work of the Department for General Surgery, Trauma Surgery and Neurosurgery at the Knappschaftskrankenhaus in Bochum-Langendreer until 1948, when he became chairman of the newly created Chair of Neurosurgery in Cologne. Here, with his peculiar dynamism, he built up his new clinic according to his high rank as a clinician, scientist and teacher. Here he exerted his undefatigable and fruitful activity until his retirement as Emeritus in 1968. Patients and pupils from all over the world came to Cologne to see WILHELM TÖNNIS, a testimony of his unequalled qualities as physician and teacher. The teacher-pupil relationship between OLIVECRONA and TÖNNIS became a firm friendship, the expression of which is the "Handbuch der Neurochirurgie", jointly edited by both masters and their pupils. During the highly fruitful years to follow, TÖNNIS concentrated his efforts on the classification of cranial traumas, on the symptomatology, diagnosis and therapy of tumors and vascular malformations of the brain. Simultaneously, he invested much time and personal engagement in the task of making neurosurgery a well-known and independent specialty, and in helping to found the German Society of Neurosurgery, which owes him so much. Today TÖNNIS can proudly contemplate the fruits of his undefatigable activity. More than words, the numerous homages from all over the world give a vivid testimony of his merits. WILHELM TÖNNIS is an honorary member of numerous national and international Medical Societies, doctor honoris causa of several foreign universities, and carrier of the OTFRID FOERSTER-Medal, the ERB-Medal, the HARVEY CUSHING-Medal, the PARACELSUS-Medal and the WALTER POPPELREUTER-Medal.

With veneration, gratitude and affection, his pupils and friends, as well as the members of our Society, wish the man who is frequently considered as, and in fact constitutes, the "Father of German Neurosurgery", good luck, health and joy of life for many years to come!

KURT SCHÜRMANN

To the 70th Birthday of Arist Stender

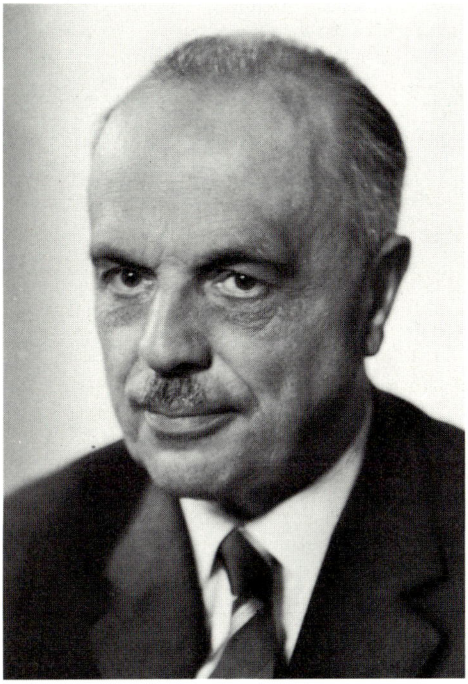

On April 12, 1973, Professor Dr. A. STENDER, retired professor of neurosurgery and former director of the Neurological-Neurosurgical University Hospital Berlin-Westend, completed the 70th year of his life. The German Neurosurgeons extend to him their sincere wishes of fortune and blessing.

ARIST STENDER has earned outstanding merits during the stormy development of neurosurgery during the past 50 years. He belongs to those neurosurgeons, who always paid special attention to the neurological part of his specialty. His teachers MAX NONNE, HEINRICH PETTE and later, OTFRID FOERSTER, exerted great influence on him. He had his surgical training with BRÜTT. Additionally, he worked for some time with the American Neurosurgeons CUSHING and BAILEY.

In 1939, he became the neurosurgical successor of OTFRID FOERSTER in Breslau.

During the War, he dedicated himself successfully to the care of peripheral nerve injuries, systematically enlarging the basic knowledge created by OTFRID FOERSTER. Following the War, when he was forced to give up the directorship of his hospital in Breslau, he immediately succeeded in founding a Neurological-Neurosurgical Department at the University Hospital of Westend in Berlin-Charlottenburg, which very soon became one of the leading hospitals in teaching and research.

In 1950, he was one of the prominent founders of the German Society of Neurosurgery, in 1969, he became one of its Honorary Members. The planning of the two recently inaugurated Neurosurgical Clinics in Berlin-Westend and Berlin-Steglitz conceived according to the most modern aspects, was largely his work.

The German Neurosurgeons wish him good luck and health for many more years.

HELMUT PENZHOLZ

Bestowing of the OTFRID FOERSTER-Medal Upon HUGO KRAYENBÜHL

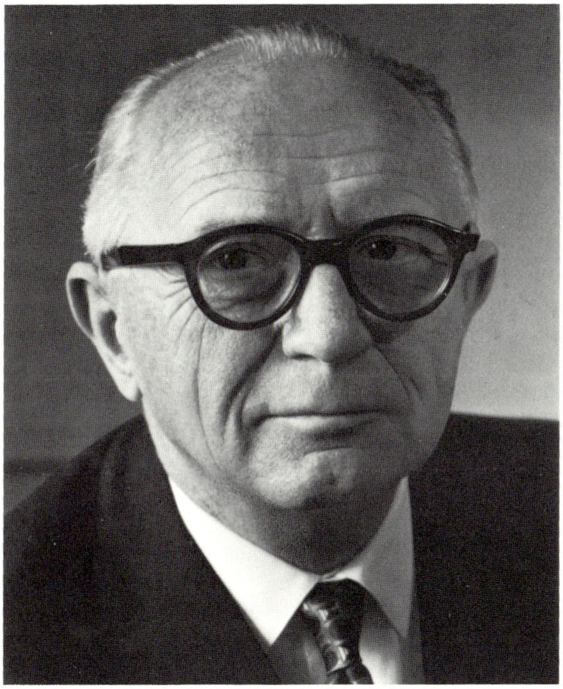

"Idee und Erfahrung werden in der Mitte nie zusammentreffen, zu vereinigen sind sie nur durch Kunst und Tat"

GOETHE to SCHOPENHAUER (1816)

When the German Society of Neurosurgery instituted the FEDOR KRAUSE- and the OTFRID FOERSTER-Medals in 1950, it was led by the scope of keeping alive in our Society the memory of these two German pioneers in Neurosurgery. The bestowing of one of these medals is celebrated by a Memorial Lecture and constitutes the highest honor, bestowed by the German Society of Neurosurgery to one of the most outstanding Neurosurgeons of today.

On his 100th birthday OTFRID FOERSTER is alive in our memories as the ingenious interpreter of his surgical experiences enriching Neurophysiology and Neuropathology. Thus, what was more appropriate, than to confer the medal in his honor to, and have his Memorial Lecture held by HUGO KRAYENBÜHL, a neurosurgeon, scientist and teacher ranking among the most prominent neurosurgeons in the world. The bestowing upon KRAYENBÜHL of the highest honor of our Society , honors our Society itself. As WILDER PENFIELD expressed it,

KRAYENBÜHL ranks equally with HARVEY CUSHING, WALTER DANDY, CHARLES FRAZIER, ERNEST SACHS and his own teacher, Sir HUGHES CAIRNS. Nothing is left to add, since KRAYENBÜHL gathers in a unique way in his work and personality the synthesis made by GOETHE in his letter to SCHOPENHAUER, as cited above.

Mainz, May 3, 1973

In the name of the
Deutsche Gesellschaft für Neurochirurgie

KURT SCHÜRMANN

Otfrid-Foerster Memoral Lecture
The Treatment of Intramedullary Spinal Cord Tumors and Cervical Syringohydromyelia

H. KRAYENBÜHL

It is a great honour and pleasure for me to deliver a Memorial Lecture to the memory of OTFRID FOERSTER in the year of his 100th birthday and thus also to be able to express my hearfelt thanks to the German Neurosurgical Society.
I regard this highest distinction of the German Neurosurgical Society as the climax of my academic career. At the same time, I am now able to repay a debt of gratitude to the leading German neurologist and, neurosurgeon, who was my friend ever since the memorable meeting of the Society of British Neurological Surgeons and the German Neurosurgeons in the year 1937 in Breslau. Because at this meeting the treatment of intramedullary tumors, among other topics, was discussed and OTFRID FOERSTER had in 1917 already reported on the first successfully operated intramedullary spinal cord tumor, it is a great pleasure for me to comment on these questions which are always absorbing to neurosurgeons and to report on the operative results obtained since FOERSTER's time.

The case reported in 1917 was that of a 40-year-old female patient with an advanced motor and sensory tetraplegia. It is remarkable that the level diagnosis was made exclusively from a neurological point of view and a radical extirpation of a solid intramedullary glioma from C_5-D_2, was accomplished by careful morcellation of the tumor with an excellent functional result. The patient was capable of walking again by herself with only a moderate ataxia, and the paretic muscle groups of the arms became practically completely functional. Truly a sensational result: In two further cases reported in 1920 one enormously long tumor from C_2-L_4 could not be radically removed, and the second patient died from pneumonia after a radical extirpation of the tumor from D_8 to the medulla oblongata. In 1935 FOERSTER reported together with GAGEL a success rate of 30% in 20 intramedullary tumors with operative mortality of 15 %. This result obviously did not satisfy the Master Neurosurgeon as he wrote pessimistically with BAILEY in 1936 in "A Contribution to the Study of Gliomas of the Spinal Cord with Special Reference to their Operability": "Finally one may attempt to dissect out the tumor at the first operation. Our own experience and a study of the literature make us inclined to think this procedure rarely advisable".

Also CAIRNS and RIDDOCH wrote in 1931 that the best method of treatment of the different types of intramedullary tumors was still an open question. In the following years the different authors occupied themselves with the question as to whether the suitable therapy was surgical, X-ray or a combination of both. GREENWOOD presented by far the most important contribution (1954, 1963, 1967) in that he indicated the outstanding significance of employing bipolar coagulation forceps in the shelling out of the tumor because bipolar coagulation under constant saline irrigation cannot damage the spinal cord tissue surrounding the tumor. Also the advantage of using fairly strong magnifying eyeglasses during the operation was established.

GREENWOOD accomplished the radical removal of nine ependymomas with good to very good late functional results, while in his series only one astrocytoma could be radically removed. In 1967 I have, together with YASARGIL, indicated the advantages of the microsurgical technique which, under stereoscopic view and with fine instruments permits, one to handle and spare the tissues in the best possible manner. As to how far these expectations have been fulfilled in the surgery of intramedullary tumors, I wish to set forth in today's paper on the basis of our material of 80 cases in the period from 1940 to the beginning of 1973. The differing methods of treatment are weighed against one another and from this discussion I will try to ascertain which type of treatment, of those which are today at our disposal, appears to me to be the most successful for the patients.

Case Material of Intramedullary Spinal Cord Tumors

In Table I the 80 cases are recorded according to the histological classification which I have studied with ANGST and OBERBECKMANN. It is evident that the ependymomas and the astrocytomas are most frequent and the spongioblastomas and the gliomas, which are not classified more exactly, rank next. I will comment upon the results of treatment in 64 cases of these types of tumor in order to form a definite opinion as to the best indications for treatment. Because of time limitation, I cannot discuss the rarer types of tumors; in these the problems of treatment are the same as with the more frequent tumors.

Table I. Follow-up study on 80 intramedullary tumors of the spinal cord from the Neurosurgical Clinic of Zürich in the period 1940 - 1973

Spongioblastoma	13 cases
Astrocytoma	21
Ependymoma	20
Glioma, unclassified	10
Medulloblastoma	2
Neurinoma	2
Papilloma	1
Angioreticuloma	4
Melanoma	1
Dermoid	2
Lipoma	2
Metastases (Hypernephroma)	2
	80 cases

Table II. Summary of 13 patients with spongioblastoma

Patients	age at opera-tion	sex	Course of Illness and Survival duration in months			Localization of Tumor	Treatment			
			preoperative course	postoperative course	alive in year:(if surviving)		E	E+ X-ray	D	D+ X-ray
1. K. C.	8y	M	84	24	1972	D6-11				x
2. B. H.	13y	F	48	12	+	C1-6		x		
3. K. M.	14y	F	1 1/2	4 1/2	+	D2-4	M			
4. S. O.	19y	F	3	41	1972	D3-5	m			
5. B. O.	22y	F	18	165	+	C2-D1				x
6. P. L.	43y	F	2	16	+	C5-7				x
7. A. O.	44y	M	96	108	1972	C2-6	X			
8. Z. O.	45y	M	132	300	1972	C2-5		X		
9. R. E.	46y	F	48	50	1972	C4-7	M			
10. M. H.	12y	M	1	1day	+	Med-D2			x	
11. R. F.	31y	M	96	36	1972	Med-C3				x
12. V. J.	17y	F	12	120	1972	C5-7	X			
13. S. M.	21y	M	6	6	+	C2-5	m			

X = total removal with ordinary surgical techniques
x = partial removal with ordinary surgical techniques
M = total removal with microsurgical techniques
m = partial removal with microsurgical techniques
\+ = death
E = extirpation
D = decompression

Intramedullary Spongioblastoma

Table II refers to the treatment of 13 patients with spongioblastoma. There were four types of treatment, namely extirpation (E), extirpation combined with X-ray treatment (E+X-ray), decompression with tumor biopsy (D) and decompression with tumor biopsy with subsequent X-ray treatment (D+X-ray). In group E case 3 died of cerebral metastasis of the glioma despite radical extirpation with microsurgical technique and case 13 with subtotal resection died as a result of increase of tetraparesis postoperatively with intercurrent illness. The remaining four cases showed a substantial improvement of the preoperative paretic signs, of whom the three undergoing radical operation were able to walk normally (i.e. 100 %).

As an example, case V.J., a 17-year-old female student is mentioned. 10 years after radical removal of the tumor (Fig. 1) she is fully capable of carrying on her daily activities; she displays slight weakness of the right hand, atrophy of the small hand muscles and analgesia and anesthesia in the right eighth cervical dermatome. The microsurgical subtotal extirpation of the tumor in case 4 brought about an improvement of motor function of the left leg after a transiently increased paraplegia.

In the group E+X-ray case 2 showed a transient improvement only; and died of a tumor extension into the ventricular system after one year. On the other hand, case 8 can walk by himself with a cane 25 years after operation with marked spasticity in the right arm and leg as before operation. As to how much the X-ray treatment contributed in this long catamnesis is doubtful in the assessment of the radical tumor extirpation. In case 10 of group D decompression led to death immediately after operation. The tumor was localized in the upper cervical cord up to the medulla oblongata.

In group D+X-ray two cases died; case 5 showed an improvement over many years with complete working capacity after a transient decline. Finally, however, because of progressive worsening, 13 years later, she underwent reoperation with subtotal tumor resection during which cardiac arrest led to exitus. The second case (case 6) died of cachexia after progressively getting worse. In case 1 an amazing improvement of the neurological symptoms is maintained provisionally over two years and in case 11 over three years in that there is subjective absence of symptoms with slight neurological signs.

In this comparison of the types of treatment, it is seen that radical tumor extirpation affords the best results; success with radiation over years is probable only in cases 1 and 11. It is notable that the best operative successes were obtained with the tumors localized in the middle and lower cervical cord.

Intramedullary Astrocytoma

Table III relates to intramedullary astrocytomas. With 21 patients the tumor was radically removed 8 times and the spinal cord radiated three times in addition. In 3 further cases a subtotal extirpation of the tumor was carried out. Of these cases, five (cases 2, 3, 8, 18, 19) showed a good to very good result (i.e. 80-100 % =gait normal). Case 9 is of particular interest; at present there is a twenty-year catamnesis with complete ability to work and only bilateral Babinski reflexes and reduction of vibratory sensation in both lower legs as neurological signs. In case 19 this 11-year-old boy underwent a radical removal of a cystic and solid astrocytoma of the entire spinal cord from C_1 - L_2 in three laminectomies (Fig. 2) employing

Table III. Summary of 21 patients with astrocytoma

Patients			Course of Illness and Survival			Localization of Tumor	Treatment			
	age at operation	sex	duration in months preoperative course	postoperativ course	alive in year:(if surviving)		E	E+ X-ray	D	D+ X-ray
1. W.R.	5y	F	48	20 1/2	+	Med-lumb			x	
2. K.M.	6y	M	4	56	1972	D8-L1	M			
3. A.W.	16y	M	8	58	1972	C2-D2	M			
4. C.V.	22y	F	1	84	+	D2-8		x	x	
5. R.R.	23y	M	156	360	+	C7-D4		X		
6. H.A.	24y	F	2	108	1972	D10-12		X		
7. W.M.	28y	F	48	314	1972	D7-10			x	
8. K.Z.	31y	F	216	27	1972	Obex-C7				x
9. H.A.	33y	M	12	240	1972	C7-D1	X			
10. L.A.	34y	M	6	11 1/2	+	D7-12		x		
11. H.M.	36y	M	84	64	+	C1-D2				x
12. P.A.	38y	M	10	11	+	D8-10		x		
13. W.E.	42y	F	18	103	+	D1-6				x
14. P.R.	44y	F	66	264	+	C7-D3	x			
15. S.F.	49y	M	1/2	36	1972	D9-11	m			
16. O.M.	64y	F	36	66	+	D11-L1		X		
17. G.O.	54y	F	72	24	+	C3-4			x	
18. M.F.	30y	F	12	6	1972	C2-5	X			
19. W.R.	11y	M	18	36	1973	C1-L2	M			
20. W.R.	7y	F	48	1day	+	C2-D2			x	
21. B.H.	13y	F	48	12	+	C2-4	m			

microsurgical techniques. The patient could walk and normal movements of the arm were, attained postoperatively; on the other hand, disturbances of micturation and defecation remained. Only in case 15 did subtotal resection of the tumor result in a satisfactory result in that the patient has practically a normal gait 3 years after operation. With a 13-year-old female, B.H. (case 21), the intramedullary glioma with unclear boundaries was subtotally removed with microsurgical technique. The illness led to death 3/4 of a year later as a result of tumor extension from the third ventricle to the conus terminalis. In group E+X-ray, only in cases 5 and 6 was the result (with unchanged paraparesis of the legs) satisfactory by means of excellent rehabilitation therapy. In the remaining 4 cases the result remained poor because of progression of the illness and finally death. Decompression alone has practically always failed; only in case 7 has the preoperative paraplegia remained stationary during 26 years; the patient was fully rehabilitated. At operation a biopsy for tumor diagnosis was obtained by aspiration. The result in 3 cases with decompression and X-ray therapy remained unsatisfactory; the illness worsened progressively until death after years of illness in case 11 and 13. In case 3 the possibility of X-ray damage to the spinal cord remains in that 2 months after the application of a second X-ray series the neurological picture rapidly deteriorated. In case 8, following decompression, no change in the neurological deficit appeared; on the other hand, radiation of the tumor in a foreign clinic showed, after a probable initial improvement, a progressive worsening until tetraplegia occurred.

As we look over the results of the astrocytoma group there is no doubt that the best results were attained with radical removal of the tumor. Decompression and partial tumor removal with and without radiation gave almost exclusively disappointing results.

Intramedullary Ependymoma

Table IV summarizes the 20 patients treated who had intramedullary ependymoma and shows that in the great majority of cases radical extirpation of the tumor was the goal. Radical extirpation was attained completely 13 times. Of these, a good to excellent functional result was attained in 6 cases (5, 10, 12, 15, 18, 20) in which the neurological deficits largely or completely disappeared so that all were completely employable. As examples two cases are mentioned. Case 5, a dentist, who suffered preoperative left arm pain and weakness of finger abduction of the left hand, showed after extirpation of a partly cystic and partly solid ependymoma at the level of C_{6-7} (Fig. 3 a-c) only a diminution of vibratory sensation from D_2. He has been completely capable of working in his profession for over 9 years. Case 18 (Fig. 4 a-c), who is also completely employable, suffered postoperatively for two years only from slight spasms in the legs after he had shown preoperatively a severe spastic paresis of the legs with hypesthesia from C_6/C_7. In 7 patients the result of operation was unsatisfactory in that a more or less severe paresis of the legs remained. In this group one death is to be regretted. In case 1, a 19-year-old patient after a decompression and radiation carried out abroad without inhibition of the progressing paresis, a 15-cm-long partially solid, partially cystic ependymoma from D_3 to the medulla oblongata was removed by microsurgical technique with a clear tendency toward improvement of the paresis over three months. Then a deterioration appeared again so that reoperation was carried out because of suspicion of hematoma or adhesions. During operation a fall in blood pressure occurred, possibly as a result of an infusion incident, and then death. In 3 cases with partial tumor extirpation (7, 14, 17) there was initially no change over the preoperative condition; then the condition visibly worsened, and finally in the course of months or a

Table IV. Summary of 20 patients with ependymoma

Patients			Course of Illness and Survival			Localization of Tumor	Treatment			
	age at operation	sex	duration in months preoperative course	postoperative course	alive in year: (if surviving)		E	E+ X-ray	D	D+ X-ray
1. S.C.	19y	M	24	11 1/2	+	Med-D3	M	x		
2. G.T.	20y	F	60	177	1972	D3-8				x
3. H.W.	30y	M	6	2	+	Med-D6			x	
4. R.J.	34y	M	48	103	1972	C4-7	X			
5. M.W.	38y	M	15	112	1972	C6-7	X			
6. M.J.	40y	M	36	39	1972	D3-7	M	x		
7. V.H.	41y	M	18	4	+	D10-12	x			
8. G.E.	42y	F	36	75	1972	C3-8	X			
9. K.E.	44y	M	6	215	+	D4-7		X		
10. B.P.	44y	M	60	139	1972	D10-L1	X			
11. B.K.	45y	M	8	1	+	D6-8			x	
12. M.X.	45y	M	12	25	1972	C7-D1		M		
13. V.D.	47y	F	96	49	1972	D9-11	M			
14. D.U.	48y	M	96	20	+	C4-D1	m			
15. M.A.	51y	F	60	60	1972	C2-D2	X			
16. W.E.	51y	M	36	15	1972	D9-10			x	
17. P.E.	52y	M	84	66 1/2	+	D9	x			
18. C.G.	56y	M	36	25	1972	C4-6	X			
19. V.J.	34y	M	6	13	1972	C4-D1	X			
20. V.G.	69y	M	18	1	1973	D9-11	M			

number of years the patient died. Of the two radically operated and radiated patients, in case 12 an excellent functional result was attained with complete employability, while case 9 died in a foreign country of cachexia after almost 18 years with a poor operative result and probably progressive worsening. In case 6 a partial tumor removal was carried out abroad and then radiation; later paraplegia occurred which could not be improved by a subsequently carried out radical extirpation under the operating microscope. Case 1 was similar. In the decompression group in case 3 preparatory to reoperation two months later, cardiac arrest occurred during intubation for anesthesia. Case 11 was not changed neurologically after operation and died as a result of pulmonary embolus after one month. Case 16 improved for more than a year and tentatively is somewhat improved compared to his condition before operation, while case 2 with decompression and radiation has remained in an unchanged poor condition for 18 years. From this compilation it is evident that the outstandingly good results with radical extirpation of the tumor are attained at the level of the middle and lower cervical cord. The worst results are found with the tumors in the middle and lower thoracic cord.

Unclassified Intramedullary Glioma

In Table V, ten cases of glioma which cannot be classified more exactly are summarized. This was either because only a rapid section of the tumor during operation was carried out with the diagnosis glioma, or the biopsy material permitted no clear differentiation of the glioma. Immediately after operation 5 patients showed a deterioration of their condition; 4 were unchanged compared to their preoperative status and one patient showed an improvement. The latter is case 6, in which two months after operation the postoperative tetraplegia diminished partially, and over two years the patient was well rehabilitated. The 3 cases with decompressive laminectomies alone had all progressively worsened and finally died. Of these, case 4 is particularly striking because of his long survival of 13 years with complete tetraplegia and finally death with cardiac insufficiency. In the decompression and radiation group case 1 and case 8 showed a slight improvement during some weeks and months, but then more or less rapid progression of the paresis until death. The remaining 6 cases did not respond at all to the treatment and have progressively worsened in the course of months. Case 5 is notable insofar as he showed at a later repeated laminectomy, after 3 postoperative radiation series, a completely necrotic spinal cord over 8 segments, probably the sequel of late radiation effect. This radiated case demonstrates emphatically the problem of radiation treatment of intramedullary spinal cord tumors. BODEN showed in 1948 for the first time on the basis of 10 well documented and proven cases the possible complications of radiation-induced myelitis of the spinal cord and published the first radiation tolerance curves. BOUCHARD (1966) emphasized correctly that with the intramedullary gliomas a diseased spinal cord is involved whose blood supply is compromised to a certain degree and whose narrow, long structure makes it a highly vulnerable organ. On the basis of our case material we determined that postoperative radiation after spinal cord decompression by the so-called inoperable gliomas can lengthen the survival time of the patient but that a decrease of the neurological deficit is not attained with certainty. Also postoperative radiation does not appear to offer protection from recurrence or a renewed tumor growth.

Table V. Summary of 10 patients with unclassified glioma

Patients			Course of Illness and Survival			Localization of Tumor	Treatment			
			duration in months							
	age at operation	sex	preoperative course	postoperative course	alive in year:(if surviving)		E	E+ X-ray	D	D+ X-ray
1. L. W.	9y	M	12	6 1/2	+	Med-C7				x
2. U. M.	19y	M	3	12	+	C3-4				x
3. F. W.	23y	M	12	20	+	C3-7			x	
4. Z. E.	29y	M	24	156	+	C2-5			x	
5. I. W.	32y	M	30	153	1972	D7-11				x
6. A. P.	33y	M	12	26	1972	C3-7		x		
7. C. A.	45y	M	12	48 1/2	+	C3-5				x
8. M. M.	45y	F	45	112	+	D8-10				x
9. G. L.	52y	F	180	40	+	L2-S3				x
10. G. O.	54y	F	72	30 1/2	+	C3-7			x	

Discussion and Conclusion

In Table VI the therapeutic results are summarized in relation to the different types of treatment. There is no doubt that total removal attains the best functional result by far, that is 57 % in comparison to the group decompression and radiation with only 14 %. Within the single types of tumor the success quota with astrocytoma is 38 %, with spongioblastoma 30 % and with unclassified glioma 10 %. I am aware of the relativity of these small comparative figures; despite this they give us an idea of the best treatment possibilities for these tumors.

On the basis of our clinical material, it does not follow that with microsurgical methods better results are attained than with the classical neurosurgical methods of operation. Despite this I have not abandoned this new technique of operation because it gives us greater security for radical tumor removal thanks to the maximal preservation of the spinal cord tissue surrounding the tumor and the vessels.
I must emphasize the relativity of the tissue-sparing operative technique under the microscope. The use of the bipolar coagulator, used by GREENWOOD and improved by MALIS permits one to grasp the finest structures with very fine forceps, to isolate them and to section them without any heating effects in the surrounding tissue because the current with continuous irrigation with RINGER's solution flows only through the inner surface of the points of the forceps. This technique appears to me to be of greatest importance in that the coagulation takes place always on the surface of the tumor and not on the spinal cord. In the discussion of the individual groups I have indicated that the results with respect to function are best with localization of the tumor in the middle and lower cervical cord and worst in the middle thoracic area. This is no doubt related to the vascularization of the spinal cord which, according to LAZORTHES, is most ample in the cervical cord and most sparsely developed in the middle thoracic area. It is precisely for this reason that coagulation of the fine vessels leading the tumor itself is so important so that the spinal vascular structures are spared. The blood supply of the tumor usually occurs from the central structures of the spinal cord; thus it is so much more important to spare the blood supply of the spinal cord itself by coagulating the vessels on the tumor. Naturally the removal of the tumor and the preservation of the tissue structures is substantially simplified when the tumor is cystic, and demonstration and removal of the tumor from the cyst can be carried out. On the basis of our clinical material, I am not convinced that the astrocytomas have a less distinct boundary than the ependymomas, as is always emphasized in the literature. Under the microscope both types of tumor can have distinct or indistinct boundaries. Despite this, radical removal is to be attempted. The microtechnique under the microscope has proved useful to us for the removal of two lipomas also. If the radical extirpation of the tumor succeeds, especially with an ependymoma, it makes subsequent radiation superfluous, according to GREENWOOD. In the patient group with decompression of the spinal cord, postoperative radiation has prolonged survival time; however in the group with subtotal or radical extirpation it has no clear influence on survival time.

If our results which we have attained up to now are still not satisfying, this is due above all, to the fact that on the average tumor patients come to us at a very late stage; that is to say, only after some years. In our case material the preoperative duration of illness was 3 1/2 years! As a result of this many cases have a functionally unsatisfactory postoperative result because the severe pre-existing paresis can no longer be appreciably reversed. This is the reason why our results are still not satisfying; as with acoustic neurinomas here also early diagnosis is required.

Table VI. Summary of the results of the different types of treatment

Type of Treatment	Number of Cases	Positive Result	Negative Result	Operative Mortality	Case Mortality	Rate of Success in Percentage
E	28	16	4	1	7	57
E+X-ray	11	5			6	45
D	11	2		3	6	18
D+X-ray	14	2	3		9	14

Finally I have come to the conclusion that in the future the ideal therapy is a microsurgical radical extirpation which should guarantee the best result. However, partial excision under the operating microscope entails no advantage from the catamnestic point of view.

Cervical Syringohydromyelia

In the area of spinal neurosurgery O. FOERSTER was also interested in the operative treatment of cervical hydromyelia and syringomyelia. KUHLENDAHL in 1936 collected the case material of FOERSTER and was of the opinion that with syringomyelia and hydromyelia there was a similar, even if pathogenetically different disturbance of development involved. In syringomyelia there was predominantly a destructive process with secondary cavity formation so that no improvement could be attained by operation. In hydromyelia, however, a high-grade widening of the central canal is involved in which the liquid stands under high pressure so that the operative prospects are more favourable. Thus FOERSTER, in one of four cases of hydromyelia, made an incision 3-4 cm in length in the paper-thin posterior wall of the cervical cord, and a substantial and sustained improvement of the patient's condition was attained. In the remaining three cases the operative results were disappointing, and the slow advance of the illness could not be inhibited. Thus we have come to the view that long-term success is to be expected only in rare cases of pure hydromyelia. This opinion remained in the neurological literature until very recently. SCHLIEP and RITTER in their review (1971) made the comment that the surgical treatment of syringomyelia was only of historic interest!

The embryological basis

Even when LEYDEN in 1876 presented the hypothesis that hydromyelia and syringomyelia show the same pathogenesis and indeed "that both cavitations proceed from the central canal and are due to a pathological distention of the same origin", it was the great contribution of GARDNER to have shown that in these forms of illness a malformation in the sense of an obstruction of the cerebrospinal fluid circulation exists at the level of the foramina of the fourth ventricle. According to this concept, the cavity formation with syringomyelia occurs predominantly through the pulsatory cerebrospinal fluid pressure surges from the fourth ventricle into the central canal. He connected this malformation with an embryonical disturbance in the regression of the physiological hydrocephalomyelia in the eighth fetal week when the formation of the foramina of Magendie and Luschka in the roof of the fourth ventricle does not occur. "If the foramen of Magendie remains closed by an elastic membrane, the pressure of the cerebrospinal fluid can form a cystic widening of the fourth ventricle (DANDY-WALKER malformation). If the membrane is inelastic, the fourth ventricle is forced downward (ARNOLD-CHIARI malformation). The outlet of the fourth ventricle is therefore bridged with a permeable membrane that funnels the pulsations of the ventricular fluid into the central canal of the cord". If sufficient permeability of the roof of the fourth ventricle takes place later, a lower than usual position of the cerebellar tonsils can occur without hydrocephalus. These are the rare cases of ARNOLD-CHIARI malformation without noticeable hydrocephalus.

Clinical and Operative Experience

Considering this pathogenetic hypothesis, GARDNER presented the opinion that surgical therapy must aim at a correction of the cerebrospinal fluid course. He recommended therefore exploration of the posterior fossa with opening of the foramina of the fourth ventricle and closure of the connection between the fourth ventricle and the syrinx with a muscle transplant under the obex. The publications of GARDNER, HANKINSON, LOGUE, MAEDER et al., HADJ-DJILANI and ZANDER, van den BERGH et al. have contributed convincing results of this type so that we have operated 26 cases of cervical hydromyelia and syringomyelia since 1969. Because the operative opening of the posterior fossa and the upper cervical cord still involves a certain risk, we have in 19 cases employed the ventriculo-atrial shunt operation according to PUDENZ-HEYER or SPITZ-HOLTER for relieving the pressure in the syrinx. Preceding the operation we established by myelography the widening of the spinal cord, by Pantopaque myelography in prone position, the dependency of the tonsils, absence or existence of a slight hydrocephalus by the lumbar pneumoencephalogram or complete lack of demonstration of the cerebral ventricles. Of these 19 cases, 13 are substantially to very much improved, and in particular the atrophies, the weakness in the arms or - when present - the pyramidal tract symptoms in the legs have improved or even disappeared. In 4 cases the sensory findings have normalized and in one case edema of the arms has disappeared. In 6 cases the condition remained stationary or further deteriorated because the ventriculo-atrial drainage was no longer patent so that a second operation the exposure of the occipital foramen magnum and an upper cervical laminectomy had to be carried out. Of these patients, two have improved insofar as their pains disappeared; on the other hand, the condition in 3 cases remained stationary or progressed, and one case died at this second operation because of respiratory paralysis. In 2 cases only a cervical laminectomy with splitting of the syrinx was carried out without thereby attaining any influence on the symptoms. In 5 cases primarily, the occipital-cervical junction was dissected with the patient in sitting position. The adhesions were sectioned, the fourth ventricle was opened, and in 3 cases the connection between the syrinx and the fourth ventricle was obliterated with a muscle transplant. In 4 of these cases an improvement, in part very considerable, was attained. The spastic paraplegia of the legs diminished or disappeared; in one case of syringobulbia the aphonia and the dysphagia decreased. To some extent the atrophy in the region of the small muscles of the hand diminished, and the dissociated sensory disturbance disappeared in some patients incompletely and in some completely. In 2 cases the neck pain vanished and in one case the fasciculations. In one patient a postoperative respiratory paralysis occurred and led to death.

As an example, Fig. 5 shows a characteristic ARNOLD-CHIARI malformation and widening of the upper cervical cord of a 53-year-old male patient. The spastic paraparesis of the legs disappeared postoperatively; on the other hand the spasticity remained unchanged in the arm. In another case, a 34-year-old patient a very much thickened pial and arachnoidal transverse band and herniation of the tonsils were present in the foramen magnum with a symptomatology of one year. Following the lysis of these cord-like adhesions the patient, after 2 months of artificial respiration, expired from respiratory paralysis. The autopsy showed syringobulbia and hydromyelia. In Fig. 6 a+b a modification of the GARDNER operation may be recognized. From the opened syrinx on the left side I have pushed the muscle transplant upwards to close the communication between the fourth ventricle and the syrinx. The approach produced an excellent improvement of the neurological findings. In this 49-year-old female patient the muscle atrophy, claw hand and temperature disturbance existing for 7 years have completely disappeared, leaving a slight dissociated disturbance of sensation of the left hand. Similarly excellent progress was attained by a 32-year-old patient with a 16-year anamnesis. In this severe ARNOLD-CHIARI malformation, opening the fourth ventricle was considered too dangerous so that here the connection from the syrinx to the entrance of the fourth ventricle was closed with a muscle plug. Gross strength in the right arm and the sensation in the right leg have substantially improved, and the atrophy of the right hand muscles has disappeared. On the other hand, the slight flexion spasticity in the left hand remains. Finally in a DANDY-WALKER malformation the membrane of the cyst was resected so that the fourth ventricle, between the narrow tonsils which were herniated into the foramen magnum, was opened widely. The numerous transverse adhesions could be sectioned satisfactorily so that closing the communication between the fourth ventricle and the syrinx could be dispensed with. The patient recovered quickly from the left-sided spasticity and from the dissociated anesthesia in the right arm.

Conclusion

In summary it may be stated that, in contradiction to the still widely disseminated pessimistic attitude to the surgical treatment of cervical syringomyelia and hydromyelia, a certain optimism for the future is justified. At the present time the evaluation of the definitive therapy for this disorder clearly belongs in the realm of neurosurgery, and I trust that I have presented this approach in the sense in which the problem was understood by OTFRID FOERSTER.

REFERENCES

1. ANGST, A.: Katamnestische Untersuchung über den Einfluss der postoperativen Bestrahlungstherapie bei primären intramedullären Rückenmarksgliomen. Inaugural-Dissertation Zürich, 1973
2. BENINI, A. und H. KRAYENBÜHL: Ein neuer chirurgischer Weg zur Behandlung der Hydro- und Syringomyelie. Schweiz. med. Wschr. 99, 1137-1142 (1969)
3. BODEN, G.: Radiation myelitis of the cervical cord. Brit. J. Radiol. 21, 464-469 (1948)
4. BOUCHARD, J.: Radiation Therapy of Tumors and Diseases of the Nervous System. Philadelphia, Lea and Febiger, 1966
5. CAIRNS, H. and G. RIDDOCH: Observations on the treatment of ependymal gliomas of the spinal cord. Brain 54, 117-146 (1931)
6. FOERSTER, O.: Fall von intramedullärem Tumor, erfolgreich operiert. Berl. Klin. Wschr. 54, 338 (1917)
7. FOERSTER, O.: Diagnostik und Therapie der Rückenmarkstumoren. Berl. Klin. Wschr. 58, 818-819 (1921)
8. FOERSTER, O.: Zur Diagnostik und Therapie der Rückenmarkstumoren. Dtsch. Z. Nervenheilk. 70, 64-74 (1921)
9. FOERSTER, O. und O. GAGEL: Klinik und Pathohistologie der intramedullären Rückenmarkstumoren. Dtsch. Z. Nervenheilk. 136, 239 (1935)

10. FOERSTER, O. and P. BAILEY: A Contribution to the Study of Gliomas of the Spinal Cord with Special Reference to their Operability. Pp. 9-67 in: Jubilee Vol. for Davidenkov, Leningrad, State Inst. for Publ. Biol. and Med. Literature 1936

11. GARDNER, W. J.: The dysraphic states, from syringomyelia to anencephaly. Excerpta Medica Amsterdam, 1973

12. GREENWOOD, J. Jr.: Total removal of intramedullary tumors. J. Neurosurg. 11, 616-621 (1954)

13. GREENWOOD, J. Jr.: Intramedullary tumors of spinal cord. A follow-up study after total surgical removal. J. Neurosurg. 20, 665-668 (1963)

14. GREENWOOD, J. Jr.: Surgical removal of intramedullary tumors. J. Neurosurg. 26, 276-282 (1967)

15. HADJ-DJILANI, M. et E. ZANDER: Les syringo-hydromyélies cervicobulbaires et leur traitement. Schweiz. Arch. Neurol. Neurochir. Psychiat. 111, 353-361 (1972)

16. HANKINSON, J.: Syringomyelia and the surgeon. In: Modern Trends in Neurology. Vol. 5, 127-148 (1970). Editor: D. Williams. Butterworths, London

17. KRAYENBÜHL, H. und M. G. YASARGIL: Die Anwendung des binokulären Mikroskopes in der Neurochirurgie. Wiener Z. Nervenheilk. 25, Heft 2-4 (1967)

18. KRAYENBÜHL, H. and A. BENINI: A new surgical approach in the treatment of hydromyelia and syringomyelia. The embryological basis and the first results. J. Roy. Coll. Surg. Edinb. 16, 147-161 (1971)

19. KUHLENDAHL, H.: Die operative Beeinflussbarkeit der Hydromyelie und Syringomyelie. Dtsch. Z. Nervenheilk. 140, 1-27 (1936)

20. LAZORTHES, G.: Vascularisation et Circulation Cérébrales. Masson & Cie., p. 41, Fig. 21, 1961

21. LEYDEN, E.: Ueber Hydromyelus und Syringomyelie. Virchow's Arch. path. Anat. 68, 1-20 (1876)

22. LOGUE, V.: Syringomyelia: A radiodiagnostic and radiotherapeutic saga. Clin. Radiol. Vol. 22 (1971)

23. MAEDER, R. P., M. MUMENTHALER und H. MARKWALDER: Symptomatische zervikale Syringomyelie. Diagnostik und chirurgische Therapie anhand von acht eigenen Beobachtungen. Dtsch. med. Wschr. 95, 164-168 (1970)

24. MALIS, L. J.: In "Microvascular Surgery". ed. R. M. P. Donaghy and M. G. Yasargil. St. Louis: C. V. Mosby Co. (1967)

25. OBERBECKMANN, Ch.: Diagnose, Therapie und Katamnese intramedullärer Rückenmarkstumoren. Schweiz. Arch. Neurol. Neurochir. Psychiat. 109, 1-49 (1971)

26. SCHLIEP, G. und U. RITTER: Klinik der Syringomyelie. Fortschr. Neurol. Psychiat. 39, 53-82 (1971)

27. Van den BERGH, R. and I. DEHAENE: New concepts in the neurosurgical treatment of syringomyelia. Acta Neurochir. 26, 352 (1972)

28. ZÜLCH, K. J.: Otfrid Foerster, Arzt und Naturforscher. Springer Verlag, Berlin, Heidelberg, New York, 1966

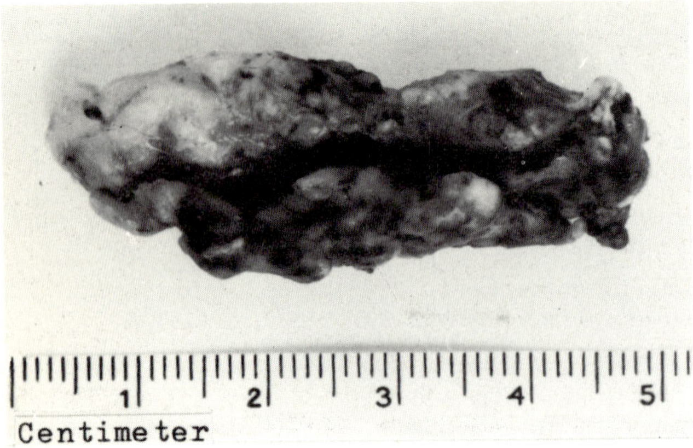

Fig. 1. Case 12 of Table II. Complete removal of a solid intramedullary spongioblastoma extending from C_5 to C_7, about 5 cm long

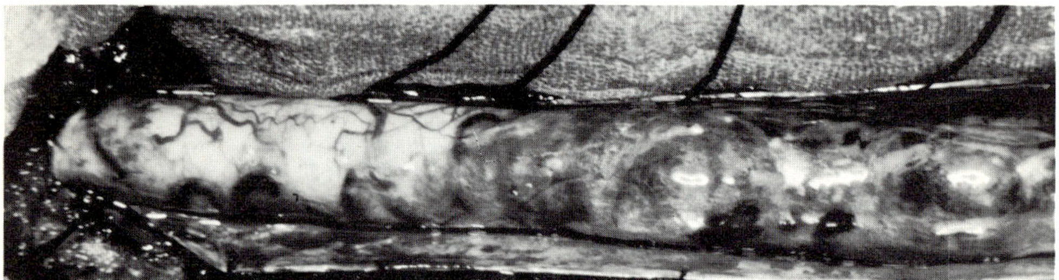

Fig. 2a and b. Case 19 of Table III. Total removal of a partly cystic, partly solid intramedullary astrocytoma, leaving a clean cavity in the lower thoracic and in the lumbar spinal cord

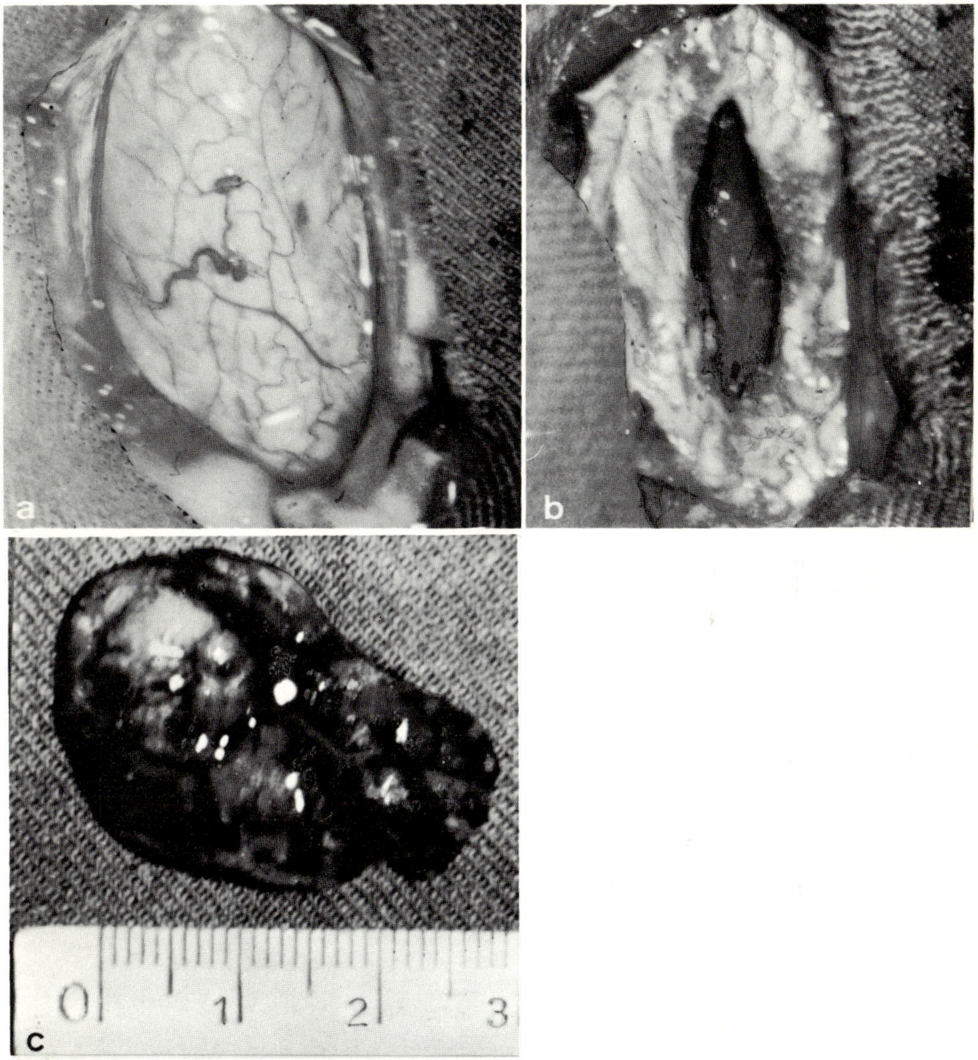

Fig. 3a-c. Case 5 of Table IV. Complete removal of a solid intramedullary ependymoma at the level of C_6 to C_7, leaving a clean cavity in the spinal cord

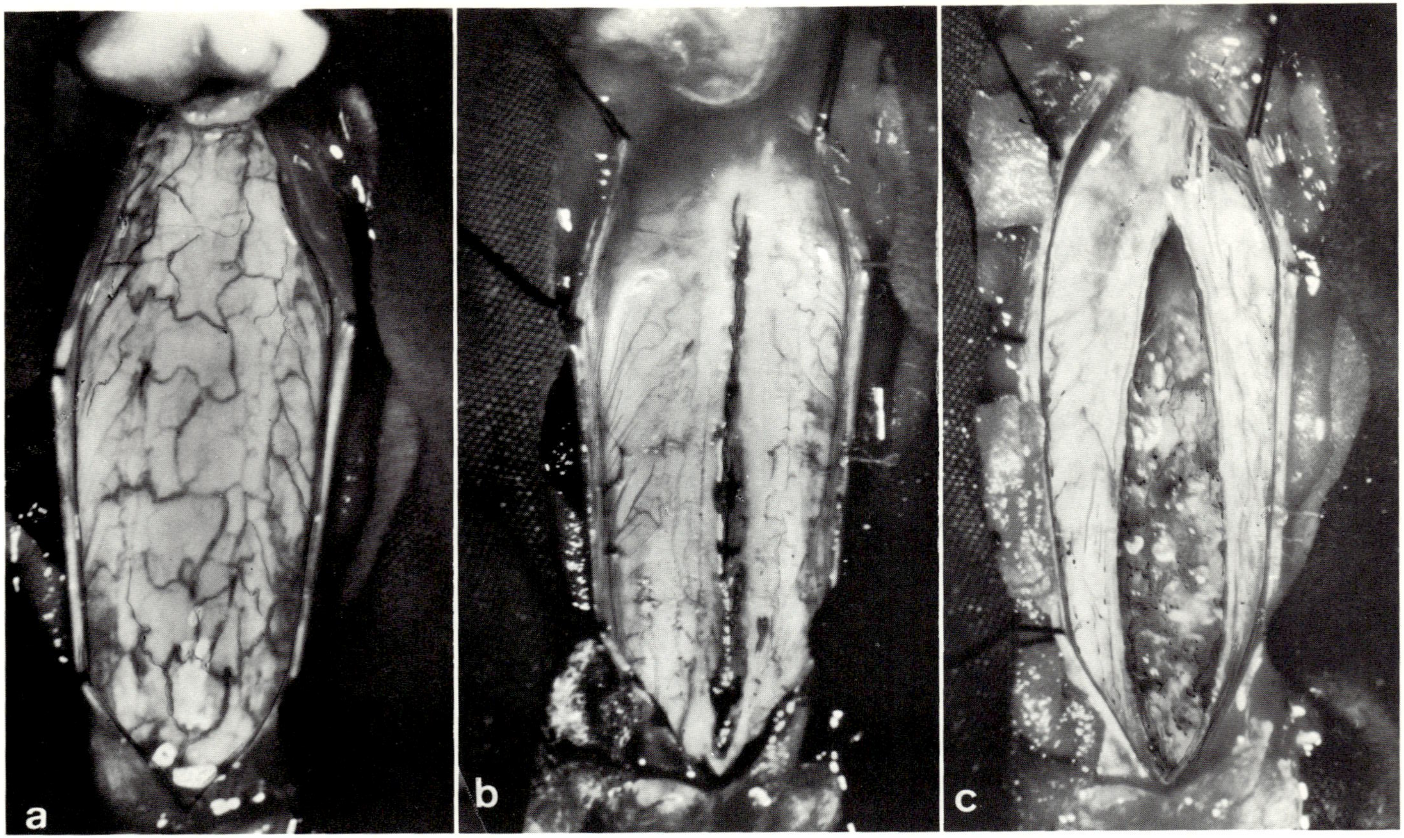

Fig. 4a-c. Case 18 of Table IV. Solid intramedullary ependymoma extending from C_4 to C_6. Total removal of the tumor through an incision in the midline of the posterior spinal cord, leaving a clean cavity in the spinal cord

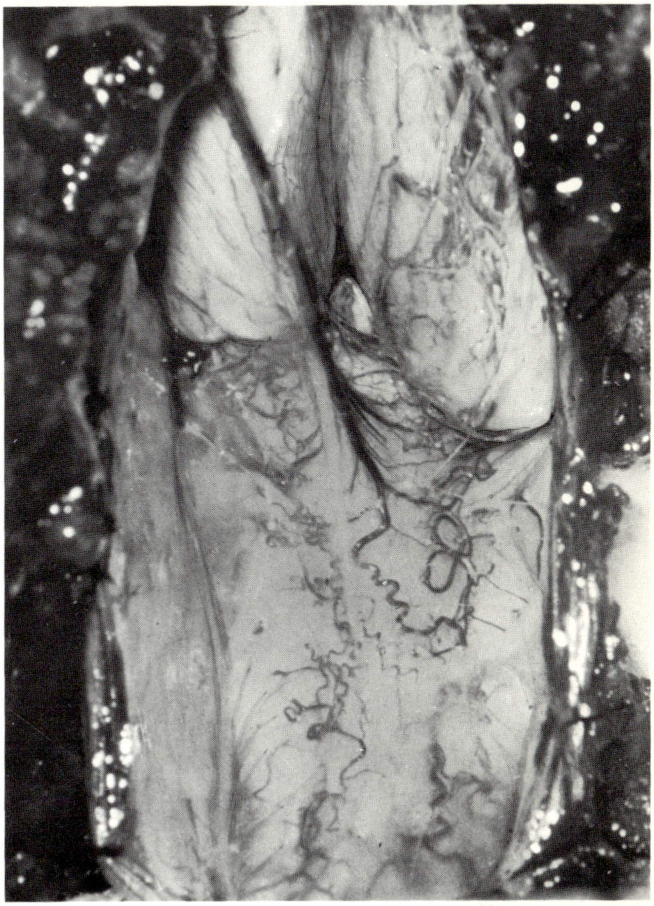

Fig. 5. A case of syringomyelia. The tonsils are protruding through the foramen magnum (Arnold-Chiari malformation) and the spinal cord is distended.

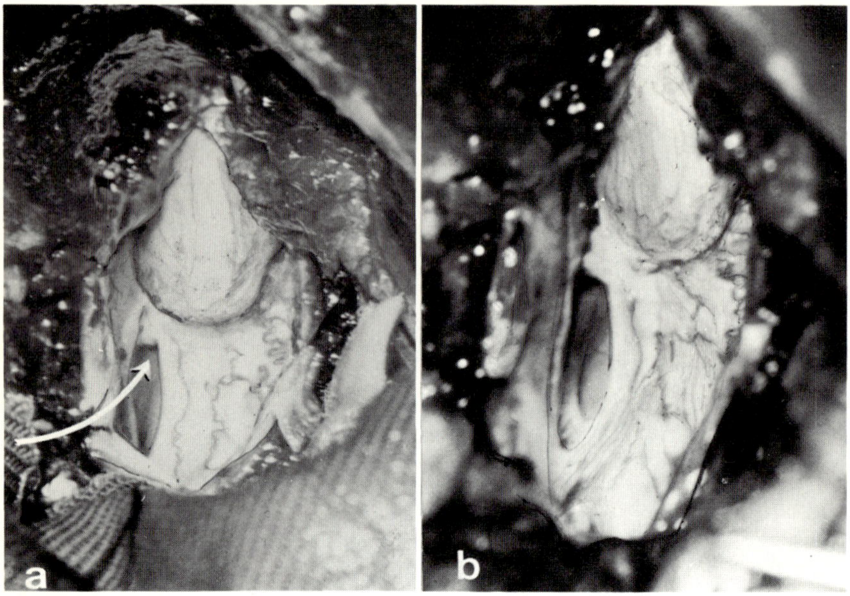

Fig. 6a-b. A case of syringo-hydromyelia.
a. Herniation of the left tonsil and distention of the cervical cord. Syrinx incised on the left side. A bit of muscle is impacted through the syrinx in the funnel-shaped opening of the central canal beneath the obex (arrow)
b. Cervical cord is collapsed after insertion of the muscle plug

Index

S. L. Palay / V. Chan-Palay

By Dr. Sanford L. Palay, Bullard Professor of Neuroanatomy, Harvard Medical School, Boston, Mass.

and Dr. Victoria Chan-Palay, Assistant Professor of Neurobiology, Harvard Medical School, Boston, Mass.

Cerebellar Cortex

Cytology and Organization

With 267 figures incl. 195 plates
Approx. 400 pages. 1973
Cloth DM 156,–; US $64.00
ISBN 3-540-06228-9

Prices are subject to change without notice

Distribution rights for Japan: Igaku Shoin Ltd., Tokyo

Contents
Preface.
Introduction.
The Purkinje Cell.
Granule Cells.
The Golgi Cells.
The Lugaro Cell.
The Mossy Fibers.
The Basket Cell.
The Stellate Cell.
Functional Architectonics without Numbers.
The Climbing Fiber.
The Neurological Cells of the Cerebellar Cortex.
Methods.

This book deals with the fine structure and organization of the cerebellar cortex of the rat. Each of the cell types and afferent fibers in the cerebellar cortex is taken up in turn and described. Both optical and electron microscopy are used and copiously illustrated. A careful study of the cerebellar cortex with these two methods indicates that considerable reliance may be placed on the Golgi technique for the general architecture and the three-dimensional form of the cells and fibers. All of the known synaptic junctions are characterized and their function is discussed from the anatomical point of view. The authors have drawn freely upon the results and insights derived from neurophysiology. All the drawings are original india ink tracings made with the aid of a camera lucida at high magnification and prepared especially for this book. The electron micrographs are also originally designed for this volume.
This book is the only comprehensive volume on the cerebellar cortex of a mammal, studied at the cytological level. It also reviews the history of our present concepts about the cellular organization of the cerebellar cortex and enunciates new principles of organization derived from the cytology of this cortex.

■ **Prospectus on request!**

Springer-Verlag
Berlin Heidelberg New York

München Johannesburg London New Delhi Paris Rio de Janeiro Sydney Tokyo Wien

K.J.Zülch
Atlas of the Histology of Brain Tumors

Title and text in six languages (English, German, French, Spanish, Russian, and Japanese)

With 100 figures. XVI, 261 pages. 1971
Cloth DM 78,–; US $32.00
ISBN 3-540-05274-7
(Distribution rights for Japan: Nankodo Company Ltd., Tokyo)

Contents: Introduction. – Tumors of Nervous and Adjacent Tissues: Nerve Cells. Neuroepithelium. Eye. Glia. Peripheral Nerves and Nerve Sheaths. Meninges, Vascular Structures of the Central Nervous System and Connective Tissue. Pineal and Pituitary Glands, Craniopharyngeal Duct. Paraganglia. Various Tissues. – References. – Subject Index.

This atlas shows the growth pattern of the intracranial tumors, their frequent variations and the typical changes occurring as a result of regressive changes. Therefore, it guides one in the art of making a correct classification. There is also a discussion concerning the prognosis based on "genuine growth" in which Kernohan's grading system is further developed and adapted for daily use. It is hoped that this atlas forms a solid basis for the morphological diagnosis of brain tumors.

Cerebral Circulation and Stroke

Editor: **K. J. Zülch**
71 figures. XII, 222 pages. 1971
Cloth DM 59,–; US $24.20
ISBN 3-540-05060-4
(Distribution rights for Japan: Nankodo Company Ltd., Tokyo)

A review of current research in cerebral circulation and stroke by contributors who are particularly active and original clinicians and researcher in this field.

K.J.Zülch
Atlas of Gross Neurosurgical Pathology

Approx. 371 figures. Approx. 320 pages. 1973
In preparation
ISBN 3-540-06480-X

Contents: Introduction. – Generalised and Local Increased Intracranial Pressure and its Consequences, Mass-Movements and Hernias: General Rules for Displacement due to Space-Occupying Lesions. The Obstructive Hydrocephalus. – References. – Subject Index.

Designed for the practicing neurosurgeon, neuroradiologist, neuropathologist and neurologist, this atlas sets out to depict very exactly the size, shape and preferred site of the main space-occupying lesions of the brain, thus principally tumors, with an indication of prognosis. Such knowledge is essential for diagnosis, differential diagnosis, surgery and radiotherapy. The accompanying text is brief but informative.

Proceedings in Echo-Encephalography

International Symposium on Echo-Encephalography, Erlangen, Germany, April 14th and 15th, 1967
Editors: **E. Kazner, W. Schiefer, K. J. Zülch**
Translator: M. Lewke
278 figures. XI, 258 pages. 1968
Cloth DM 68,–; US $27.90
ISBN 3-540-04300-4
(Distribution rights for U.K., Commonwealth, and the Traditional British Market (excluding Canada): John Wright & Sons Ltd., Bristol)

Experts in the use of the method assembled from all over the world to provide a picture of the present state and future potential of ultrasonics in the diagnosis of brain disease.

Prices are subject to change without notice

Springer-Verlag Berlin Heidelberg New York
München Johannesburg London New Delhi Paris Rio de Janeiro Sydney Tokyo Wien